CREATIVE ARTS AND PLAY THERAPY FOR ATTACHMENT PROBLEMS

Creative Arts
and Play Therapy
for Attachment
Problems

Edited by

Cathy A. Malchiodi
David A. Crenshaw

THE GUILFORD PRESS
New York   London

© 2014 The Guilford Press
A Division of Guilford Publications, Inc.
370 Seventh Avenue, Suite 1200, New York, NY 10001
www.guilford.com

Paperback edition 2015

Chapter 11 © 2014 Richard L. Gaskill and Bruce D. Perry

Printed in the United States of America

This book is printed on acid-free paper.

Last digit is print number: 9 8 7 6 5

The authors have checked with sources believed to be reliable in their efforts to
provide information that is complete and generally in accord with the standards
of practice that are accepted at the time of publication. However, in view of the
possibility of human error or changes in behavioral, mental health, or medical
sciences, neither the authors, nor the editors and publisher, nor any other party
who has been involved in the preparation or publication of this work warrants
that the information contained herein is in every respect accurate or complete,
and they are not responsible for any errors or omissions or the results obtained
from the use of such information. Readers are encouraged to confirm the
information contained in this book with other sources.

Library of Congress Cataloging-in-Publication Data

Creative arts and play therapy for attachment problems / edited by
Cathy A. Malchiodi, David A. Crenshaw.
    pages cm. — (Creative arts and play therapy)
  Includes bibliographical references and index.
  ISBN 978-1-4625-1270-6 (hardback : acid-free paper)
  ISBN 978-1-4625-2370-2 (paperback : acid-free paper)
  1. Attachment disorder in children. 2. Art therapy. 3. Play
therapy. I. Malchiodi, Cathy A. II. Crenshaw, David A.
  RJ507.A77C74 2014
  618.92′891653—dc23
                                                      2013031210

About the Editors

Cathy A. Malchiodi, PhD, ATR-BC, LPAT, LPCC, is an art therapist, creative arts therapist, and clinical mental health counselor, as well as a recognized authority on art therapy with children, adults, and families. She has given more than 350 presentations on art therapy and has published numerous articles, chapters, and books, including *Understanding Children's Drawings*; *Handbook of Art Therapy, Second Edition*; and *Creative Interventions with Traumatized Children*. Dr. Malchiodi is on the faculty of Lesley University and is a visiting professor at universities in the United States and internationally. She is also founder of the Trauma-Informed Practices and Expressive Arts Therapy Institute and has worked with a wide variety of community, national, and international agencies, particularly on the use of art therapy for trauma intervention, disaster relief, mental health, and wellness. The President of Art Therapy Without Borders, a nonprofit organization supporting international art therapy initiatives and service, Dr. Malchiodi is the first person to have received all three of the American Art Therapy Association's highest honors: Distinguished Service Award, Clinician Award, and Honorary Life Member Award. She has also received honors from the Kennedy Center and Very Special Arts in Washington, DC.

David A. Crenshaw, PhD, ABPP, RPT-S, is Clinical Director of the Children's Home of Poughkeepsie, New York, and Faculty Associate at Johns Hopkins University. He is a Fellow of the American Psychological Association and of its Division of Child and Adolescent Psychology. Dr. Crenshaw is Past President of the Hudson Valley Psychological Association, which honored him with its Lifetime Achievement Award, and of the New York Association for Play Therapy. He serves on the editorial board of the *International Journal of Play Therapy* and has published numerous journal articles, book chapters, and books on child therapy, child abuse and trauma, and resilience in children. Co-Chair of the board of directors of Astor Services for Children and Families and an advisory board member of the Courthouse Dogs Foundation in Seattle, Dr. Crenshaw has been a passionate advocate for legislative proposals to enhance children's rights. He is a frequent presenter at statewide and national conferences on play therapy.

Contributors

Jennifer N. Baggerly, PhD, Department of Counseling and Human Services, University of North Texas at Dallas, Dallas, Texas

Kira Boesch, BA, Doctoral Program in Clinical Psychology, City University of New York at City College, New York, New York

Phyllis B. Booth, MA, The Theraplay Institute, Evanston, Illinois

David A. Crenshaw, PhD, ABPP, RPT-S, Children's Home of Poughkeepsie, Poughkeepsie, New York

Christina Devereaux, PhD, Dance/Movement Therapy and Counseling Program, Department of Applied Psychology, Antioch University New England, Keene, New Hampshire

Teresa Dias, BA, Drama Therapy Master's Program, Division of Expressive Therapies, Lesley University, Cambridge, Massachusetts

Athena A. Drewes, PsyD, Astor Services for Children and Families, Rhinebeck, New York

Richard L. Gaskill, EdD, Department of Counseling, Educational Leadership, and Educational and School Psychology, Wichita State University, Wichita, Kansas

Eliana Gil, PhD, Gil Institute for Trauma Recovery and Education, Fairfax, Virginia

Jessica Gorkin, MEd, Doctoral Program in Clinical Psychology, City University of New York at City College, New York, New York

Eric J. Green, PhD, Department of Counseling and Human Services, University of North Texas at Dallas, Dallas, Texas

Henry Kronengold, PhD, Doctoral Program in Clinical Psychology, City University of New York at City College, New York, New York

Jennifer Lee, PhD, Columbia University College of Physicians and Surgeons, New York Presbyterian Hospital, New York, New York

Sandra Lindaman, MA, MSW, The Theraplay Institute, Evanston, Illinois

Cathy A. Malchiodi, PhD, ATR-BC, LPAT, LPCC, Division of Expressive Therapies, Lesley University, Cambridge, Massachusetts; Trauma-Informed Practices and Expressive Arts Therapy Institute, Louisville, Kentucky

Christen Pendleton, EdS, Department of Graduate Psychology, Combined–Integrated Program in Clinical and School Psychology, James Madison University, Harrisonburg, Virginia

Bruce D. Perry, MD, PhD, Child Trauma Academy, Houston, Texas; Department of Psychiatry and Behavioral Sciences, Feinberg School of Medicine, Northwestern University, Chicago, Illinois

Jacqueline Z. Robarts, MA, Nordoff Robbins Music Therapy Centre, London, United Kingdom

John W. Seymour, PhD, Department of Counseling and Student Personnel, Minnesota State University, Mankato, Mankato, Minnesota

Cynthia C. Sniscak, LPC, RPT-S, Beech Street Program, LLC, Carlisle, Pennsylvania

Anne Stewart, PhD, Department of Graduate Psychology, James Madison University, Harrisonburg, Virginia

Madeleine Terry, BA, Doctoral Program in Clinical Psychology, City University of New York at City College, New York, New York

Glade L. Topham, PhD, Department of Human Development and Family Science, Oklahoma State University, Tulsa, Oklahoma

Steven Tuber, PhD, Doctoral Program in Clinical Psychology, City University of New York at City College, New York, New York

Risë VanFleet, PhD, Family Enhancement and Play Therapy Center, Playful Pooch Program, Boiling Springs, Pennsylvania

William F. Whelan, PsyD, The Virginia Child and Family Attachment Center, University of Virginia, Charlottesville, Virginia

Marlo L.-R. Winstead, MSW, LSCSW, School of Social Welfare, University of Kansas, Lawrence, Kansas; Play Therapy Program, MidAmerica Nazarene University, Olathe, Kansas; The Theraplay Institute, Evanston, Illinois; Enriching Families, Tallahassee, Florida

Preface

The quality of parent–child interactions early in life has consistently been a focus in psychiatry, psychology, and the other mental health professions. More recently, leaders in the field of attachment theory have emphasized the crucial role of secure and positive early interpersonal relationships in human development. Much of our increased knowledge about attachment comes from greater understanding of neurodevelopment, the brain's responses to trauma, and how adverse events can result in disrupted, insecure, or disorganized attachment. As a result, there is now wide agreement that these findings support the idea that the quality of attachment during infancy and childhood significantly impacts emotional, cognitive, physical, and social development throughout the lifespan. We also know that nurturing, protective, and caring interactions between infants and primary caregivers not only are essential for attachment security, but also literally shape the structure and function of the child's developing brain. In particular, research and clinical findings pinpoint the central role of the right hemisphere of the brain in healthy attachment.

While there are many effective ways to treat attachment problems, we believe that there are specific, experientially based approaches that stimulate right brain activity and are important in reestablishing secure and positive attachment experiences. In particular, therapies that give young children ways to express their inner worlds through nonverbal communication are key. Additionally, the most effective approaches are those that are "user friendly" and come naturally to children.

We believe that the creative arts and play therapy have a natural affinity with attachment problems in children. Creative arts therapies (art, music, and dance/movement) and play therapy are approaches that capitalize on "right-brain-to-right-brain" connections between the child client and therapist. When early attachment experiences are disrupted by trauma, neglect, physical and sexual abuse, loss, separation from caregivers, or other factors, it becomes essential to use interventions that use forms of expression and processing to initiate and stimulate reparative processes in a brain-focused way. These experiential, sensory approaches are corrective experiences for the child even when the critical periods in early development are compromised. Through intensive, sequential, and repetitive play and creative arts therapy, child clients can successfully recapitulate and repair early sensorimotor, somatic, cognitive, and psychosocial experiences missed at earlier developmental junctures.

Creative Arts and Play Therapy for Attachment Problems is about that vital healing and reparative process, emphasizing a wide range of play therapy and creative arts therapy approaches. It is also the first volume in a new Guilford Press series, "Creative Arts and Play Therapy." As series editors, it is our privilege to bring theory, practice, and pragmatic applications of play therapy and creative arts therapies to a wide range of practitioners, including psychologists, social workers, mental health counselors, marriage and family therapists, play therapists, art therapists, music therapists, drama therapists, dance/movement therapists, psychiatric nurses, child life specialists, and health care professionals.

Finally, as mental health professionals who have worked with children with attachment problems, we are particularly excited and inspired by the work and depth of knowledge and expertise presented in this book. Each chapter in this volume provides clinical wisdom, specific interventions and approaches, and clinical applications that all practitioners who work with children can use in their work. We hope that these contributions not only form a foundation for greater understanding of play therapy and creative arts therapies with young clients, but also inspire readers to apply these methods in their own work with children.

CATHY A. MALCHIODI
DAVID A. CRENSHAW

Contents

III. Clinical Applications: Approaches to Working with At-Risk Populations

PART I

Introduction

CHAPTER 1

Creative Arts Therapy Approaches to Attachment Issues

Cathy A. Malchiodi

During the last several decades, attachment theory has significantly influenced the practice of psychotherapy; this has resulted in the acceptance of early bonding experiences as essential to well-being later in life. Attachment theory is not an approach in and of itself, but it has generated a whole range of therapeutic practices and models focused on increasing an insecurely attached or traumatized individual's ability to form secure relationships, regulate affect and behavior, and emotionally and physically attune to others. Attachment research emphasizes the psychobiological aspects of communication between caregiver and child, including interactive speech, vocalizations/sounds, body language/gestures, and eye contact. The overall goal of attachment work in therapy generally involves recreating experiences that recapture what the individual may have missed in early relationships.

The creative arts therapies include the purposeful application of visual arts, dance/movement, music, and dramatic enactment within a psychotherapeutic framework. Like play therapy, they are experiential, active approaches that capitalize on engaging individuals of all ages in multisensory experiences for self-exploration, personal communication, developmental objectives, socialization, and emotional reparation. This chapter defines and explains the basic foundations of the creative arts therapies, with an emphasis on the psychobiological and neurodevelopmental aspects of these sensory-based approaches to attachment work. It also explores how these therapies are used to treat disrupted or insecure attachment, and to enhance and support the development of secure attachment, particularly in children who have experienced multiple traumatic events or losses.

3

What Are the Creative Arts Therapies?

While many play therapists, counselors, and psychologists use one or more of the arts in their work with clients, the creative arts therapies emerged in the 20th century as distinct approaches with various theoretical and methodological frameworks. These approaches have been used to address a variety of emotional, behavioral, social, and physical disorders in individuals of all ages (Malchiodi, 2005; Warren, 2004) and are defined by psychology as "action therapies" (Weiner, 1999). Art and music making, dance and drama, creative writing, and play are experiential in nature. For example, art making, even in its simplest sense, can involve arranging, touching, gluing, constructing, painting, forming, and many other active experiences. All creative arts therapies encourage clients to become active participants in the therapeutic process, and can energize the clients, redirect their attention and focus, and influence emotions.

The creative arts therapies are most commonly defined as follows:

- *Art therapy* is the purposeful use of visual art materials and media in intervention, counseling, psychotherapy, and rehabilitation; it is used with individuals of all ages, families, and groups (Edwards, 2004; Malchiodi, 2012a).
- *Music therapy* uses music to effect positive changes in the psychological, physical, cognitive, or social functioning of individuals with health, behavioral, social, emotional, or educational challenges (American Music Therapy Association, 2013; Wheeler, Shultis, & Polen, 2005).
- *Drama therapy* is defined as an active, experiential approach to facilitating change through storytelling, projective play, purposeful improvisation, and performance (Johnson, 2009; National Drama Therapy Association, 2013).
- *Dance/movement therapy* is based on the assumption that body and mind are interrelated, and is defined as the psychotherapeutic use of movement as a process that furthers the emotional, cognitive, and physical integration of the individual and influences changes in feelings, cognition, physical functioning, and behavior (Goodill, 2005; National Dance Therapy Association, 2013; Payne, 2013).
- *Poetry therapy* and *bibliotherapy* are terms used synonymously to describe the intentional use of poetry and other forms of literature for healing and personal growth (Micozzi, 2011; National Association for Poetry Therapy, 2013).

The terms *expressive therapies* or *expressive arts therapies* are sometimes used interchangeably with the term *creative arts therapies*. However, the term *expressive therapies* is usually used in reference to a variety of creative methods and experiential approaches involving, but not limited to, all the arts therapies and various forms of play therapy (props, games, and sandplay). The *integrated arts approach* or *intermodal therapy* (also known as *multimodal therapy*) involves the use of two or more expressive therapies in an individual or group session. Intermodal therapy distinguishes itself from its closely allied disciplines of art therapy, music therapy, dance/movement therapy, and drama therapy by focusing on the interrelatedness of the arts. It is based on a variety of orientations, including arts as therapy, art psychotherapy, and the use of arts for traditional healing (Knill, Barba, & Fuchs, 2004).

In subsequent sections of this chapter, the relationship between attachment work and art, music, dance/movement, and drama therapies is explained within the context of attachment theory (Bowlby, 1988/2005; Schore, 2003), psychobiology and neurodevelopment (Perry, 2009; Siegel, 2012), and trauma-informed expressive arts therapies (Malchiodi, 2012a, 2012c). In order to explain how trauma-informed expressive arts therapy is used in the treatment of attachment, a brief case vignette is presented and used to illustrate key applications of creative arts therapies with attachment challenges. Specific applications of the creative arts therapies to support and enhance attachment are covered in more detail with case examples in other chapters of this book.

Creative Arts Therapies and the Brain

Just as attachment theory continues to be informed by the growing understanding of the brain, applications of the creative arts therapies are being clarified within the context of neuroscience and psychobiology. This section reviews five key areas in creative arts therapies and attachment work: (1) sensory-based interventions, (2) nonverbal communication, (3) right-hemisphere dominance, (4) affect regulation, and (5) relational interventions.

Sensory-Based Interventions

First and foremost, the creative arts therapies provide sensory experiences; that is, they are predominantly activities that are visual, kinesthetic, tactile, olfactory, and/or auditory in nature. In fact, each creative arts therapy is multisensorial; for example, music therapy not only involves sound, but also includes vibration, rhythm, and movement. Dramatic enactment may include vocalization, visual impact, and other sensory aspects. Dance/movement therapy encompasses a variety of body-oriented sensations, and art therapy is not limited to images because it also provides a variety of tactile and kinesthetic experiences.

Research on attachment disorders underscores the importance of sensory-based approaches in treatment that encourage active participation and include multisensory qualities. Perry (2008) presents a neurodevelopmental perspective: He describes the essential role of sensory-based experiences in early childhood, and discusses how they enhance secure attachment, affiliation with others, empathy, and self-regulation. He observes that our history as a human species has always included wellness practices such as holding each other; engaging in dance, song, image creation, and storytelling; and sharing celebrations and family rituals. These actions were used in early healing practices and, according to Perry, are now known to be effective in altering neural systems involved in stress responses and developing secure attachment. Similarly, the arts therapies are normalizing experiences for children and trauma-informed practices, in that they involve experiences that children in all cultures recognize (Malchiodi, 2008).

Siegel (2012) offers another perspective that clarifies the role of the creative arts therapies in treating attachment disorders from a sensory perspective. He cites the importance of "critical micromoments" of interaction with a client; these include the client's tone of voice, postures, facial expressions, eye contact, and motion, which Siegel believes provide clues to the individual's psychobiology. These sensory-based cues become particularly important in identifying and formulating strategies for addressing disrupted, insecure, or disorganized attachment. Siegel also proposes the use of experientially based methods such as drawing to help individuals become aware of sensations, emotions, images, and relationships.

Nonverbal Communication

Nonverbal communication is our most basic form of communication, and it is how caregiver and infant initially connect in the infant's first years of life (Schore, 2003). Although most creative arts therapies involve talk, they are also defined as nonverbal approaches because self-expression through an activity becomes a major source of communication. For children in particular, nonverbal means of communication are an important part of any therapy, because children do not always have the words to convey feelings and experiences accurately.

Because thoughts and feelings are not strictly verbal and are not limited to storage as verbal language in the brain, expressive modalities are particularly useful in helping individuals communicate aspects of memories and stories that may not be readily available through conversation. Memories in particular have been reported to emerge through touch, imagery, or carefully guided body movements (Rothschild, 2000). For some individuals, conveying a memory or story through one or more expressive modalities is more easily tolerated than verbalization. For example, children who have been severely traumatized may repeat experiences through play or art activity when the trauma memories are particularly complex or overwhelming (Gil, 2006; Malchiodi, 1997, 2008). In addition, nonverbal expression through a painting, play activity, imaginative role play, or movement may be a corrective experience in and of itself for some individuals.

Right-Hemisphere Dominance

In the field of attachment, it is widely accepted that what happens early in life in terms of relationships affects brain development and is essential to secure attachment (Perry, 2009). *Neuroplasticity* (also called *brain plasticity*) is the brain's ability to renew and, in some cases, even to rewire itself to compensate for deficits or injuries (Doidge, 2007). Brain plasticity is greater early in life—a fact underscoring the importance of appropriate intervention with young children in order not only to enhance attachment, but also to support the development of appropriate affect regulation, interpersonal skills, and cognition.

The right hemisphere of the brain is particularly active during early interactions between very young children and caregivers, and it stores the *internal working model* for attachment relationships and affect regulation (Klorer, 2008; Schore, 2003). Siegel (2012) and Schore (2003) note that interactions between baby and caregiver are right-brain-mediated, because during infancy the right cortex is developing more quickly than the left. Siegel (2012) also observes that just as the left hemisphere requires exposure to language to grow, the right hemisphere requires emotional stimulation to develop properly. He proposes that the output of the right brain is expressed in "non-word-based ways," such as drawing a picture or using a visual image to describe feelings or events.

Research on the impact of trauma proposes that highly charged emotional experiences are encoded by the limbic system and right brain as sensory memories (van der Kolk, 2006). Consequently, expression and processing of these memories on a sensory level are important parts of successful intervention (Rothschild, 2000; Steele & Malchiodi, 2012). Current thinking about trauma supports the effect of childhood trauma on integration of the hemispheres (Teicher, 2000), and it suggests that sensory-based interventions may be effective because they do not rely on the individual's use of left-brain language for processing (Klorer, 2008) and are predominantly right-brain-driven.

Affect Regulation

Hyperarousal is a common response in individuals whose attachment is insecure, disorganized, or disrupted; in particular, young clients who have experienced traumatic events have understandable difficulties with affect regulation. Children who have been victims of interpersonal violence are particularly at risk for problems with affect regulation, including hyperarousal and dissociation. On an implicit level, these children's worldviews include feelings of abandonment and lack of safety; in order to stay safe, they may often react with rage at anyone who is perceived as a threat, or may become disengaged from adults because they come to feel that caregivers abandon or hurt children.

The treatment of attachment difficulties begins with regulation of emotions, stress reduction, and restoration of feelings of safety. Fortunately, specific applications of the creative arts therapies can be used to activate the body's relaxation response. Depending on the individual, experiences with art making, music, and/or movement can have a comforting and calming affect that decreases anxiety or fear. For example, even simple activities such as drawing a picture of a pleasant time or hearing a soothing, familiar song, story, or rhyme are effective because of the imagination's capacity to recall sensory memories and details of positive moments (Malchiodi, 1997, 2008). Creative arts activities may stimulate the placebo effect through mimicking self-soothing experiences of childhood and inducing relaxation (Malchiodi, 2012a). A well-known example of affect regulation via mimicry is the child who strokes a blanket or toy in a way that mimics a caregiver's comfort. Creative arts therapies, especially with attachment disorders, seek to help individuals find activities that are effective in tapping positive sensory experiences, that can be practiced over time, and that eventually become resources for regulating overwhelming emotions. Repetition of pleasurable experiential activities can become a source of self-soothing, and as Gladding (2005) notes, the arts often allow people to experience themselves differently and in positive ways. Through carefully chosen opportunities for self-expression, individuals are able to exhibit and practice novel and adaptive behaviors, including the ability to induce calm feelings and self-soothe.

Relational Interventions

Interpersonal neurobiology (Badenoch, 2008; Siegel, 2012) refers to an overarching theory that weaves together many strands of knowledge, including attachment research, neurobiology, and developmental and social psychology. It is based on the idea that social relationships shape how our brains develop, how our minds perceive the world, and how we adapt to stress throughout the lifespan. In the field of counseling, the creative arts in counseling are defined as inherently "relational" approaches to treatment (Gladding, 2005). *Relational therapy* is historically defined as an approach that empowers individuals with the skills necessary to create productive and healthy relationships. In a broad sense, all psychotherapy and counseling are relational approaches, because the outcome of intervention is dependent on the core relationship between the therapist and client. Most therapy also addresses disruptions in relationships, such as acute or chronic trauma, loss, or attachment disruption.

Creative arts therapies are inherently relational therapies because they involve an active, sensory-based dynamic between practitioner and individual. All creative arts therapies are relational approaches to treatment that may involve mirroring, role play, enactment, sharing, showing, and witnessing (Malchiodi, 2005, 2012a). They may be helpful in repairing and reshaping attachment through experiential and sensory means, and may tap those early relational states that existed before words became dominant, allowing the brain to establish new, more productive patterns (Malchiodi, 2012b; Riley, 2002). In addition, being an attuned and focused witness to a child's efforts to complete a hands-on task, and assisting those efforts when appropriate, mimic the neurobiological relationship between a caring adult and a child. For some children, repetitive experiential and self-rewarding experiences that include a positive and attuned witness are central to repairing disrupted attachment and developing a sense of security and confidence (Perry, 2009). In brief, reparative enactments of secure attachment experiences, co-created by therapist and client, are fundamental to positive change.

Although all the creative arts therapies can be used with a goal of enhancing relationship, dance/movement therapy is most often used to address attachment issues, because it focuses on the body. For example, *mirroring* is commonly used to establish and enhance the relationship between the individual and the therapist. The goal of mirroring is not merely to have the client imitate movements, postures, facial expressions, and gestures, but to achieve a sense of connection and understanding between the client and practitioner. This is also a form of nonverbal, right-hemisphere communication that naturally occurs in secure attachment relationships through shared gestures, postures, and facial expressions between a caregiver and child. (For more information on dance/movement therapy, see Devereaux, Chapter 6, this volume).

Relational aspects are evident in art, music, and drama therapy also. In art therapy, a therapist is a provider of materials (nurturer), an assistant in the creative process, and an active participant in facilitating visual self-expression (see Malchiodi, Chapter 4, this volume). These are experiences that emphasize interaction through experiential, tactile, and visual exchanges, not just verbal communication, between the client and therapist. Music therapy (see Robarts, Chapter 5, this volume) provides similar experiences through interaction with music making; it also has the potential to tap social engagement and communication when collaboration or simultaneous playing of instruments is involved. Porges (2010) notes that vocalizations are particularly effective in stimulating a sense of affiliation and relationship, and that experiences involving specific music can inherently calm and self-regulate. Finally, drama therapy (see Gil & Dias, Chapter 7, this volume) offers multisensory ways to establish relationship through role play, mirroring, and enactment, and often includes other creative arts and play to support and enhance attachment.

Trauma-Informed Expressive Arts Therapy

Exposure to traumatic events is recognized as a significant factor in the development of attachment disorders (Oppenheim & Goldsmith, 2007). Freud (1920/1955) himself observed that traumatic experiences shatter the "protective shield" and threaten the core of the attachment relationship. Crises or loss disrupt parent–child dynamics and cause stress reactions in both the child and adult; these disruptions hinder the child's ability to find security from the caregiver, and may compromise the parent's ability to provide needed reassurance and comfort to the child. Insecure, disrupted, or disorganized attachment is often related to chronic traumatic experiences early in life. In general, these trauma experiences are encoded implicitly as sensory memories that are kinesthetic, auditory, olfactory, visual, and/or affective in nature. They influence relationships with caregivers and others, because individuals respond from lower-brain and limbic systems rather than from cortical areas (executive functions) of the brain.

Trauma-informed expressive arts therapy is one model for intervention that integrates neurodevelopmental knowledge and the sensory qualities of all the arts in trauma intervention, including attachment issues (Malchiodi, 2012a, 2012c). In brief, this approach takes into consideration how the mind and body respond to traumatic events; recognizes that symptoms are adaptive coping strategies rather than pathology; and helps individuals move from being "survivors" to becoming "thrivers" (Malchiodi, 2012c). Trauma-informed expressive arts therapy is based on the idea that the creative arts therapies are helpful in reconnecting implicit (sensory) and explicit (declarative) memories of trauma and in the treatment of post-traumatic stress disorder (PTSD) (Malchiodi, 2012a). In particular, it is an approach used to improve an individual's capacity to self-regulate affect and moderate the body's reactions to traumatic experiences to set the stage for eventual trauma integration and recovery.

Trauma-informed expressive arts therapy is also a means to address and enhance attachment, particularly in children who have experienced multiple traumas and losses. It includes a neurosequential approach that capitalizes on the expressive therapies continuum (Lusebrink, 2010) as a framework for applying appropriate creative arts therapies interventions (see Table 1.1). In attachment work, an emphasis is placed on arts-based experiences that reinforce a sense of safety through reconnection to positive attachment and self-soothing. The creative arts therapies are also used as ways to build strengths through experiences of mastery that normalize and enhance resilience. In brief, this means providing various opportunities for the individual to engage in creative experimentation that integrate experiences of unconditional appreciation, guidance, and support—experiences found in families with secure attachment relationships. In work with either a child or an adult, the goal is to help the individual recover the "creative

TABLE 1.1. Neurodevelopment and Arts Therapies

Area of brain	General functions	ETC level	Art therapy interventions
Brainstem	• Focus • Attunement to others • Attachment to others • Stress responses	Kinesthetic/ sensory	• Sensory use of art materials • Texture and tactile elements • Self-soothing arts experiences (visual, music, movement) • Experiences of connection and approval • Rituals/structure in presentation
Midbrain diencephalon	• Motor skills • Coordination • Stress responses • Attunement to others • Attachment to others	Kinesthetic/ sensory	• Physically oriented activities (cross the midline; engage body) • Learning skills via art and play • Self-soothing arts experiences (visual, music, movement) • Experiences of connection and approval • Rituals/structure in presentation
Limbic system	• Affect regulation • Pleasure • Relationships • Attunement • Attachment	Perceptual/ affective	• Masks, puppets for projection and relational play • Arts and crafts for creative expression and skill enhancement • Group art therapy/family art therapy • Self-soothing arts experiences (visual, music, movement) • Rituals/structure in presentation
Cortex	• Cognition • Executive function • Self-image • Social competency • Communication	Cognitive/ symbolic	• Cognitive-based methods possible, but sensory and affective methods may still be needed • Bibliotherapy with arts and play • Arts for skill enhancement and self-esteem • Teamwork in group art therapy • Problem-solving skills

Note. Based on the expressive therapies continuum (ETC) in Lusebrink (2010), Malchiodi (2012c), and Perry (2006). From Malchiodi (2012b). Copyright 2012 by The Guilford Press. Reprinted by permission.

life" (Cattanach, 2008), and to gain or regain a sense of well-being in one-self and in relationship to others.

In order to illustrate some of the key aspects of a trauma-informed expressive arts therapy approach with an attachment focus, the following brief case vignette is presented.

Case Vignette: Joanne, a Survivor of Multiple Traumas

Background and Early Sessions

Joanne, age 10, was referred to therapy after she witnessed her father beating her mother, Marie, on three occasions and was herself the victim of repeated physical abuse by her father. Marie did not report the incidents of child abuse or domestic violence until protective services removed Joanne and her younger brother Mark, age 5, from the home when their mother became unconscious due to a drug overdose. Joanne found her mother lying on the floor of their apartment and called the police, while Mark knelt screaming next to his mother's inert body. Although their mother recovered, social services felt it was in the children's best interests to stay at a residential treatment facility for the short term.

When I first visited Joanne at the facility, she was hypervigilant and unable to concentrate for very long. But she did like to draw and paint, and wanted to make a picture of her family because she missed her mother very much. When I asked Joanne to tell me more about the drawing, she said it was a picture of herself, Mark, and "my mommy." There were three human figures in the picture, each drawn appropriately for Joanne's age range (Figure 1.1). I asked, "Is there anyone else in the picture?" Joanne replied, "Well, I forget about my daddy a lot. He was mean to my mommy and hurt her all the time. He hit me and Mark, too."

Joanne's statement did not surprise me. Child abuse and domestic violence affect attachment relationships; children feel fearful that the violent parent or parental figure will cause injury or put them in danger. In order to resolve her difficult relationship with an abusive father, Joanne simply left him out of the picture. In subsequent art therapy sessions with Joanne, I also learned more about the complexities of her relationship with her mother: Joanne had increasingly become frightened and often angry at her mother, feeling abandoned during numerous incidents when Marie passed out from drug overdoses. In Joanne's case, attachment was also disrupted by Marie's neglect, indifference, or unresponsiveness; it shattered Joanne's trust that Marie would protect her from harm. Marie and Joanne both reported that Joanne was often anxious (hyperaroused) and also experienced sleep problems (nighttime anxiety and nightmares). In addition, Joanne's school counselor observed that she had difficulty with comprehension, focus, and attention, as well as with impulsively acting out (e.g., hitting other children or yelling at her classroom teacher).

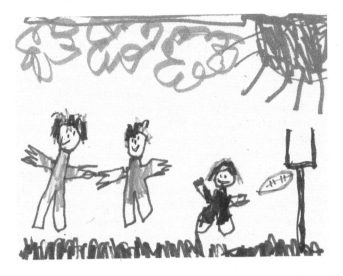

FIGURE 1.1. Joanne's drawing of her family, including her mother and younger brother but excluding her father.

Joanne's responses to me during our initial sessions mirrored her fear and anger about her primary caregivers. For example, she generally demanded my undivided attention when she was engaged in art making or play—particularly in the creative arts therapy group sessions, when she competed for attention with other child participants. On one occasion, she had a violent tantrum when I did not have enough clay on hand for her to complete a project; at another time, she scolded me for being a few minutes late for a session. It was easy to see that Joanne feared abandonment and had a difficult time self-regulating her emotions when confronted with situations she could not completely control or circumstances that felt unsafe.

In Joanne's case, the abuse by her father and a sense of abandonment by her mother both contributed to her attachment difficulties. Her attachment role also became disorganized because she had to assume the role of the caregiver when Marie's drug addiction prevented her from providing appropriate parenting to her children. In the art and play therapy room, Joanne often took on an adult persona, caring for other children and insisting on having a "helper" role during sessions.

A "Brain-Wise" Framework for Creative Intervention

In my work with Joanne, creative arts therapies interventions were guided by the five principles outlined in the earlier section on creative arts therapies and the brain, and by a trauma-informed expressive arts therapy framework. In brief, Joanne would benefit most from arts-based activities that addressed her emotional reactions and stress responses, create a sense of safety, and (to some extent) teach attunement to others and social awareness. She also would benefit from experiencing a positive relationship with me through sensory activities that recapitulated early attachment experiences via nonverbal and right-hemisphere interventions.

Initially, Joanne was able to show me easily through drawings that she felt detached from her abusive father by literally leaving him out of the picture. When working with children like Joanne, I generally start with arts experiences that are neurodevelopmentally related to lower parts of the brain (brainstem, midbrain, and limbic system) and designed to be self-soothing and self-regulating. Although Joanne was 10 years old, I introduced a few activities that I might use with much younger children, such as listening to various soothing rhythms, playing drums and percussion instruments together, and recalling favorite songs from preschool days. I introduced felt markers with different smells of familiar foods for drawing activities, as well as a variety of tactile materials for art making. In doing so, I took on the role of someone who provided materials for creative self-expression and accepted this self-expression with unconditional regard. At other times, I taught Joanne some child-friendly yoga poses, including ones that made us laugh because we enjoyed being "silly" together. We practiced deep breathing together, and I taught Joanne several child-appropriate mindfulness activities, such as balancing a long peacock feather on the tip of her finger and a colorful, self-created butterfly on the tip of her nose (Figure 1.2). All of these interventions were selected to support self-soothing experiences; in addition, I was making a "right-brain-to-right-brain" connection with Joanne by communicating with her through hands-on activities rather than words alone (the left hemisphere) and by using creative interventions to build a relationship.

Although it took many weeks before Joanne could engage in these initial sessions without angry or anxious feelings, she eventually began to feel safe in our relationship. She began to let me know what activities she enjoyed instead of communicating through tantrums, and even made suggestions indicating that she felt comfortable collaborating with me (e.g., asking if we could "make cookies together" or use materials "to build a house for a mother bird and her baby birds"). At this point in our relationship, I asked Joanne to share her feelings with me through art expression. She felt safe enough to respond with colors, lines, and shapes when I asked her "how your body feels when you worry" and "where in your body you feel worry, fear, and anger." I also introduced her to some simple musical instruments (drums, rattles, kazoo, and various percussion instruments) and encouraged her to make sounds to communicate feelings to me without words; Joanne began to use this activity as a way to convey to me how she was feeling at the beginning of each session. With my help, she was also able to begin to recognize situations when she felt these emotions and what types of situations caused her to become distressed.

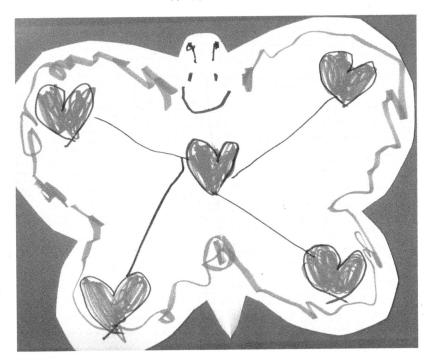

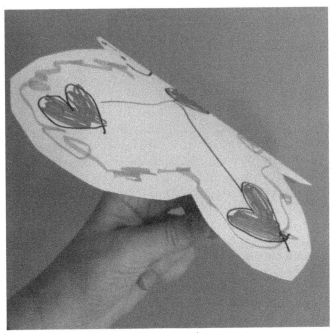

FIGURE 1.2 Two views of the butterfly Joanne created for use in a mindfulness activity.

My repetitive role as a provider of sensory means of self-expression, with unconditional positive regard for the outcome, became the bridge for Joanne to experience secure attachment with an adult. We made a good deal of progress in building a relationship before Joanne was moved to foster care in another town along with her brother, Mark. Her therapy continued for another year with another therapist after my work with her ended. However, before we terminated our sessions together, Marie was allowed to begin reestablishing her parenting role with Joanne and was asked to participate in several mother–child creative arts therapies sessions with us.

Because a trauma-informed expressive arts therapy approach applies to individuals of all ages, and particularly those who may be in need of trauma or attachment intervention, I repeated several of the activities I had used earlier with Joanne with Marie as a participant. For example, Marie herself was in need of self-regulation through other means than drugs; because she had been in a violent relationship with her husband for most of their married life, she understandably needed some self-soothing experiences as well. In particular, I focused on some simple self-soothing creative activities that Marie could initiate with Joanne at home, such as quiet times for drawing, scrapbooking pictures, and collage work. More importantly, I was able to introduce some experiences of collaborative, attachment-enhancing activities, such as building a dollhouse together from shoeboxes and making puppet families from socks. Although I do not know the ultimate outcome of our work together, I do know that Joanne, Mark, and Marie were eventually reunited, and that Marie, with the help of addictions counseling, has been able to maintain a drug-free existence.

Conclusion

With many child clients like Joanne and parents like Marie, we have a limited number of sessions to accomplish attachment goals that may or may not be retained over time. Despite the challenges of these types of situations, I believe that we do make an impact on the individuals we seek to help by using creative arts as part of therapy, for one key reason: The creative arts therapies are "brain-wise" interventions. When used in purposeful ways, these approaches are compatible with what we currently understand about the brain and attachment; they capitalize on nonverbal and right-hemisphere communication, active participation, and the self-soothing nature of creative expression through images, sound, movement, and enactment. Most importantly, the creative arts are a way to experience a secure relationship with a helping professional that resonates on a sensory level in both mind and body, and in a place within each of us where attachment is most authentically recognized, integrated, and appreciated.

REFERENCES

American Music Therapy Association. (2013). *About music therapy.* Retrieved February 25, 2013, from *www.musictherapy.org/about/musictherapy*

Badenoch, B. (2008). *Being a brain-wise therapist: A practical guide to interpersonal neurobiology.* New York: Norton.

Bowlby, J. (2005). *A secure base.* New York: Routledge. (Original work published 1988)

Cattanach, A. (2008). *Play therapy with abused children.* London: Kingsley.

Doidge, N. (2007). *The brain that changes itself.* New York: Penguin.

Edwards, D. (2004). *Art therapy.* Thousand Oaks, CA: Sage.

Freud, S. (1955). *Beyond the pleasure principle.* In J. Strachey (Ed. & Trans.), *The standard edition of the complete psychological works of Sigmund Freud* (Vol. 18, pp. 7–64). London: Hogarth Press. (Original work published 1920)

Gil, E. (2006). *Helping abused and traumatized children.* New York: Guilford Press.

Gladding, S. (2005). *Counseling as an art: Creative arts in counseling* (3rd ed.). Alexandria, VA: American Counseling Association.

Goodill, S. (2005). *Introduction to medical dance/movement therapy.* London: Kingsley.

Johnson, D. R. (2009). *Current approaches in drama therapy.* Springfield, IL: Thomas.

Klorer, P. G. (2008). Expressive therapy for severe maltreatment and attachment disorders: A neuroscience framework. In C. A. Malchiodi (Ed.), *Creative interventions with traumatized children* (pp. 43–61). New York: Guilford Press.

Knill, P., Barba, H. N., & Fuchs, M. (2004). *Minstrels of the soul: Intermodal expressive therapy.* Toronto: EGS Press.

Lusebrink, V. (2010). Assessment and therapeutic application of the expressive therapies continuum: Implications for brain structures and functions. *Art Therapy, 27*(4), 168–177.

Malchiodi, C. A. (1997). *Breaking the silence: Art therapy with children from violent homes* (2nd ed.). New York: Brunner-Routledge.

Malchiodi, C. A. (Ed.). (2005). *Expressive therapies.* New York: Guilford Press.

Malchiodi, C. A. (Ed.). (2008). *Creative interventions with traumatized children.* New York: Guilford Press.

Malchiodi, C. A. (2012a). Art therapy and the brain. In C. A. Malchiodi (Ed.), *Handbook of art therapy* (2nd ed., pp. 17–26). New York: Guilford Press.

Malchiodi, C. A. (2012b). Developmental art therapy. In C. A. Malchiodi (Ed.), *Handbook of art therapy* (2nd ed., pp. 114–129). New York: Guilford Press.

Malchiodi, C. A. (2012c). Trauma-informed art therapy with sexually abused children. In P. Goodyear-Brown (Ed.), *Handbook of child sexual abuse: Prevention, assessment, and treatment* (pp. 341–354). Hoboken, NJ: Wiley.

Micozzi, M. (Ed.). (2011). *Fundamentals of complementary and alternative medicine* (4th ed.). St. Louis, MO: Saunders/Elsevier.

National Association for Poetry Therapy. (2013). *National Association for Poetry Therapy.* Retrieved February 25, 2013, from *www.poetrytherapy.org/index.html*

National Dance Therapy Association. (2013). *About dance/movement therapy.* Retrieved February 25, 2013, from *www.adta.org/About_DMT*

National Drama Therapy Association. (2013). *What is drama therapy?* Retrieved February 20, 2013, from *www.nadt.org/what-is-drama-therapy.html*

Oppenheim, D., & Goldsmith, D. (Eds.). (2007). *Attachment theory in clinical work with children.* New York: Guilford Press.

Payne, H. (Ed.). (2013). *Dance movement therapy: Theory, research and practice.* New York: Routledge.

Perry, B. (2006). The neurosequential model of therapeutics: Applying principles of neuroscience to clinical work with traumatized and maltreated children. In N. B. Webb (Ed.), *Working with traumatized youth in child welfare* (pp. 27–52). New York: Guilford Press.

Perry, B. (2008). Foreword. In C. A. Malchiodi (Ed.), *Creative interventions with traumatized children* (pp. ix–xi). New York: Guilford Press.

Perry, B. (2009). Examining child maltreatment through a neurodevelopmental lens. *Journal of Trauma and Loss, 14,* 240–255.

Porges, S. W. (2010). Music therapy and trauma: Insights from the polyvagal theory. In K. Stewart (Ed.), *Symposium on music therapy and trauma: Bridging theory and clinical practice.* New York: Satchnote Press.

Riley, S. (2002). *Group process made visible.* New York: Taylor & Francis.

Rothschild, B. (2000). *The body remembers.* New York: Norton.

Schore, A. (2003). *Affect regulation and the repair of the self.* New York: Norton.

Siegel, D. (2012). *The developing mind* (2nd ed.). New York: Guilford Press.

Steele, W., & Malchiodi, C. A. (2012). *Trauma-informed practices with children and adolescents.* New York: Routledge.

Teicher, M. H. (2000). Wounds that won't heal: The neurobiology of child abuse. *Cerebrum, 2*(4), 50–62.

van der Kolk, B. (2006). Clinical applications of neuroscience research in PTSD. *Annals of the New York Academy of Sciences, 1071*(4), 277–293.

Warren, B. (2004). *Using the creative arts in therapy: A practical introduction* (2nd ed.). New York: Routledge.

Weiner, D. (1999). *Beyond talk therapy: Using movement and expressive techniques in clinical practice.* Washington, DC: American Psychological Association.

Wheeler, B. L., Shultis, C. L., & Polen, D. W. (2005). *Clinical training guide for the student music therapist.* Gilsum, NH: Barcelona.

CHAPTER 2

Play Therapy Approaches to Attachment Issues

David A. Crenshaw

The need to explicate the role of play therapy and the creative arts therapies with attachment issues was vividly brought to my attention when I searched the index of the often consulted and acclaimed second edition of the *Handbook of Attachment* (Cassidy & Shaver, 2008). In this comprehensive volume of 1,020 pages, I found only four separate references to page numbers in the index for play, and none for play therapy, art therapy, creative arts therapy, or expressive arts therapy. I should note that the four selections of page numbers in the index referring to play were important ones, briefly detailing (1) the role of attachment security in social play repertoires; (2) the critical importance of attachment for the quality of play; (3) the dependence of "play-mothering" and later caregiving capacity on the experience of maternal care; and (4) the facts that exploratory behavior is playful and that play only develops in a secure context. In spite of this lack of attention until recently among attachment theorists and play therapy researchers, there is a long history of play therapy approaches dedicated to treating attachment problems.

Early Roots of the Focus on Attachment in Play Therapy

The crucial role of favorable early attachment was recognized and written about extensively by the early psychoanalysts. A consensus in psychoanalytic writing from the earliest days was that human infants need unconditional love in order to develop in a healthy way what one analyst called "non-obligating solicitude" (Bonime, 1989). The psychoanalyst Erich Fromm (1947) expressed it eloquently:

> Motherly love does not depend on conditions which the child has to fulfill in order to be loved; it is unconditional, based only upon the child's request and the mother's response. No wonder that motherly love has been a symbol of the highest form of love in art and religion. (pp. 99–100)

Freud (1909/1959) also weighed in on the incomparable role of early attachment figures:

> For a small child his parents are the first and the only authority and the source of all belief. The child's most intense and most momentous wish during these early years is to be like his parents (that is, the parent of his own sex) and to be big like his father and mother. (p. 237)

Lili Peller (1946) understood that this love needs to come from those with whom the infant is biologically bonded—a fact that has led to immeasurable heartbreak for children and parents in the foster care system. Peller wrote:

> The child's greatest need is for love from the persons to whom he is attached, and not merely from persons who chance to be near him. 'Persons of his environment,' his teacher or nurse or a kind-hearted aunt, may offer this love amply to the child—yet he profits but little. We can assume that many foster-children have been offered love and affection to no avail. (p. 415)

The psychoanalyst Edward Edinger (1972) beautifully described the gift enjoyed by recipients of unconditional love in infancy: "The sense of innate worth prior to and irrespective of deeds and accomplishments is the precious deposit that is left in the psyche by the experience of genuine parental love" (p. 167).

Early roots of play therapy's focus on attachment and attachment trauma can also be found in the writings of Donald Winnicott (1971), as detailed by Tuber, Boesch, Gorkin, and Terry in Chapter 13 of this volume. Tuber (2008) has explained in an earlier publication that Winnicott (1971) identified a tolerable window of infant distress when the mother (primary caregiver) is absent; when this window is exceeded in duration, or the infant undergoes emotional duress, the experience for the infant is one of confusion and disorganization. Interestingly, nearly two decades later the term *disorganized attachment* was introduced by Main and Solomon (1990) to describe the effects of severe attachment trauma.

Winnicott became interested in attachment issues and the corollary experiences of separation and loss during World War II. Winnicott, along with John Bowlby, Anna Freud, and other prominent British and European analysts, worked hard to resettle children in the countryside so that they could escape the incessant bombings in London. In a letter written in 1939 to the *British Medical Journal* and titled "Evacuation of Small Children," Bowlby and Winnicott, along with the analyst Emanuel Miller, stated:

> It is quite possible for a child of any age to feel sad or upset at having to leave home, but . . . such an experience in the case of a little child can mean far more than the actual experience of sadness. It can in fact amount to an emotional "black-out" and can easily lead to a severe disturbance of the development of the personality which may persist throughout life. (Bowlby, Miller, & Winnicott, 1939, pp. 1202–1203)

Thus, in the midst of the horror of World War II, these early analysts described what we now consider *attachment trauma* and what is sometimes called in children *developmental trauma*.

What Is Attachment Trauma?

Attachment trauma is one of the terms intended to address the growing consensus that posttraumatic stress disorder (PTSD) does not adequately describe what happens to people when they suffer interpersonal trauma. This is especially true when the trauma ruptures relationships with primary attachment figures. PTSD—a diagnostic classification in the third, fourth, and now fifth editions of the American Psychiatric Association's (1980, 1994, 2013), *Diagnostic and Statistical Manual of Mental Disorders* (DSM-III, DSM-IV, and DSM-5 respectively)—describes a cluster of symptoms that tend to ameliorate in time (often in 3 months) and are responsive to evidence-based treatments, most notably cognitive-behavioral therapy. What the diagnosis of PTSD does not adequately detail is the often enduring relational impact when trauma intrudes into the interpersonal life of any person, but especially a child. If, for example, a child is abused by the very person(s) responsible for his or her well-being, safety, and nurture, the insidious effects on the capacity to trust, to risk closeness with another, and to envision a positive future are common enduring sequelae not addressed by the PTSD classification of symptoms; nor can they be addressed adequately in brief treatment models.

The inadequacy of the PTSD diagnostic criteria has long spurred a debate among some of the leading trauma researchers and clinicians. Judith Herman (1992) offered the term *complex trauma* to delineate trauma that involves repeated and chronic abuse, instead of a single traumatic event that can cause PTSD symptoms. Previously, Lenore Terr (1990) distinguished between *Type 1* and *Type 2* traumas. Type 1 represents single-event trauma, whereas Type 2 refers to repeated or chronic trauma and often multiple traumatic factors (such as growing up in poverty, exposure to abuse, and/or exposure to domestic or community violence). Herman also decried the use of what she considered demeaning diagnostic labels that are used to characterize the complexity of symptoms resulting from repeated exposure to trauma, such as borderline personality disorder. More recently, Bessel van der Kolk (2005) has offered the term *developmental trauma* to describe complex trauma in childhood, because of its potentially devastating impact on the course of the unfolding developmental process.

Allan Schore (2012) has written eloquently about *relational trauma*. Schore emphasizes the impact of unfavorable early attachments (during the first 18 months of life) on the development of the right hemisphere of the brain. Schore has demonstrated that ruptures and lack of repair of the attunement process between the infant and the primary caregiver result in impaired development of the right hemisphere. One of the major effects is the inability to regulate emotions adequately, and another is impaired relational capacity.

There was a time some 20 years ago when the work of attachment researchers and the work of clinicians in therapy rooms ran on separate tracks, with little collaboration between the two groups. All of that changed when the writings of two master integrators from the University of California at Los Angeles (UCLA), Daniel Siegel and Allan Schore, became widely read. Siegel's (1999, 2012) *The Developing Mind* opened the eyes of many to the possibilities of making use of attachment theory and research findings in therapeutic work. His development of the interpersonal neurobiological approach not only combined attachment research with psychotherapy theory and research, but added the contributions of neuroscience to our understanding of how attachment and psychotherapy change the structure of the brain. As noted above, Schore (1994, 2003a, 2003b, 2012) is the other UCLA researcher and clinician who has been able to synthesize findings from psychoanalytic and attachment theory with neuroscience research to highlight the pivotal role of favorable early attachments in the proper development of the right hemisphere of the brain, which in turn critically influences the development of emotional regulation. Schore has also delineated the important implications of his work for psychotherapy, since emotional dysregulation is a key feature of most childhood and adult psychiatric disorders. This exciting work has not validated the concept of infantile determinism, because neuroscience research has demonstrated that new brain connections can be made throughout life, but it has affirmed the Freudian emphasis on early parent–child relationships and the critical periods for secure attachments coinciding with the incredible rate of brain development in the first 2 years of life.

Bruce Perry (Perry & Szalavitz, 2006), another key contributor to our understanding of the neurobiological underpinnings of emotional and relational development, has explained that if critical periods in the early attachment process are missed, a child is not doomed; however, when repair is attempted later in development, it will take much longer and require much repetition of favorable experiences with attachment figures. The good news is that children possess impressive innate capacities for self-reparative and healing processes, combined with security in relationships with caregivers. The bad news is that if the healthy innate forces combined with favorable attachment experiences come later in the developmental sequence, it will take much more time to effect the positive changes.

Jon Allen (2013) is another seminal theorist and clinician; his work builds on the attachment research of British theorists, particularly Peter Fonagy (Fonagy & Target, 1997). Fonagy and his colleagues used the term *attachment trauma* to refer not only to trauma that takes place in the context of attachment relationships, but also to the damaging impact of such trauma on the capacity to develop secure attachment. Allen views *neglect* (defined as the lack of psychological attunement) as central to attachment trauma. Allen elaborates further that "trauma stems from being left *psychologically alone in unbearable emotional pain*" (p. xxii; emphasis in original).

In addition to the lack of consensus regarding the definition of attachment trauma and the controversies surrounding inclusion–exclusion of complex PTSD and developmental trauma disorder in DSM-5 (they were ultimately excluded), there is lack of agreement on variations of attachment disorders. Beginning with DSM-III, and followed by DSM-IV and DSM-IV-TR, reactive attachment disorder (RAD) was the only recognized attachment disorder included in this official diagnostic classification manual of the American Psychiatric Association. RAD is a rare form of attachment trauma suffered primarily by children who have been institutionalized in early life and/or severely abused. There were two recognized forms of this disorder: (1) the emotionally withdrawn/inhibited form, in which there is a failure to respond to comfort when offered and failure to seek comfort when distressed from a preferred attachment figure; and (2) the disinhibited/indiscriminately social type, in which the child is overly interested in interacting with and sometimes seeking affection from unfamiliar adults, without distinction. These more severe forms of attachment disorder are seen in some children in residential treatment centers, as well as in some (but certainly not all) cross-cultural adoptions of previously institutionalized children.

DSM-5 split the previously existing category of RAD into two separate diagnoses. Reactive attachment disorder is now defined as a lack of or incomplete formation of preferred attachments to familiar people, with a dampening of positive affect that resembles internalizing disorders (e.g., anxiety). Disinhibited social engagement disorder is the other diagnosis.

Play therapists may work with children with RAD in their private offices, clinics, or residential treatment center playrooms, but far more frequently play therapists see children with less severe problems of insecure attachment, and the goal is to increase attachment security. Even more advantageous are the prevention programs that can head off such relational problems by intervening early.

How Does Play Therapy Address Attachment Trauma?

Since the value of all psychotherapy rests on the foundation of the therapeutic relationship, play therapy, with its emphasis on the dyadic relationship, offers the possibility of greater attachment security for a child who has suffered interpersonal trauma. In addition, play therapy has a distinct advantage over other relationship therapies, in that one of the therapeutic powers of play is attachment formation (Schaefer, 1993; Schaefer & Drewes, 2014). Schaefer explains that secure attachment can be facilitated in children by replicating the positive parent–child relationship through sensory–motor play. Schaefer (1993) has observed, "Playful interactions involving touch and smiling are perhaps the most natural and enjoyable ways to form an attachment with a child in the playroom" (p. 11).

Theraplay

An early form of play therapy that preceded the seminal volumes on loss and attachment by Bowlby was a focused attachment process called Theraplay (Jernberg, 1979). In 1967, Ann Jernberg was appointed the director of the Head Start program in Chicago. She recruited Phyllis Booth as one of her assistants (see Booth, Lindaman, & Winstead, Chapter 9, this volume). Jernberg did not feel that referring the numerous children who needed intervention to existing crowded mental health clinics was an adequate solution; instead, she developed her own program. In order to meet the enormity of the need, she designed her program to make use of paraprofessionals working under the supervision of mental health professionals. Theraplay is a model of play therapy that is based on healthy parent–child interactions and draws partly on the work of Austin Des Lauriers (1962) and Viola Brody (1997). As a result of this pioneering work with Head Start, the Theraplay Institute was formed in 1971, and children from the community were referred for treatment. From this modest beginning in Chicago in the late 1960s, Theraplay is now practiced in over 36 countries around the world.

Filial Therapy

Filial Therapy (FT), developed by Bernard and Louise Guerney in the late 1950s, has considerable research support and has developed as a powerful family therapy and play therapy intervention (B. G. Guerney, 1964; L. F. Guerney, 2003; L. F. Guerney & Ryan, 2013; VanFleet, 2013). It has a specific focus on attachment and treating forms of insecure attachment, along with more severe cases of attachment trauma (see Topham, VanFleet, & Sniscak, Chapter 8, this volume). One of the compelling advantages of FT in the treatment of attachment trauma is the presence of the primary attachment figure(s) in the treatment. Attachment security is being built between the child and one or more primary caregivers even as the trauma is being addressed.

The Circle of Security

In addition to the attachment formation power of play, play enhances the relationship of the child not only with the play therapist but with others who may participate in the play therapy, such as the primary caregiver(s) in FT, in developmental play therapy (Brody, 1997), and in prevention programs like the Circle of Security (see Stewart, Whelan, & Pendleton, Chapter 3, this volume). The Circle of Security program specifically teaches parents to recognize when children need encouragement to explore and to move away from the parent, and to provide support and a secure base to return to when the child needs a safety net. The playful interactions combined with the sensitive attunement of the parent's empathic responding to the child's needs greatly enhances the attachment bonds. Schaefer (1993) has written: "The role of play in facilitating a positive relationship is related to the nature of playful interactions that are fun filled and concerned with enjoyment rather than achievement" (p. 12). The most effective way to build an attachment or enhance a relationship with a child is to create safe, trusting, and gratifying experiences with an adult, and play is an effective and natural medium to facilitate the process.

The Neurosequential Model of Therapeutics

As noted earlier, one of the pioneers in the neurobiology of attachment is Bruce Perry (Perry, 2009; Perry & Szalavitz, 2006), who has articulated the Neurosequential Model of Therapeutics. This model involves many play components, including sensory–motor play to help soothe the brainstem (see Gaskill & Perry, Chapter 11, this volume). The Neurosequential Model of Therapeutics has brought new understanding to the work of the play therapist in addressing disruptions of early attachments. Perry explains that what we do in therapy sometimes doesn't matter as much as when we do it. Timing and sequence are essential in addressing attachment trauma, and Gaskill and Perry offer a map to guide us.

Case Vignette: Play Therapy for Attachment Trauma

Individual Play Therapy Sessions

Jason, a 6-year-old boy constantly in trouble at school, entered the playroom and immediately headed for the plastic tubs of puppets. Puppets went flying in all directions until he found one that appealed to him. He finally settled on an alligator, with unusually sharp and long teeth; he then threw in the direction of the therapist a rather defenseless puppet, a beaver. Before the therapist was able to get his hand fully into the beaver puppet, Jason, with a startling roar, pounced on the beaver and locked him in a vise-like grip with amazing strength for such a young child. What were striking about the alligator's aggression were the intensity and the affect behind it. At one point, the therapist had to set a limit, because the viciousness of the attacks caused physical pain. To prevent injury to child and therapist, Jason was told, "It is OK for the alligator to be angry and attack the beaver, but it is not OK for either of us to get hurt, so you need to be not quite so rough." It was the only time that a limit was needed: Jason, while still expressing considerable rage in the alligator's attacks on the beaver in the remainder of that session and in subsequent sessions, always stopped short of inflicting pain on the therapist or causing injury to himself. The individual play sessions that followed were active, largely focused on the theme of aggression and revenge, but there was a gradual, nonlinear reduction in the intensity of the affect expressed as well as symbolized through the action of the play. Also, accurately depicting the pain of Jason's life situation, the alligator always acted alone. There were no companions or friends.

The rage expressed by this first-grade boy in the form of a vengeful, attacking alligator puppet accurately symbolized his internal inferno, stemming from multiple factors—most obviously the sudden death of his father, who had died of a heart attack while running a marathon 6 months earlier. Of the four children, Jason, the second-born, had experienced the most conflictual relationship with his father and carried the heaviest burden following his sudden death. Jason's attachment with his father had been insecure/ambivalent, and there was no longer an opportunity to make it more secure. Jason's father had been harder on him than on his two sisters and his younger brother. The paternal grandmother observed that Jason's father had had similar impulse and externalizing problems when he was Jason's age. Jason's mother had tried to protect Jason and thought her husband was truly too hard on him, but she surmised that her husband mostly had good intentions and didn't want Jason to have the same hard struggles that he had experienced as a child.

Although the father's intentions were probably good, the effect on Jason was to make him feel that he could never please his father, in spite of desperately wanting his approval. Jason experienced his father's concern more sharply as massive rejection. In addition, Jason struggled with neurodevelopmental challenges. His impulsivity was a component of his attention-deficit/hyperactivity disorder (ADHD), which made it hard for him to function without alienating his siblings or his peers at school and in sports. Whether with his siblings or his peers, he always was determined to be first and was quite willing to push others out of line if they were ahead of him. He was far more than a "rough-and-tumble boy" on the playground, sometimes hitting peers broadside at full speed, and occasionally causing injury (as well as alarm on the part of school officials and worried parents of other first graders). The play therapist attended frequent meetings with the mother and his teachers and school officials at his elementary school because of Jason's bullying, aggressive, and intimidating behavior. Behavioral plans were developed and implemented, with temporary improvements but no lasting change, because the underlying issues were complicated and would take time to work through adequately.

What Jason had experienced as a core part of his attachment trauma was a deep hurt shared by many children whose attachments are traumatically ruptured; it took the form of identification as a "child who does not fit." Jason "did not fit" in his family because of his dysregulated behavior associated with ADHD and his hostility stemming from his perception of rejection by his father. Jason "didn't fit" in school for the same reasons, plus his attempts to compensate for his lack of acceptance by becoming hypercompetitive. His extreme competitiveness further alienated his peers—not only in school, but when he played soccer or baseball. Jason always had to be captain, always win, and always be first, or else he would explode in anger. Any experience that symbolized "loss" in the slightest way triggered a huge emotional reaction, almost always taking the form of blind rage. James Garbarino (1999) has noted that the closest thing to a psychological malignancy is social rejection in childhood. When the rejection is perceived within a child's family as well as in his or her social world, the malignancy is particularly potent and often accompanied by the most profound forms of rage.

Jason shared another psychodynamic constellation with other children who suffer attachment trauma. Clinical experience indicates that anger/rage is experienced by children as an empowering emotion, whereas sorrow leaves them feeling vulnerable and exposed. Underneath Jason's burning rage was the far more delicate and vulnerable feeling of profound sorrow. The loss of his father was sudden and final, leaving him no opportunity to make amends or to resolve the struggle and conflict with his father. The wound was anything but clean, and healing would be complicated by the permanent absence of his father.

The individual play therapy sessions helped build trust in the therapist and enhanced the therapeutic relationship. Jason was able to displace safely, within the symbolism of the aggressive play (the alligator puppet's attacking the beaver and other defenseless animal puppets), the burning rage stemming from his unresolved loss and grief and from his social rejection. The play sessions allowed him to modulate his rage as he gave full expression to its intensity in a safe and controlled environment, and then, over a period of 10 subsequent sessions, exercised more conscious and safer control over different levels of intensity of affective expression. The individual play therapy, however, could not provide all of the ingredients needed for healing such a severe rupture in Jason's attachments. The play therapist needed to shift approaches to enlist the resources of the family system.

Focused Family Therapy Sessions

Although the play therapist would not have credibility in convincing Jason that there could be another meaning to his father's harshness, his mother, paternal grandmother, and aunts were in a more favorable position to do so. Basically, what Jason needed was a phase of cognitive work focused on modifying his belief that his father had never accepted him or loved him. The play therapist knew that it was going to take more than one person and more than one session to make a dent in his strongly held belief that his father "hated him," which he repeatedly stated. The play therapist decided to call on one family resource at a time. In the first session, his mother was invited to join with the therapist in talking with Jason about her belief that although Jason's father had been strict and tough on him, he did so because he loved him and he didn't want his son to get into trouble repeatedly, the way he had done himself. The play therapist primarily played the role of "silent witness" (Gil, 2010), but did amplify the alternative way of understanding the father's intention. When the mother stated her view of what the father was trying to do, the play therapist said, "Oh, that's a new way of looking at how your father felt about you. He was hard on you because he loved you, and he didn't want you to go through the hard times he went through." Jason was attentive but seemed skeptical.

Next the play therapist called on the paternal grandmother, who, in spite of her own considerable grief resulting from the death of her only son, did a remarkable job of sharing with conviction her belief that Jason's father had loved him and wanted to teach him lessons that he himself had had to learn the hard way. What seemed to intrigue Jason the most were the many examples his grandmother gave him of how his father had gotten into trouble when he was Jason's age. Some of them, like the time his father poured glue on his first-grade teacher's wooden chair, made him laugh. He seemed relieved that he was not the only "black sheep" in the family, and he also gained a sense of solidarity with his father. His mother's argument that his father had only been trying to straighten him out and keep him out of trouble seemed to gain more credibility with every story of misbehavior that the grandmother told.

Family Play Therapy

The final stage of Jason's therapy took the form of family play therapy (Gil, 1994), with the goal of restoring connections with his mother and siblings. In one quite poignant session with the mother and all four of her children, the children decided that the eagle puppet had a broken wing.

This was a powerful metaphor. Until the sudden, traumatic death of the father this had been an "all-American" type of family. The family members were all quite active, into sports and outdoors activities, but now they were grounded and having trouble getting airborne again. In the beginning, Jason refused to participate with his siblings. He sat next to his mother, but turned away from the other children. Jason was literally enacting in the session the destructive identity that he had embraced of "the child who did not fit—did not belong." His primary attachments had been disrupted not only by the unexpected death of his father, but by the alienation of his siblings and his peers. Jason enacted in the session the pattern that he doggedly enacted in his daily life, making sure that he was the "child who did not belong." His unspoken credo was "I will reject you before you will even get the opportunity to reject me." Yet beneath this maladaptive defensive pattern was the hunger that all humans share for acceptance and belonging.

The therapist recognized this as a critical moment in the family play therapy. Would everyone together—mother, siblings, and therapist—be able to convince Jason that he had an important place in the family, or would he choose to remain outside the circle of the family in his lonely, painful self-imposed exile? His mother expressed in a heartfelt way her wish for Jason to join the family and participate in the family play of the "eagle with a broken wing." Each of his siblings also tried their best to convince Jason to join them, but he still was holding out. The therapist then said to Jason, "We need you, Jason. We will not be able to heal the eagle's broken wing without you." The therapist then handed him the doctor's kit. Everyone in their room held their breath until Jason sprang to his feet and came over and began attending to the eagle, which was tenderly held by one of his sisters. This was a turning point. Jason finally was able to accept that he no longer had to be the "child who did not belong." His family had been convincing, and he was invested from that point on in the family play drama of healing the eagle's broken wing.

A particularly interesting feature of Jason's empathic attending to the eagle as a doctor with his various instruments of healing was singing to the eagle. Only a few weeks later, in a meeting with his mother, did I learn the significance of the singing. His mother told me that an important breakthrough had occurred at home in the week before the pivotal session. The loving and empathic mom had always gathered the children at bedtime and sung to them a song they all loved. After the death of the father, Jason in his anger would not tolerate his mother's singing. In the week prior to the "eagle's wing" session, Jason had come to his mom and asked her if he could sing the song that she had formerly sung before bedtime to the children. Jason did sing it and remembered all the words. This was part of the reparative movement toward reunion with his family, his acceptance of his father's death, and his willing to embrace the love of his family and perhaps for the first time enter into a heartfelt sense of belonging.

Conclusion

Play therapy has rich and enduring early roots in attachment theory, and some early work in attachment-focused play therapy even predates attachment theory. Not only did the early child psychoanalysts regard the parent–infant bond as a primary focus, but Theraplay—with its emphasis on enhancing attachment and bonding through playful interactions between primary caregivers and their babies—was launched in Chicago in the late 1960s, before the major writings of John Bowlby (who is most often identified as the pioneer of attachment theory) were published. Donald Winnicott, as an early analyst and pediatrician, used play therapy as a way of strengthening attachment, and collaborated later with Bowlby on projects during World War II to deal with the disrupted attachments of children evacuated from the bombings of London. More recently, the work of Allan Schore, Daniel Siegel, and Bruce Perry, grounded in the science of neurobiology, has greatly expanded our understanding of the neurobiology of early attachments; these researchers have shown how favorable consistent interactions are essential for infants to develop gradually the capacity for affect regulation, and how the timing of our interventions needs to be informed by new understandings of brain development. It is an exciting time to be a play therapist.

REFERENCES

Allen, J. G. (2013). *Restoring mentalizing in attachment relationships: Treating trauma with plain old therapy.* Arlington, VA: American Psychiatric Publishing.

American Psychiatric Association. (1980). *Diagnostic and statistical manual of mental disorders* (3rd ed.). Washington, DC: Author.

American Psychiatric Association. (1994). *Diagnostic and statistical manual of mental disorders* (4th ed.). Washington, DC: Author.

American Psychiatric Association. (2000). *Diagnostic and statistical manual of mental disorders* (4th ed., text rev.). Washington, DC: Author.

American Psychiatric Association. (2013). *Diagnostic and statistical manual of mental disorders* (5th ed.). Arlington, VA: Author.

Bonime, W. (1989). *Collaborative psychoanalysis: Anxiety, depression, dreams, and personality change.* Cranbury, NJ: Associated University Presses.

Bowlby, J., Miller, E., & Winnicott, D. W. (1939, December 16). Evacuation of small children [Letter]. *British Medical Journal, ii*(4119), 1202–1233.

Brody, V. (1997). *The dialogue of touch: Developmental play therapy.* Northvale, NJ: Aronson.

Cassidy, J., & Shaver, P. R. (Eds.). (2008). *Handbook of attachment* (2nd ed.). New York: Guilford Press.

Des Lauriers, A. (1962). *The experience of reality in childhood schizophrenia.* New York: International Universities Press.

Edinger, E. F. (1972). *Ego and archetype.* New York: Putnam.

Fonagy, P., & Target, M. (1997). Attachment and reflective function: Their role in self-organization. *Developmental Psychopathology, 9,* 679–700.

Freud, S. (1959). Family romances. In J. Strachey (Ed. & Tran.), *The standard edition of the complete psychological works of Sigmund Freud* (Vol. 9, pp. 235–242). London: Hogarth Press. (Original work published 1909)

Fromm, E. (1947). *Man for himself: An inquiry into the psychology of ethics.* New York: Rinehart.

Garbarino, J. (1999). *Lost boys: Why our sons turn violent and how we can save them.* New York: Anchor Books.

Gil, E. (1994). *Play in family therapy.* New York: Guilford Press.

Gil, E. (2010). Children's self-initiated gradual exposure: The wonders of post-traumatic play and behavioral reenactments. In E. Gil (Ed.), *Working with children to heal interpersonal trauma: The power of play* (pp. 44–63). New York: Guilford Press.

Guerney, B. G., Jr. (1964). Filial therapy: Description and rationale. *Journal of Consulting Psychology, 28,* 303–310.

Guerney, L. F. (2003). The history, principles, and empirical basis of Filial Therapy. In R. VanFleet & L. F. Guerney (Eds.), *Casebook of Filial Therapy* (pp. 1–19). Boiling Springs, PA: Play Therapy Press.

Guerney, L. F., & Ryan, V. M. (2013). *Group Filial Therapy: A complete guide to teaching parents to play therapeutically with their children.* Philadelphia, PA: Kingsley.

Herman, J. (1992). *Trauma and recovery: The aftermath of violence—from domestic abuse to political terror.* New York: Basic Books.

Jernberg, A. (1979). *Theraplay: A new treatment using structured play for problem children and their families.* San Francisco: Jossey-Bass.

Main, M., & Solomon, J. (1990). Procedures for identifying infants as disorganized/disoriented during the Ainsworth Strange Situation. In M. T. Greenberg, D. Cicchetti, & E. M. Cummings (Eds.), *Attachment in the preschool years: Theory, research, and intervention* (pp. 121–160). Chicago: University of Chicago Press.

Peller, L. E. (1946). Incentives to development and means of early education. *Psychoanalytic Study of the Child, 2,* 397–415.

Perry, B. D. (2009). Examining child maltreatment through a neurosequential lens: Clinical application of the Neurosequential Model of Therapeutics. *Journal of Loss and Trauma, 14,* 240–255.

Perry, B. D., & Szalavitz, M. (2006). *The boy who was raised as a dog: And other stories from a child psychiatrist's notebook.* New York: Basic Books.

Schaefer, C. E. (Ed.). (1993). *The therapeutic powers of play.* Northvale, NJ: Aronson.

Schaefer, C. E., & Drewes, A. A. (Eds.). (2014). *The therapeutic powers of play: 20 core agents of change* (2nd ed.). Hoboken, NJ: Wiley.

Schore, A. N. (1994). *Affect regulation and the origin of the self: The neurobiology of emotional development.* Hillsdale, NJ: Erlbaum.

Schore, A. N. (2003a). *Affect dysregulation and disorders of the self.* New York: Norton.

Schore, A. N. (2003b). *Affect regulation and the repair of the self.* New York: Norton.

Schore, A. N. (2012). *The science of the art of psychotherapy.* New York: Norton.

Siegel, D. J. (1999). *The developing mind: How relationships and the brain interact to shape who we are.* New York: Guilford Press.

Siegel, D. J. (2012). *The developing mind: How relationships and the brain interact to shape who we are* (2nd ed.). New York: Guilford Press.

Terr, L. (1990). *Too scared to cry: Psychic trauma in childhood.* New York: Harper & Row.

Tuber, S. (2008). *Attachment, play and authenticity: A Winnicott primer.* Lanham, MD: Aronson.

van der Kolk, B. A. (2005). Developmental trauma disorder. *Psychiatric Annals, 35,* 401–408.

VanFleet, R. (2013). *Filial Therapy: Strengthening parent–child relationships through play* (3rd ed.). Sarasota, FL: Professional Resource Press.

Winnicott, D. (1971). *Playing and reality.* London: Tavistock.

PART II

Clinical Applications: Approaches to Working with Attachment Issues

CHAPTER 3

Attachment Theory as a Road Map for Play Therapists

Anne Stewart
William F. Whelan
Christen Pendleton

> We are here concerned with nothing less than the nature
> of love and its origins in the attachment of a baby to his
> mother. . . . Attachment originates in a few specific patterns
> of behavior, some of which are manifest at birth and some of
> which develop shortly afterward. . . . Attachment is manifested
> through these patterns of behavior but the patterns do not
> themselves constitute the attachment. Attachment is internal.
> —AINSWORTH (1967, p. 429)

Attachment theory proposes that important behavior systems in all humans serve to maintain proximity between children and caregivers (Ainsworth, Blehar, Waters, & Wall, 1978; Bowlby, 1969, 1973, 1980). The Circle of Security (COS) is one of the most recent models expressing the therapeutic dimensions of attachment theory. The COS model helps illustrate the power of attachment theory to build secure relationships through sensitive everyday interactions. In this chapter, we describe the attachment-theory-based COS model; explain the major features of the COS; and provide a case vignette to illustrate the ways the COS may be used as a "roadmap" to guide play therapists' work. We first provide a brief introduction to the foundations of attachment theory and to major findings from field research. We then show the relationship between attachment theory and COS, and we share research supporting the importance of secure attachments in the lives of the children we serve as play therapists.

Overview of Attachment Theory and Findings
from Field Research

According to the theory, children's *attachment behavior system* leads them to seek proximity to their caregivers in times of distress—whether the distress is mild or severe, momentary or long-standing. The caregivers, in turn, are prompted by their *caregiving behavior system* to serve as a safe haven of protection for their children, and as a secure base for children to use as they explore their world. The attachment and caregiving systems thus serve the biological functions in humans (as in other species), of ensuring protection in dangerous surroundings and promoting exploration and learning (Bowlby, 1969, 1982, 1988). Mary Ainsworth's innovative field and laboratory research, in the context of John Bowlby's theory, brought a scientific approach to the study of development (Ainsworth & Bowlby, 1991).

In 1954, Ainsworth set out for Kampala, Uganda, to begin her field studies in infant development, with special attention to the growth of attachment and the developmental pathway of bonding (see Ainsworth, 1967). What she found most often among the Ugandan babies and mothers, and later replicated in her famous Baltimore study (Ainsworth et al., 1978), was a predominant pattern of secure behavior. The pattern included the infant's increased differential responding toward the mother (as compared to other people) over time; exploration of the environment with the mother's support; contentment; returning to the mother for rest and refueling; and lower anxiety compared to other children.

Attachment Theory and the COS Model

Ainsworth (1967) summarized her findings by describing two distinct but related phenomena: the secure child's growing ability to use the caregiver effectively as (1) a secure base for exploration (of the social and physical environment) and (2) a haven of safety when tired or distressed. Over 30 years later, a graphic depiction of this summary was created, called the COS (Marvin, Cooper, Hoffman, & Powell, 2002)—and, along with it, an intervention for supporting the development of secure attachment–caregiving patterns (Marvin et al., 2002). This chapter extends these ideas and interventions to the child–therapist relationship in the context of play therapy. We illustrate how the use of the COS can enrich a play therapist's conceptualization of a child's needs, promote effective filial therapy and parent consultation, and enhance the healing benefits of the child's relationship experience with the play therapist. Let's consider the importance of a secure attachment for children's emotional well-being and learn how attachment relationships grow.

The Benefits of Secure Attachment

Why should we play therapists be concerned about the quality of a child's attachment? How can promoting more secure attachments benefit the children with whom we work? One compelling reason to use an attachment-based perspective like the COS is that when children come to us with behavioral and emotional problems, they are experiencing corresponding difficulties in their relationships with parents, teachers, or peers. In addition, many of the problems for which children are referred for treatment reflect basic difficulties in regulation of behavior, thoughts, and feelings. Disturbances in relationships and disruptions in regulation are central concerns addressed in the attachment-based COS approach and interventions.

Evidence Supporting the Importance of Secure Attachment for Child Outcomes

The secure pattern of relationship development is the attachment pattern most associated with resilience and positive outcomes in the childhood years and in adulthood (Grossmann, Grossmann, & Kindler, 2005; Sroufe, 2005). While secure attachment patterns do not ensure good outcomes across the lifespan, or protect individuals from all forms and levels of stress, children with secure attachments tend to have more effective and satisfying relationships with parents, friends, and teachers than children with nonsecure patterns do. They are better at social problem solving and the repair of relationship upsets, are more successful academically, have fewer behavior problems, are at lower risk for psychiatric problems and trouble with the law than their nonsecure peers, and are themselves more successful parents (e.g., Sroufe, 2005; Sroufe, Egeland, Carlson, & Collins, 2005).

Children with a secure pattern tend to send clear emotional cues to their parents (and play therapists) during times of mild to moderate arousal and stress, and their cuing tends to be robust. Their behavior usually fits the circumstances and clearly communicates their emotional needs, making it relatively easy for adults to perceive their cues correctly, make accurate inferences about their needs, and respond appropriately to those needs. During occasional moments of miscuing, when a child needs a parent but behaves as if there is no need or as if the parent is not important to him or her, parents of secure children are generally able to read through the miscue and address effectively the child's underlying need.

From a practical point of view, as well as an evolutionary one, the immediate outcome of this pattern is that the child's needs are usually correctly identified and met in the moment-to-moment emotional and behavioral episodes of the day. The longer-term outcome is that the child's brain builds an increasingly sophisticated structure of neural connections and subroutines—a structure that results in effective rhythms of soothing;

co-regulation of thoughts, emotions, and behavior; abilities for self-control; and behavioral and social competence (Schore, 2001, 2005).

Building Blocks of Secure Attachments

Our readers may have already deduced a remarkable discovery: Attachment patterns are built one interaction at a time, over time. This is good news for parents and play therapists. Indeed, it appears both from research (Dozier, 2005) and from our clinical practice that although caregivers with secure patterns cannot meet all their children's needs all of the time, they are able, through their own accurate perceptions and sensitivity to the children's emotional signals, to help the children form healthy attachment relationships through day-to-day interactions. This is a lovely and wonderful process to witness. Such caregivers, including birth parents, foster parents, teachers, and play therapists, provide an emotional environment that is sensitive, flexible, adaptive, and generally able to fine-tune itself to meet the needs of a particular child.

Children with histories of disturbed family relationships, interpersonal violence, and emotional and physical maltreatment tend to have nonsecure and usually high-risk (disorganized, disoriented, controlling, etc.) patterns of interaction. Compared to their secure peers, children with nonsecure patterns of attachment often exhibit underdeveloped abilities for co-regulation (i.e., little ability to make use of caregivers for regulation of emotion and behavior), for rhythms of soothing and self-control, or for effective partnership behavior. In this regard, and through no fault of their own, children with nonsecure attachment patterns provide fewer clear cues about their emotional and relationship needs in the moment. It is no wonder that caregivers often describe difficulty in developing relationships with these children, and often experience the children's behavior and emotions as enigmatic and unpredictable.

The COS Model

Attachment-based play therapy helps reorder and organize a child's emotional experiences through attuned and responsive interactions with a play therapist, so that the child's relationships and behaviors will become more satisfying, coherent, and rewarding. The COS helps the play therapist focus on meeting the child's basic relationship needs through play-based interactions (Stewart, Whelan, Gilbert, & Marvin, 2011).

Dimensions of the COS

In the COS model, the two basic dimensions are divided into top-of-the-Circle and bottom-of-the-Circle needs (see Figure 3.1). In the therapeutic

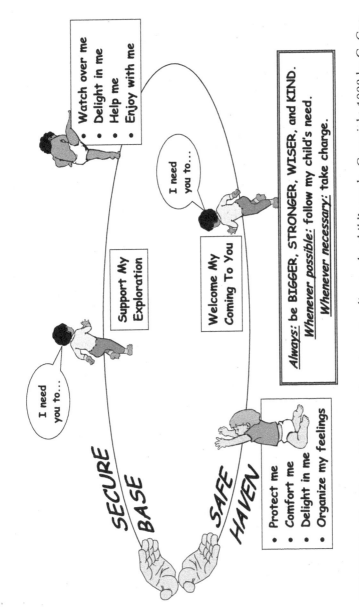

FIGURE 3.1. The Circle of Security: Caregiver attending to the child's needs. Copyright 1998 by G. Cooper, K. Hoffman, R. Marvin, and B. Powell. *circleofsecurity.org*. Reprinted by permission.

play relationship, *needs* are the child's needs from the therapist, in the moment, within the context of their growing relationship. Using this perspective, the therapist learns to ask the question "What does the child need from me?" rather than "Why is the child behaving this way?" The child's needs at the top of the Circle include *support my exploration, watch over me, help me, delight in me*, and *enjoy with me*. A child's needs at the bottom of the Circle include *welcome my coming to you, protect me, soothe me, organize me*, and *delight in me*.

The Importance of Observation

From a COS perspective, accurately observing interactions within an empirically supported theory is the foundation of understanding and helping. In this regard, identifying what the child's body is doing in interactions is initially more important for the therapeutic work than asking why it is happening. The therapist notices the child's body orientation, proximity, movement, physical contact, tone of voice, content of speech, body language, and feelings expressed. The therapist alters his or her behavior in the playroom from moment to moment according to the child's needs, and makes judgments about when to actively follow the child's needs versus when to take charge of the child's emotional experience and behavior in order to lead or protect the child. The result is that the therapist can use the COS to differentiate diagnosis and treatment of the child (Cooper, Hoffman, Powell, & Marvin, 2006). When the child's needs are met in a responsive, contingent manner, this helps to build neurological subroutines and abilities in the child and to generate patterns for soothing; coregulation of emotion, thinking, and behavior; partnership behavior; and abilities for self-regulation and competence (Hoffman, Marvin, Cooper, & Powell, 2006; Whelan & Marvin, 2011).

As shown in Figure 3.1 and noted above, there are five primary needs at the top of the Circle:

1. *Support my exploration* refers to the child's need to experience support from the therapist to explore the playroom materials and activities—and, most importantly, to explore the relationship with the therapist. Encouragement for exploration is provided by the play therapist's affect, tone of voice, and body language, and is conveyed through attuned interactions and comments. Memories, worries, and fears, as well as past trauma, loss, and maltreatment, may be addressed in developmentally appropriate creative arts and expressive activities, in discussions, and of course in the context of imaginative play.

2. *Watch over me* reflects to the child's need for the therapist to make accurate observations of his or her behavior, so that accurate inferences and conclusions can be drawn about the child's needs. Given the charge to maintain the physical and psychological safety of the playroom, the

therapist must determine whether the child's actions reflect accurate emotional cuing or miscuing.

3. *Delight in me* concerns the positive emotional affect and acceptance the therapist communicates to the child. Delight can convey strength, safety, love, hope, and/or forgiveness—all in a well-timed reflection, gaze, or tone of voice. Delight is quickly lost in times of stress and is the only need to appear at both the top and the bottom of the Circle, due to its vital role in healing. Play therapists can promote healing through brief but genuine delight-filled interactions in the playroom, and in filial therapy through helping a caregiver experience delight in his or her child.

4. *Help me* refers to the play therapist's scaffolding the child's exploration of toys, play themes, emotions, and their relationship in the playroom.

5. *Enjoy with me* denotes the child's need for the therapist to convey how much the therapist simply enjoys the child's company and likes sharing activities with him or her. The child benefits by experiencing reciprocal and moment-to-moment partnership behavior, as well as the warmth and support inherent in relationships without conditions.

At the bottom of the Circle, there are also five primary needs:

1. *Welcome my coming to you* refers to accepting the child's uncertainty, distress, confusion, rudeness, rejection, sadness, aggression, misattributions, and poor judgments. Importantly, this does not mean approving of or reinforcing misbehavior, but rather welcoming whatever the child brings in order for the child to experience the therapist as being bigger, stronger, wise, and kind.

2. *Protect me* concerns the child's need for physical and emotional protection, including protection from events in the playroom, as well as from negative or overwhelming memories and emotions that become activated in the play therapy.

3. *Comfort me* includes the therapist's attempts to absorb and regulate the child's pattern of overarousal or inhibition and to soothe the child's anxiety and distress, without dismissing the child's upset.

4. *Delight in me* refers to sharing brief, playful moments of joy in the child, especially through interactions and activities that are fun and meaningful for both child and therapist. Expressing genuine pleasure at the presence of another person is one of the best ways to reassure children or adults that they are valued.

5. *Organize my feelings* refers to ways in which the therapist takes charge of the child's emotional experience, and sets the emotional tone to lead the child in a healthier interaction during times of upset. This is done via the therapist's presence and sensitivity, tone of voice and demeanor, body language, verbal expression, and physical movement. The therapist gives the child practice in the experience of having another person lead him or her through emotional arousal and distress, and helps the child

experience the safety and rest that comes in relying on the strength and security of one who is bigger, stronger, wiser, and kind.

Therapists who have the most success implementing the COS model have the ability to reflect on their own thoughts and feelings regarding a therapeutic relationship with the child, and to wonder how their thoughts, feelings, and behavior affect the child. They also exhibit the ability to see things kindly and empathically from the child's point of view and from a developmental standpoint, and to alter their own therapeutic caregiving behavior in the moment according to the child's changing needs. They are able to take charge and be bigger, stronger, wiser, and kind as needed. Importantly, this kind of therapeutic caregiving includes keen sensitivity not only to the child's cues, but also to the child's miscues (e.g., Marvin et al., 2002).

COS Cues and Miscues

In the COS model, *cuing* refers to behavioral and emotional signals from the child that, directly or indirectly, indicate the child's needs "around the Circle." *Miscuing* refers to behavioral and emotional signals from the child that point away from what the child actually needs at that time. Common examples of a child's miscues in relation to a therapist (or in relation to a parent or teacher) include anxious/avoidant behavior such as looking away, walking away, hiding his or her face, not responding to overtures, leaving the room, refusing to engage or collaborate, and rejecting the therapist's attempts at co-regulation. Miscues can also include behaviors such as rudeness, aggression, lying, stealing, or fire setting. For other children, common miscues include babyish behavior and exaggerated or overly bright affect; for still others, they include attempts to organize or take charge of interactions with the therapist or caregiver, attempts to take care of the adult, or punitive or bossy behaviors (i.e., role-reversed behaviors). Something all of these behaviors have in common is that they tend to push the therapist away or distract the therapist, at times when the child is otherwise clearly in need of adult help somewhere on the Circle. Such miscuing obscures the child's underlying relationship needs of the therapist around the Circle, and makes it more difficult for the therapist to identify them accurately. If these behaviors are not identified as miscues, then it is likely that the therapist will attempt to treat the miscues (or symptoms) and be led astray from the child's relationship needs in the therapy. From this point of view, a clue that important miscues may have been missed occurs when a target problem fails to improve with intervention, or when new problems continually pop up to replace the old ones. A way for a therapist to determine whether he or she has been chasing miscues, rather than meeting the child's needs (and thereby missing opportunities to shape the child's emotions and behaviors toward health), is that the emotional and behavioral problems do not improve or simply mutate over time rather than resolve. (Of course there are other reasons why things may not improve, including illness or the presence of stress or trauma in the child's life of which the therapist is not yet aware.) As one would expect, the therapist needs to reflect continually on the child's movement around the Circle, as well as on his or her own behavior and feelings, during interactions with the child.

Case Vignette: A COS-Informed Intervention

The COS as a Roadmap for Play Therapy

The COS helps play therapists conceptualize and meet a child's emotional needs by guiding how they intervene in the playroom. Here is an example of applying the COS model of observing the child's behavior, making inferences about where the child is on the Circle, inferring the child's needs, and responding in an individual play therapy format.

Malik was a 7-year-old child from a multistressed background. He was raised for the first 4 years of his life by his birth mother and father, who both struggled with substance abuse problems. Malik's childhood was marked by neglect, chaos, and domestic violence. Malik's parents frequently engaged in physical altercations in his presence, and although they tried to address his physical needs, they were often unavailable to provide for his emotional needs. At age 4, Malik was removed from his parents and was raised by relatives for the subsequent 3 years. Once he was removed from their care, Malik saw his parents only sporadically and was disappointed when they did not follow through with promises to attend family functions and holidays. The year Malik turned 7, his birth mother separated from his father, completed a drug rehabilitation program, and began working toward reunification with Malik. She started to engage in supervised visits with him and was completing court-ordered therapy as part of her reunification plan. Malik's relatives, who maintained physical custody of him, supported the reunification efforts and cooperated in assisting with supervised visitations. Therapy was arranged by child protective services for Malik, who exhibited unpredictable emotional reactions, such as aggression, defiance, difficulty separating, and clinginess with his mother. Malik's therapist, Laura, began by meeting individually with Malik for play therapy. As their work progressed, Laura engaged in filial therapy and consultation with Malik's biological mother and with the extended relatives who maintained physical custody. Laura used the COS as a roadmap to build her conceptualization of Malik's emotional needs, to guide her interactions with Malik in the playroom, and to guide her interactions and discussions with his caregivers.

During her initial sessions, Laura welcomed Malik by following his needs in the playroom, using the COS to guide her thinking about how to help him and make use of her to regulate his behavior. As Laura carefully observed Malik, she noticed that he engaged in more aggressive play with the dollhouse, banging the parent figures. When he was speaking for the figures, Malik's voice became louder and more pressured; his body tensed as he made the father and mother figures yell at one another and banged them together. Laura noticed that his language also became more violent than she had previously heard. Malik angled his body slightly away from Laura as he placed a young boy figure sitting in the corner of the dollhouse.

LAURA: I see that one is over there all alone. Maybe he is watching those two yelling.

MALIK: Yeah, they are always yelling and hitting. He doesn't wanna hear it.

LAURA: Ah, so he hears a lot of yelling and sees a lot of hitting. I wonder what he is thinking and feeling.

MALIK: Errrr-ow-ow-ow. (*Makes a low rumbling sound as his shoulders tense. He suddenly throws the dollhouse chair at the boy figure.*) He is bad, and that's why his mommy is leaving him there!

Although Laura was alarmed at the dramatic change in Malik's demeanor, she remained calm and close to him. She noticed that his breathing was shallow and rapid, and that tears sprang to his eyes as he toppled the rest of the furniture in the dollhouse. Using the COS, Laura understood how Malik's toppling of the furniture and threatening growl were miscues, fueled by his tendency to become dysregulated when enacting family scenes. Actually, his reaction made sense to her when she considered the chaotic and unpredictable nature of his first 4 years, coupled with the sense of abandonment he experienced at being removed from his parents' custody, shuffled among relatives, and repeatedly disappointed. Laura understood that Malik's sympathetic nervous system was activated and overburdened—something that had happened all too often as he witnessed verbal and physical aggression. From her observations, Laura knew that Malik was at the bottom of the Circle, and that his needs were for protection, comfort, and help with organizing his feelings.

Laura inferred that Malik was experiencing intense feelings that he could not make sense of by himself. Furthermore, she knew that this type of behavior often pushed away caregivers and peers, and elicited punitive or disciplinary responses from his parents and teachers. She could tell that Malik was feeling sad, vulnerable, scared, anxious, and angry, and his behavior conveyed to her, "I am overwhelmed and don't know what to do with the all the strong feelings that I am experiencing." Laura thus recognized Malik's need for welcoming and protection from his intense feelings, comfort to feel valued, and help in organizing his jumbled emotions. She also recognized that when he was this upset, assistance would be hard for Malik to accept. She understood that even though he needed her help, he was not used to getting help from adults, and that this would be a large part of their therapeutic work together. Laura offered her composed presence and a few calm but strongly stated (and nonjudgmental) comments, to let Malik know that his feelings would be accepted and that she would not be misled by miscues. She reflected, "It is so hard for him to know what to do! He feels so many big feelings all at the same time—the feelings all come out as throwing chairs and tables."

Since this was not the first time this kind of interaction had occurred, Laura's interaction demonstrated to Malik that she would consistently respond to his needs in a patterned way. Malik's shoulders eased slightly as he turned toward Laura. She leaned in toward Malik and inched a bit closer to him. Malik nodded slowly and relaxed slightly, looking up at Laura briefly as he began setting up the dollhouse furniture. Later in the session, Laura completed a drawing activity with Malik. On a gingerbread person outline,[1] Malik named four feelings the boy in the house might be feeling, matched colors with the feelings, and then drew where in his body he experienced those feelings. Laura and Malik talked about when Malik had feelings like the boy in the dollhouse, and what or who helped him feel better. After a few moments of talking, Malik began to crawl slowly around the playroom. He approached Laura, pretending to lick his hands.

MALIK: I'm a cat (*making purring sounds*).

LAURA: Oh, so you are a cat—a cat with a big motor for purring!

MALIK: You can pet my head if you want to. I am a friendly cat.

LAURA: You are a friendly cat, all comfy and safe, ready for some pats on your head (*patting Malik gently*).

MALIK: Yeah, and you can make me some milk, and then I'll take a nap here.

Laura observed that Malik's breathing had slowed, and that his face was relaxed as he crawled toward Laura and sat next to her legs. Laura recognized Malik's movement toward her and the content of his speech as cues that he needed her to welcome his coming and provide him caregiving within this play; she followed his needs and recognized that in doing so she was helping him at the bottom of the Circle. In this moment of interaction, his body had a chance to practice and experience what it felt like to bring some of his needs directly to her.

Malik lay down quietly at Laura's feet, which she recognized as a time of emotional refueling in the safe haven that she had provided him. After a few deep breaths, Malik opened his eyes, stretched his arms, and looked around at the toys across the room. Laura was able to see that her work in

---

[1]The gingerbread person drawing activity is based on an activity developed by Athena A. Drewes. (See Drewes, Chapter 12, this volume.)

attending to Malik's bottom-of-the-Circle needs had helped to co-regulate his emotions, and that he was feeling recharged and was moving toward the top of the Circle.

> LAURA: You are waking up from your nap and feeling better (*smiles*), and stretching your legs and paws and looking around at the toys. I'm so glad you took a nap here with me. Now there is so much to see in the playroom.

Malik eyed the trucks across the playroom and began to crawl toward them, but turned back to look at Laura midway, his eyes looking as if he wanted to make sure that she was still watching him. Laura recognized that Malik was now at the top of the Circle, as indicated by his calmer presence and his willingness to venture away from her. She understood his need for her to support his exploration.

> LAURA: I am still here, watching you. It looks like you have a plan as to what you might like to play with.
>
> MALIK: (*Smiles and crawls more rapidly this time to the trucks.*) I want to drive us! (*Faces Laura and moves toward her with the truck in his hand.*)

Laura smiled, delighting in Malik and moving in his direction to enjoy with him. Laura joined Malik on the carpet, sitting next to him and allowing him to direct their play as she remained attuned to his needs. She noticed that his relaxed body posture, his close proximity to her, his affect, and the content of his speech were all consistent and indicative of Malik's position on the top of the Circle. Laura sat next to Malik, pretended to buckle her seatbelt, and said, "You are going to take us for a ride. You know how to drive this truck!" She beamed back at Malik, reflecting his own look of delight. As Malik reached out and turned an imaginary steering wheel, Laura leaned slightly to the right, noting, "We are going around a curve." Malik giggled, leaning into Laura's shoulder in the same direction. They swayed in similar directions as he drove. Laura was able to meet Malik's top-of-the-Circle needs while co-regulating their body movements and emotions as Malik took them for a ride.

The COS as a Roadmap for Filial Work and Parent Consultation

The COS graphic (Figure 3.1) and approach can also guide filial work and parent consultation. Malik's case provides an illustration of how COS can be applied to these intervention formats.

As therapy progressed, Malik's mother and at times his extended relatives were invited to participate in therapy and receive consultation to learn about the COS dimensions and use the COS to think about Malik's needs. Using problem behaviors brought in by the caregivers, Laura helped them apply the COS to discover how Malik was communicating (and miscommunicating) his needs to them. Laura worked with Malik's mother and relatives to recognize, understand, and respond to his needs around the Circle with play-based interventions.

On the day that Malik's mother presented for their filial session, Laura invited her to the room, keeping in mind the ways in which the COS could also be used to welcome his mother and understand her needs in this new situation. As Malik and his mother entered the room, his mother hung back, looking nervous and unsure. Laura noticed the look of uncertainty on Malik's mother's face and determined that she was likely to be feeling out of place, vulnerable, and worried about what Laura would think of her.

LAURA: We are so happy to have you here today in the playroom. We've been talking about this special visit for a few weeks now. Malik and I talked about the different feelings that he might have today, and the way that people can feel nervous and excited all at once.

MALIK'S MOTHER: (*Smiles shyly and nods.*)

MALIK: Yeah, when I feel nervous in my tummy, like there are butterflies in there, I do balloon breathing to help calm down.

LAURA: Malik, you are remembering the balloon breathing that we learned in the playroom. (*To Malik's mother*) He is a real expert in using balloon breathing—taking deep breaths—to relax.

Malik beamed, looking at Laura and his mother. Laura modeled for his mother a response to his top-of-the-Circle needs, enjoying his skill and delighting in his demonstration of breathing skills. She noticed the way in which both Malik and his mother seemed to relax as they moved toward one another, sat down close together, and touched one another's stomachs as they engaged in the deep breathing technique. Laura also noticed the happiness on their faces as Malik taught his mother the technique, and the delight that his mother was able to convey as she and Malik breathed in tandem and laughed as they imagined balloons in their stomachs. As the demonstration ended, Laura noticed that both Malik and his mother looked to her with a "What's next?" expression. Laura took charge to lead the session by suggesting that they engage in a "reading and feelings identification" activity. She invited Malik's mother to read a story aloud, explaining that Laura and Malik would work to identify the feelings that the story characters were experiencing.

Laura pointed to the page that Malik's mother was reading, and wondered with Malik how the bear in the story was feeling and how they might be able to figure it out. She helped Malik notice what the bear was doing and saying.

MALIK: The bear is yelling 'cause he's mad (*in a tentative voice.*)

LAURA: Hmmm, it makes sense to you that when someone is yelling, they may be mad. That makes sense to me too. What about you, Mom?

MALIK'S MOTHER: Yes, and the story said that the bear's toys were taken away by the other animals, and I can imagine that that might make him feel mad.

LAURA: Well, Malik, it looks like you were right. You knew that this bear was feeling mad. I wonder how this bear's roar might sound when he is feeling so mad?

MALIK: I don't know. (*Giggles and looks up at his mother.*)

MALIK'S MOTHER: What do you think?

MALIK: Like this. Rooooaaarrr!

LAURA: Oh, wow! That was a big roar! (*Smiles at Malik and delights in his enthusiasm.*) I wonder if I can try one.

MALIK: Yeah, do it!

Malik giggled as Laura roared and then laughed with him. Laura was even more pleased when Malik's mother asked if she should try. The adults enjoyed the activity with Malik and delighted in him as he let out the final and loudest roar. Laughing, they agreed that they could continue with the story and could help each other to determine the bear's feelings. As they generated clues about the bear's feeling states, Malik inched closer to his mother and reached toward her to point to the book, letting his hand rest on her leg when it lowered. Laura recognized his need for his mother to enjoy the story with him and welcome his closeness, and she was pleased to see that his mother read his cues correctly and responded by placing her arm around him.

In a private meeting with his mother after the play session, Laura was able to point to this moment as a wonderful example of her reading his cues. She helped his mother notice the effect this had on Malik, how much he enjoyed it, and how this helped his exploration and experience of the story and his enjoyment with her. It also allowed Malik and his mother to continue to enjoy themselves together in the activity, delight in his ability to roar like a bear, and feel comfortable enough to engage in play by making animal noises together.

In a subsequent parent consultation session, Laura worked with Malik's mother on developing attunement and engaging with delight. Laura introduced and practiced an activity with Malik's mother in which she learned to face Malik directly, noticing and mirroring his facial expressions and body movements. She helped Malik's mother notice his facial expressions, body posture, movement, proximity, and tone of voice. Laura and Malik's mother practiced this activity several times before inviting Malik into the session to try it out. Malik's mother responded to his top-of-the-Circle need to be delighted in by asking him if he would like to play a game with her in which she would become his mirror. Malik giggled and said that he would. Laura explained that Malik's mother would stand opposite Malik and would mirror all of his expressions and movements for the next minute. As they engaged in the activity, Malik's mother remained affectively attuned with Malik. When the activity concluded, Malik's mother noted that she had enjoyed spending time playing with him and looked forward to playing again soon. Malik yelled, "Me too!" Laura again met privately after the session with Malik's mother to hear her experience of playing together and point out moments of co-regulation and attunement between her and her son. In this way, she helped his mother bask in the wonder of these small and powerful moments of connectedness and feel the reality of how important she was to her son.

The case of Malik and his mother is just one example of relationship healing in action—of the way little moments of intimacy can be guided to help a child and a parent experience (or awaken) the reality of their love and longing for each other. When this happens, the memory and experience will give the two a better chance of getting through difficult experiences ahead. The refueling, safety, and comfort they experience in small moments will protect them in times of trouble and make it more likely that they can stay with each other and practice rhythms of soothing, co-regulation, and forgiveness.

As the vignette illustrates, use of the COS in play therapy is not meant to be prescriptive, but rather employed as a relationship map to guide play therapists in recognizing and understanding children's needs. Play therapists are then in a better position to help shape a child's automatic patterns of thinking, feeling, and behaving toward security and resilience. Although security is characterized by resilience, buoyancy, emotional coherence, and competence, it is also robust, with a seemingly contrary (and wonderful) balance of dependence and independence. Isn't this what we wish for our children (and clients)? That is, we wish them to become strong and independent on the one hand, while also becoming connected in healthy and rejuvenating relationships on the other.

Conclusion

The COS graphic (Figure 3.1) portrays the way children move around the Circle with secure caregivers, smoothly venturing out from them to explore and returning to them for refueling and protection. Within a therapeutic relationship, the therapist attempts to be bigger, stronger, wiser, and kind, and seeks to follow the child's needs and take charge (to help, protect, and lead the child) as necessary. From an attachment perspective, the

COS can be used as a map to show how the power of attuned interactions comes through the therapist's ability to observe the child; arrive at developmentally sensitive inferences and conclusions about the child's needs; co-regulate the child's emotions, thinking, and behavior; and meet the child's needs within safe and sensitive relationship interactions. The healing power of this therapeutic relationship unfolds as the child experiences being safely held, organized, emotionally valued, and protected by the therapist at the bottom of the Circle, and effectively and delightfully supported in exploration at the top of the Circle.

We believe that the COS conceptual framework brings simplicity and direction to complex clinical situations. Therapists report feeling more confident, relaxed, and effective in their work when they employ the COS as a user-friendly map: They have many more experiences of feeling that they know what children need in various play therapy situations, and what to do to help them in the moment (i.e., in terms of welcoming the children's needs at the bottom of the Circle and supporting their exploration at the top). For these play therapists, the COS becomes an experiential, and eventually intuitive, template for developing the most secure and healing relationship possible with their child clients.

REFERENCES

Ainsworth, M. D. S. (1967). *Infancy in Uganda: Infant care and the growth of love.* Baltimore, MD: Johns Hopkins University Press.

Ainsworth, M. D. S., Blehar, M. C., Waters, E., & Wall, S. (1978). *Patterns of attachment: A psychological study of the Strange Situation.* Hillsdale, NJ: Erlbaum.

Ainsworth, M. D. S., & Bowlby, J. (1991). An ethological approach to personality development. *American Psychologist, 46,* 331–341.

Bowlby, J. (1969). *Attachment and loss: Vol. 1. Attachment.* New York: Basic Books.

Bowlby, J. (1973). *Attachment and loss: Vol. 2. Separation.* New York: Basic Books.

Bowlby, J. (1980). *Attachment and loss: Vol. 3. Loss: Sadness and depression.* New York: Basic Books.

Bowlby, J. (1982). Attachment and loss: Retrospect and prospect. *American Journal of Orthopsychiatry, 52*(4), 664–678.

Bowlby, J. (1988). *A secure base: Parent–child attachment and healthy human development.* New York: Basic Books.

Cooper, G., Hoffman, K., Powell, B., & Marvin, R. (2006). The Circle of Security intervention: Differential diagnosis and differential treatment. In L. J. Berlin, Y. Ziv, L. M. Amaya-Jackson, & M. T. Greenberg (Eds.), *Enhancing early attachments: Theory, research, intervention, and policy* (pp. 127–151). New York: Guilford Press.

Dozier, M. (2005). Challenges of foster care. *Attachment and Human Development, 7*(1), 27–30.

Grossmann, K., Grossmann, K. E., & Kindler, H. (2005). Early care and the roots of attachment and partnership representations. In K. E. Grossmann, K. Grossmann, & E. Waters (Eds.), *Attachment from infancy to adulthood: The major longitudinal studies* (pp. 98–136). New York: Guilford Press.

Hoffman, K. T., Marvin, R. S., Cooper, G., & Powell, B. (2006). Changing toddlers' and preschoolers' attachment classifications: The Circle of Security intervention. *Journal of Consulting and Clinical Psychology, 74*(6), 1017–1026.

Marvin, R., Cooper, G., Hoffman, K., & Powell, B. (2002). The Circle of Security project: Attachment based intervention with caregiver–pre-school child dyads. *Attachment and Human Development, 4*(1), 107–124.

Schore, A. N. (2001). Effects of a secure attachment relationship on right brain development, affect regulation, and infant mental health. *Infant Mental Health Journal, 22*(1–2), 7–66.

Schore, A. N. (2005). Attachment, affect regulation and the developing right brain: Linking developmental neuroscience to pediatrics. *Pediatrics in Review, 26,* 206–211.

Sroufe, L. A. (2005). Attachment and development: A prospective, longitudinal study from birth to adulthood. *Attachment and Human Development, 7*(4), 349–367.

Sroufe, L. A., Egeland, B., Carlson, E., & Collins, W. A. (2005). Placing early attachment experiences in developmental context. In K. E. Grossmann, K. Grossmann, & E. Waters (Eds.), *Attachment from infancy to adulthood: The major longitudinal studies* (pp. 48–70). New York: Guilford Press.

Stewart, A. L., Whelan, W. F., Gilbert, J., & Marvin, R. S. (2011, October). *Applying attachment theory and the Circle of Security model in play therapy.* Paper presented at the Association for Play Therapy International Conference, Sacramento, CA.

Whelan, W. F., & Marvin, R. S. (2011, April). *Caregiver patterns that moderate the effects of abuse and neglect.* Paper presenting results from the Virginia Foster Care study (NIH Award No. GC11456) at the biennial meeting of the Society for Research in Child Development, Montréal.

CHAPTER 4

Art Therapy, Attachment, and Parent–Child Dyads

Cathy A. Malchiodi

This chapter describes art-based approaches in work with parent–child dyads to build and enhance positive attachment. As defined in Chapter 1, *art therapy* is a creative approach that includes the purposeful use of art media (drawing, painting, and constructing) as an intervention for a variety of psychosocial, cognitive, and physical challenges in people of all ages (Malchiodi, 2005, 2012a). Art therapy is a somewhat different experience from play therapy, because the main goal is the creation of a tangible product to express perceptions, feelings, and imaginings.

The use of art therapy to address attachment issues is based both in concepts from object relations theory and in a contemporary understanding of neurodevelopment and neuroplasticity. These conceptual frameworks underscore that it is possible to revisit the window of opportunity for the development of secure attachment through sensory-based interventions and reinforcement of positive relationships. Art therapy is one way to engage the body and mind through experiential learning; when used as central to dyad work with parents and children, it provides opportunities for mutual *attunement*—a principle central to successful interpersonal relationship and attachment (Badenoch, 2008; Siegel, 2007). This chapter provides an overview of the importance of art therapy in attachment work with parent–child dyads, with an emphasis on why art therapy is an effective intervention and on recommended guidelines and approaches for its use to build secure attachment.

Art Therapy and Attachment

Historically, three main concepts are important in clinical applications of art therapy and attachment issues: (1) Donald Winnicott's *"good enough" parent*; (2) *transitional object* and *transitional space*; and (3) the art therapist's *third hand*. The first two concepts come from psychoanalytic and object relations theories; the third hand is an idea that originated from the field of art therapy (Henley, 1992; Kramer, 1993). In the 21st century, these concepts are being reframed through the growing understanding of the *developing mind* (Siegel, 2012) and *neurosequential development* (Perry, 2006; Perry & Szalavitz, 2006).

The "Good Enough" Parent

Winnicott (1965, 1971) was particularly interested in children's capability to be successfully with others as a prerequisite for being alone. He developed the concept of the *"good enough" mother* (referred to as the *"good enough" parent* in this chapter) who creates a relationship and environment that help the child internalize positive experiences, including secure attachment, without being overly protective. The "good enough" parent is also a way of explaining psychosocial aspects of any therapeutic relationship that model and reinforce experiences of basic comfort for an individual, with the purpose of reducing stress reactions and enhancing a sense of self-efficacy. Increased understanding of neurobiology now confirms that secure and positive relationships with adult figures are essential for children to thrive and flourish throughout life (Perry & Szalavitz, 2006; Steele & Malchiodi, 2012).

Art therapists who work with insecure or disrupted attachment in children often temporarily assume the role of "good enough" parent through their strategic use of art activities and their role as providers of creative materials (Malchiodi, 2012b). In brief, art therapists recapitulate positive relational aspects through purposeful creative experiences that offer sensory opportunities to reinforce secure attachment. In contrast to verbal counseling, art therapy engages not only the mind, but also the body in repetitive, rhythmic, tactile, auditory, olfactory, and other sensory aspects found in the early relationship between a child and parent.

Transitional Object and Transitional Space

Siegel (2012) discusses *evocative memory*, which children use to bring an image of attachment to mind. Winnicott (1953, 1971) is credited with the classic term *transitional object*, meaning an object (person, thing, or mental representation) or ritual that is used for self-soothing. In other words, a transitional object is something that helps children hold onto a representation of a parent or caregiver until they are able to do so on their own.

For example, when a parent and child take home artwork from a session, the artwork becomes the transitional object that contains the experience of their work together in art therapy. It also may be a representation of a specific experience shared in art therapy, such as a depiction of a family activity, a loss of a significant person, or some other event. Klorer (2008) notes that art expression itself functions as a transitional object, because it supports self-relationship, empowerment, and connection with the therapist and helps children to create a variety of metaphors through art that self-soothe and reduce internal conflict.

Transitional space is defined as an intermediate area of experience where there is no clear distinction between inner and outer reality (Winnicott, 1971). Art and play therapy use transitional spaces because they offer ways for individuals to bridge subjective and objective realities and to practice attachment and relationships. Transitional space is also a type of holding environment; in art therapy, the art therapist creates and facilitates a holding environment that includes a safe place where all creative expression is accepted, respected, and valued unconditionally.

The Third Hand

Art therapist Edith Kramer (1993) is credited with the concept of the *third hand* and its application to clinical work. In brief, the *third hand* refers to the art therapist's use of suggestion, metaphors, or other techniques to enhance the individual's progress in therapy. Kramer believes that an effective art therapist must have a command of the third hand to enhance a client's creativity without being intrusive, imposing the therapist's own style or artistic values, and/or misinterpreting meanings found in images. What Kramer calls the third hand in art therapy echoes what Siegel (2010) refers to as *mindsight*, a capacity for insight (knowing what one feels) and empathy (knowing what others feel). Thus third-hand interventions are provided nonintrusively (with insight and empathy), so that the therapist does not change the content of the client's art expression or inadvertently influence the individual. This stance also echoes the concept of the "good enough" parent, who supports the child's self-efficacy and sense of safety during exploration, experimentation, and learning.

There are many ways the third hand is used in art therapy to encourage attachment and demonstrate on a sensory level that the therapist is a "good enough" parent. For example, when working with a child client, I may begin a drawing for the child to complete as a way of establishing a relationship or communication. In another situation, I may prevent a child's clay figure from falling apart by showing the child how to reinforce the legs or armature. Sometimes an art therapist literally becomes the hands for an individual; for instance, a child with a debilitating medical illness may need me to help cut and arrange photos for a collage. At other times, I may make art during the session alongside a client if it is therapeutically helpful, or I may even communicate something nonverbally through an art expression rather than use words.

What Kramer defined as the third hand can also be defined as a form of attunement. *Attunement* is generally defined as a relational dynamic that helps to build a healthy sense of self in children and is a central feature of every caring relationship and secure attachment (Perry & Szalavitz, 2006; Siegel, 2012). It also refers to a parent's or caregiver's ability to respond with empathy to a child's emotions and moods. Well-attuned parents are able to detect what their children are feeling and to reflect those emotions back through sensory means, such as facial expressions, vocalizations, touch, and other behaviors; it helps children to recognize their own feelings and develop the ability to self-regulate. Perry implies that attunement is the capacity to be able to read the nonverbal communication and rhythms of others. In other words, it is not only perceiving what individuals say, but also attending to eye signals, facial gestures, tone of voice, and even breathing rate. In art therapy, it also means attending to the content of images and nonverbal cues, as reflected in how well the therapist uses the third hand in response to the client's creative process.

Dyad Art Therapy

Dyad art therapy refers to any application that includes two people (such as a parent and child or a couple) working on either individual artwork or co-created artwork during a session. The goal is to address various aspects of the dyad's relationship, including attachment issues, via creative expression and art-based directives. The concepts mentioned in the preceding section are central to applying art therapy in work with dyads, particularly parent–child dyads, to support healthy relationships and secure attachment. Dyad work also reflects the principles of interpersonal neurobiology (Badenoch, 2008; Siegel, 2007), which include empathy, attunement, and secure attachment.

Riley (2001) delineates how dyad art therapy helps to evaluate and reconstruct early attachment experiences, noting that "Learning about the interrelationship between neuronal growth and parent–child activities stimulated me to speculate if there were art therapy activities that could re-approach these bonding experiences in a manner that aroused interest between the parental/child dyad" (p. 35). Similarly, Klorer's (2008) work with children who have experienced chronic trauma and maltreatment and their parents also highlights the interconnection among neurodevelopment, art and play-based approaches, and attachment. She emphasizes that positive attachment as well as recovery from chronic trauma does not necessarily come about through a series of directives aimed at specific issues, but through the support and the creative environment provided by the art therapist.

Most of my clinical work with attachment is with parents and children who have experienced interpersonal violence, repeated traumas and losses, or lack of psychoeducation on parenting—all of which can disrupt bonding and successful parenting (Malchiodi, 1997, 2008, 2012c). In these cases, normal attachment is disrupted in many different ways, including developmental challenges, posttraumatic stress, dissociative reactions, and attention difficulties. For many, normal social and cognitive growth is halted because the parent–child focus is turned to personal safety and basic survival needs, especially in situations of interpersonal violence. The children may appear to have hyperactivity or an oppositional or conduct disorder, when in fact insecure or disrupted attachment may be the barrier to performance and affect regulation. In addition, some children adopt the role of parent within the family system—exchanging the normal role of child for one of caregiver, and thus missing experiences that contribute to appropriate attachment responses later in life.

When working with insecure, disrupted, or avoidant attachment, I see art therapy as an expressive approach to help children and parents revisit neurodevelopmental and psychosocial aspects of attachment to strengthen their relationship. It is also a way to capitalize on sensory learning to facilitate change. Engaging in art making together is not only a shared experience; it is an effective approach to learning, because creative expression is experienced on multiple sensory levels—visual, tactile, kinesthetic, olfactory, and auditory. Art therapy also sets up relational dynamics that are uniquely different from those in verbal psychotherapy and counseling. The relationship includes not only the parent–child dyad and the therapist; it also includes the art process itself and the art products created by the dyad. In work with a dyad, how a parent responds to a child's art expression and creative activity is an important part of the experience, in addition to the therapist's intervention. This provides the added opportunity for the art therapist to model and reflect being a "good enough" parent and appropriately using the third hand for the parent. Parents have the chance to learn important verbal and nonverbal responses to their children to strengthen communication, develop empathy, and build attachment (for more information on responding to art products and process, see below).

In the remainder of this chapter, I describe specific considerations and art-based approaches used in working with a parent–child dyad: 20-year-old Lisa and her 6-year-old son, John. Lisa became a single parent at the age of 14 and grew up in a home where she was physically and sexually abused by her father and brother. John's father was physically abusive to Lisa, and her pregnancy was difficult, resulting in a premature birth. Mother and child had a strained relationship from John's infancy through his preschool years, and her grandmother took over much of the caregiving. She and John were recommended for multiple sessions of individual and dyad art therapy to work on issues of attachment and chronic trauma.

Safety First

Without safety, there can be no attachment or relationship; it is also the first step toward setting the stage for successful art therapy. Therefore, initially anyone using art-based interventions must consider how to provide opportunities for creative expression in a consistent and predictable manner. This includes introducing parents and children to the art therapy room and its contents, which may include an array of materials for drawing, painting, and constructing, as well as props for creative play. In working with children and parents from violent homes and communities, I have also learned that establishing a well-organized space conducive to stress reduction and consistency is essential to successful intervention, including building attachment.

Safety also includes establishing rules for physical and emotional safety during art-making sessions, such as no verbal or physical violence in the therapy room or office, and no destroying of another individual's artwork. It also includes reinforcing the ideas that artistic talent is not necessary and that all efforts at creative expression are valued, important, and accepted. Communicating acceptance of all art expressions is particularly important, because it reflects a central principle in attachment: "I accept you for who you are, right now." This is a critical benchmark, because both a sense of trust and a sense of belonging are implicit within acceptance and invite positive attachment.

In the initial sessions of work with Lisa and John, I reinforced that unlike in an art class or classroom, it was not important for them to make "good art." I also emphasized that John in particular could benefit from hearing from Lisa that his creative work was unconditionally valued by her, without judgment or interpretation; I also knew that it would be important for me to be supportive of Lisa's participation in art therapy, because of her own insecurities and lack of an internal sense of safety. Because Lisa had not received the same unconditional regard and praise in her own childhood, I capitalized on strategic opportunities to model how to respond to John's efforts in art therapy, and to provide support for her own courage to participate in art activities.

Sensory Materials: Soothing Lower Parts of the Brain

Purposeful selection of art media that are multisensory, that are developmentally appropriate, and that stimulate creative expression in a variety of ways is essential to help recapitulate early experiences of exploration and mastery (Proulx, 2002). For dyad work with parents and children, it is important to have at least some drawing materials (crayons, felt markers, white paper, and colored paper), painting materials (finger paints, tempera paints, a variety of bristle and sponge brushes), collage materials (colored papers, fabrics, and yarn), and construction materials (Play-Doh, Model Magic clay, and spoons, forks, and other implements for making marks in clay). In particular, art activities that involve repetition and positive sensory sensations soothe the lower parts of the brain, reduce stress responses, enhance self-regulation, and slow down the sympathetic nervous system; they also nonverbally communicate that life is stable and consistent. (Therapists who are unfamiliar with the properties of art materials should consult Malchiodi, 2012a.) For example, pudding painting with one's fingers, blowing paint across a paper with straws, and modeling with soft clay often involve soothing repetition and engage the senses in pleasurable ways.

Therapists should identify what specific types of art-based experiences may be self-soothing and calming for both parents and children. In attachment-focused, trauma-informed work, asking participants about cultural preferences and any positive memories about creative activities can help guide choices of media and interventions (Malchiodi, 2012d). For example, when I asked Lisa about her previous experiences with art materials, she told me how she had always longed to have a brand-new box of crayons (the 64-color box in particular) and to have time to "just color" with her mother. This memory became a catalyst for planning a session when I presented both Lisa and John with new 64-color boxes of crayons. During the art therapy session, we spent time looking at the boxes, smelling the crayons, and practicing using them on different colored and textured papers. It was not only a time for Lisa and John to enjoy the same experience, but also a session when Lisa felt that she and John had a common bond with positive sensory memories that Lisa and her mother had never had the opportunity to enjoy. In brief, through this simple gesture I was able to help Lisa recapture and reframe a part of her life related to her own attachment issues.

Scribble Chase: Enhancing Reflective Convergence

Siegel (2007) emphasizes the importance of a parent's attunement to the internal world of a child or spouse. Attunement between parent and child or adult partners enhances feelings of happiness, mutual understanding, and trust. It is necessary for two people to "feel felt" by each other, and it literally reinforces the neural circuitry for attunement in the brain. According to Siegel, the mindful awareness of oneself and of another enhances the experience of *reflexive convergence* and promotes attunement, flexibility, and interpersonal attachment.

There are many ways to use art making as an approach to reinforce attunement. One of the first things I demonstrate to parent–child dyads when working with attachment issues is the so-called "scribble chase," or two-way scribble drawing. In brief, parent and child each choose a felt marker (markers that smell like a fruit or flower are a good choice) or crayon, and each has the opportunity to be the leader in a scribble drawing on a large piece of paper (Figure 4.1). For example, the child may be the leader of the first drawing, and while he or she scribbles with a pen on the paper, the parent follows the child's lines at the same time with his or her pen. Sometimes we reverse roles and the parent becomes the leader of the scribble, with the child following.

In many cases where insecure or avoidant attachment between parent and child exists, a parent may be unsuccessful in joining in the drawing; a child may scribble all over the parent's lines; or one or both may be unable or unwilling to make any marks at all. In coaching a parent to engage in this experience with a child, it is important to help the parent prepare the child with attachment difficulties for the activity. I often suggest to a mother, for example, that she make eye contact with her child and tell the child that they will be playing a game with crayons on paper. I also may suggest that she make some sort physical contact with her child, such as a light touch on an arm or the upper back, and to place their chairs as closely together as is comfortable for them at the table. In addition, I may model the activity with either the parent or child as co-scribbler, asking one of them to be the leader of the scribble drawing while I follow or vice versa. In essence, I am demonstrating ways to attune to another's behavior, particularly to sensory, nonverbal cues.

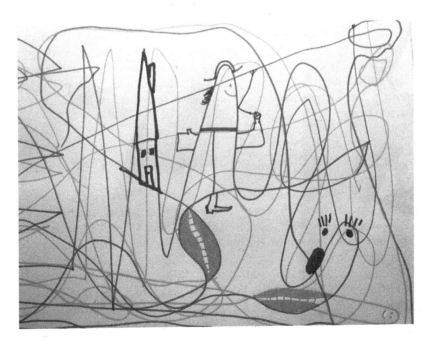

FIGURE 4.1. Example of the "scribble chase" activity.

This activity is sometimes called a "two-way conversation on paper," because many dynamics may emerge from this simple activity. For example, Lisa was eager to follow the lines scribbled by her 6-year-old son, John; however, she became immediately frustrated and angry when John was not able to follow her scribble and drew over her lines. She felt that John was doing this on purpose, and that he was being oppositional and defiant of what she thought were the rules of the scribble game. In this case, I helped Lisa understand that John's marks were not necessarily aggression toward her; they simply reflected the limited developmental motor skills of a young child who was challenged by trauma and loss. My third-hand intervention also involved ways to reframe the art experience, suggesting that perhaps John's marks were in part a positive action. I remarked that she could perhaps say to John, "I feel really happy when our lines touch. My lines are happy when your lines touched mine in the picture." My overall goal in this simple art activity is to create a sensory experience that reinforces positive relationship through tactile, visual, and physical contact and other aspects. In Lisa's case, I was able to help her start to attune to John and respond to his creative work in ways that she could carry over to other parts of the mother–child relationship to enhance positive bonding.

There is one other important aspect of a scribble chase that is also found in other art-based activities—*mirroring*. Art therapy is an approach that provides opportunities to witness another's creative expression; it also provides possibilities to introduce activities that can be imitated or learned through mirroring. As described by Gil and Dias in Chapter 7 on the integrative use of drama therapy within play therapy, mirroring is a key practice in building connection between the child and therapist; in dyad art therapy, children and parents learn through watching and interacting in similar ways. In all instances, aspects of interpersonal neurobiology are present in any shared sensory or expressive activities, including those in dyad art therapy.

The Bird's Nest Drawing and Three-Dimensional Construction

Working with a relevant metaphor through artistic expression is helpful in situations where there is insecure, disrupted, or avoidant attachment. One metaphor commonly used in art therapy is a "bird's nest." There is also an art-based assessment called the Bird's Nest Drawing (BND), which was developed to provide information about an individual's attachment security as depicted in a drawing of a bird's nest (Kaiser, 1996). The individual is asked, "Draw a picture with a bird's nest" (Figure 4.2). The BND is not a diagnostic tool per se, but a means to evoke representations of attachment, safety, and protection. Its originator, art therapist Donna Kaiser, hypothesized that the BND would encourage expression similar to that of family drawings, and that it would be less threatening to clients. Kaiser

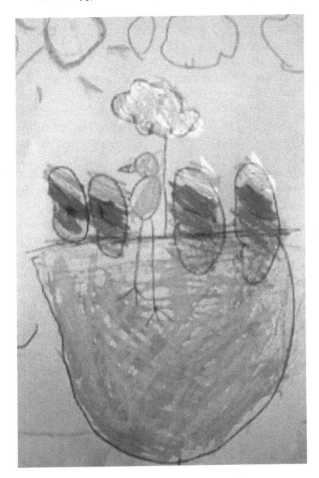

FIGURE 4.2. Drawing of a bird's nest by a child.

also developed a rating scale to measure specific graphic characteristics of secure and insecure attachment in BNDs (Francis, Kaiser, & Deaver, 2003; Kaiser & Deaver, 2009). Researchers have identified some consistent graphic elements and characteristics in these drawings that they believe are connected to attachment issues (Sheller, 2007).

Although a drawing of a bird's nest may be useful in evaluating attachment, children in particular respond positively to using a variety of art materials to create a bird's nest. In my experience, modeling clay, twigs, moss, leaves, tissue paper, and yarns have greater tactile and visual potential than drawing alone does, and they can engage children in more detailed representations. The sensory aspects of three-dimensional materials more closely approximate elements of a nest with eggs, parent birds, and baby birds, and dyads can use these more actively to express experiences of caregiving, security, and relationships through this metaphor. In dyad work, I may ask the parent and child to co-create a bird's nest together, using a variety of materials; I may also suggest that the parent allow the child to lead the way in designing the nest. I often arrange a separate session to coach the parent on ways to support the child's creative efforts for this activity, and also teach the parent about how to become a nonintrusive third hand in assisting. In addition, I use a variation of this activity that I call "creating a safe place for your duck," using a rubber duck toy that I provide as a prop.

In an individual session with Lisa, I explained to her that we would be working on a creative project on safety in an upcoming art therapy session with John, and that I would like her to try the project in advance so she could assist John. Lisa created her own "safe place" for a rubber duck on a paper plate, lining it with feathers and creating what she described as a "secure fort" for it (Figure 4.3). Without much prompting, she was quickly able to articulate her memories of fear and lack of a "safe place" as a child in a household where there was physical violence and sexual abuse. As she had observed in previous sessions, Lisa realized that these fear-based experiences compromised her own attachment to her mother, who she felt had not protected her from harm. Ultimately, Lisa's experience in creating a safe place for her duck taught her on a sensory level the importance of giving John a greater sense of safety through both actions and words. By their own mutual decision, they decided to co-create one safe place for two rubber ducks—a "Momma Duck" and a "Ducklet"—on a single paper plate (Figure 4.4).

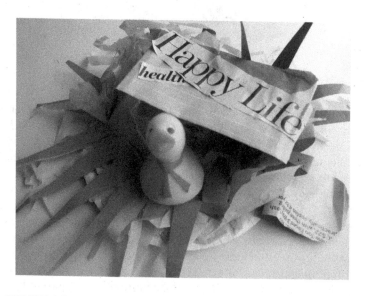

FIGURE 4.3. Lisa's construction of a safe place for a rubber duck.

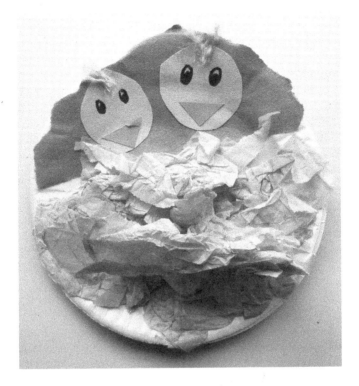

FIGURE 4.4. Lisa and John's co-created safe place for "Momma Duck" and "Ducklet."

Responding to Art Expressions

In my work with Lisa and John and with other parent–child dyads, I spend time coaching parents on what to say to their children about their art expressions rather than how to interpret their creative products. Therapists and counselors unfamiliar with art therapy often believe that it is important to be able to interpret the meaning of artwork. Although there may be visual metaphors in children's artwork that provide relevant information on trauma, loss, or other factors that may affect attachment, responding to the product and process through developmentally appropriate, "brain-wise" questions and supportive observations is much more important. Nonverbal responses are also important, including handling artwork with care and respect, and treating it with respect and value. Also, it is important to inform parents and children just how artwork will be stored between sessions if it is retained during an initial session; this can lead to a discussion of how the child's artwork that goes home should be treated or displayed. These actions reinforce a sense of safety, instill trust, and build the relationship among the therapist, parent, and child over time.

Because art therapy involves verbally responding to art expressions, practitioners can support positive attachment and attunement through their responses to art expressions, particularly those created by young clients. First and foremost, it is important not to place interpretations or judgments about the content or meaning of artwork; rather, it is much more helpful to demonstrate respect with both words and actions that art making is an important neurodevelopmental accomplishment for children. Here is a brief list of possible responses to children's creative work, which therapists can also teach parents to use when talking to their children about their art expressions:

> "I am really glad you can tell me about this and about how you feel through your drawings and artwork."
>
> "Your drawings and paintings helped me to understand how scary [sad, upset] you must have been. I get scared [sad, upset], too. It's OK to be scared [sad, upset]. I am glad that you can share these feelings through your artwork."
>
> "It doesn't matter what you draw [create]. I like watching you draw [create, play] and listening to your stories about your artwork."

In all cases, it is important to use nonverbal cues where possible and to attune these to the comfort level of clients, including eye contact, appropriate touch, and sincere gestures. Art therapy, like play therapy, provides a natural format for these attachment-building interactions, including active observation of expressive activities.

Conclusion

This brief chapter summarizes some key aspects of applying art therapy to attachment work with parent–child dyads. When art-based approaches are used to build or enhance attachment, sensory experiences that stimulate interaction and reinforce positive relationship between parent and child become the central strategies to initiate change. These sensory experiences also have the potential to recapture and restructure early experiences of bonding and attunement in both parent and child. Perry (2008) observes that "experience becomes biology" with reference to the impact of severe and recurrent trauma on attachment. Similarly, the experience of art therapy for those whose attachment has been compromised or disrupted may play a part in the recovery of what is most important to success throughout the lifespan—the experience of positive attachment and trust in secure relationships with others.

REFERENCES

Badenoch, B. (2008). *Becoming a brain-wise therapist: A practical guide to interpersonal neurobiology.* New York: Norton.

Francis, D., Kaiser, D., & Deaver, S. (2003). Representations of attachment security in the Bird's Nest Drawings of clients with substance abuse disorders. *Art Therapy: Journal of the American Art Therapy Association, 20*(3), 125–137.

Henley, D. (1992). *Exceptional children, exceptional art.* Worcester, MA: Davis.

Kaiser, D. (1996). Indications of attachment security in a drawing task. *The Arts in Psychotherapy, 23,* 333–340.

Kaiser, D., & Deaver, S. (2009). Assessing attachment with the Bird's Nest Drawing: A review of the research. *Art Therapy: Journal of the American Art Therapy Association, 26*(1), 26–33.

Klorer, P. G. (2008). Expressive therapy for severe maltreatment and attachment disorders: A neuroscience framework. In C. Malchiodi (Ed.), *Creative interventions and traumatized children* (pp. 43–61). New York: Guilford Press.

Kramer, E. (1993). *Art as therapy with children.* Chicago: Magnolia Street.

Malchiodi, C. A. (1997). *Breaking the silence: Art therapy with children from violent homes* (2nd ed.). New York: Brunner-Routledge.

Malchiodi, C. A. (Ed.). (2005). *Expressive therapies.* New York: Guilford Press.

Malchiodi, C. A. (2008). *Creative interventions with traumatized children.* New York: Guilford Press.

Malchiodi, C. A. (2012a). Art therapy materials, media, and methods. In C. A. Malchiodi (Ed.), *Handbook of art therapy* (2nd ed., pp. 27–40). New York: Guilford Press.

Malchiodi, C. A. (2012b). Psychoanalytic, analytic and object relations approaches. In C. A. Malchiodi (Ed.), *Handbook of art therapy* (2nd ed., pp. 57–74). New York: Guilford Press.

Malchiodi, C. A. (2012c). Art therapy and the brain. In C. A. Malchiodi (Ed.), *Handbook of art therapy* (2nd ed., pp. 17–26). New York: Guilford Press.

Malchiodi, C. A. (2012d). Trauma-informed art therapy and sexual abuse. In P. Goodyear-Brown (Ed.), *Handbook of child sexual abuse* (pp. 341–354). Hoboken, NJ: Wiley.

Perry, B. D. (2006). Applying principles of neurodevelopment to clinical work with maltreated and traumatized children: The neurosequential model of therapeutics. In N. B. Webb (Ed.), *Working with traumatized youth in child welfare* (pp. 27–52). New York: Guilford Press.

Perry, B. D. (2008). Foreword. In C. A. Malchiodi (Ed.), *Creative interventions and traumatized children* (pp. ix–xi). New York: Guilford Press.

Perry, B. D., & Szalavitz, M. (2006). *The boy who was raised as a dog.* New York: Basic Books.

Proulx, L. (2002). *Strengthening ties through parent–child dyad art therapy.* London: Kingsley.

Riley, S. (2001). *Group process made visible: Group art therapy.* New York: Brunner-Routledge.

Sheller, S. (2007). Understanding insecure attachment: A study using children's bird nest imagery. *Art Therapy: Journal of the American Art Therapy Association, 24*(3), 119–127.

Siegel, D. (2007). *The mindful brain.* New York: Norton.

Siegel, D. (2010). *Mindsight: The new science of personal transformation.* New York: Bantam.

Siegel, D. (2012). *The developing mind: How relationships and the brain interact to shape who we are* (2nd ed.). New York: Guilford Press.

Steele, W., & Malchiodi, C. A. (2012). *Trauma-informed practices with children and adolescents.* New York: Routledge.

Winnicott, D. W. (1953). Transitional objects and transitional phenomena. *International Journal of Psychiatry, 34,* 89–97.

Winnicott, D. W. (1965). *The maturation processes and the facilitating environment.* New York: International Universities Press.

Winnicott, D. W. (1971). *Therapeutic considerations in child psychiatry.* New York: Basic Books.

CHAPTER 5

Music Therapy with Children with Developmental Trauma Disorder

Jacqueline Z. Robarts

This chapter focuses on music therapy with children and adolescents living with unresolved attachment trauma, interpersonal violence, and/or neglect throughout early childhood, as well as high levels of stress in their homes. These children's physiological and emotional responses are affected at their core, inhibiting their psychological development and leading to *developmental trauma disorder*—an expansion of the posttraumatic stress disorder (PTSD) criteria for children with histories of complex trauma (van der Kolk, 2005). This chapter discusses music's power to affect intra- and interpersonal responses, and describes how music therapy can help children with early relational trauma. When applied with clinical perception and intent, musical improvisation and play within the therapeutic relationship can help regulate children's emotions and physiological responses, offer a wide range of sensory experiences, and encourage creative self-expression, thereby bringing about a more cohesive sense of self and continuity of being in the here-and-now.

This chapter also examines some aspects of music and *communicative musicality* (Malloch & Trevarthen, 2009; Trevarthen & Malloch, 2000), and their intrinsic *organizing* and *regulating* functions, as applied in music therapy (Robarts, 1998, 2009). From a synthesis of musical, developmental, and psychodynamic perspectives, the focus is on use of musical form as central to integrative processes of music therapy with young people whose foundations of self have been damaged by early relational trauma (Robarts, 2003, 2006, 2009).

Overview of Population

I have worked with children ages 3–18 years with attachment or early relational trauma—first during my early years as a music therapist in a music therapy department of a children's hospital with child and adolescent mental health and child development services; and later in a private music therapy center, where I specialize in this area of work with children and adults. Clinical supervision by child psychotherapists specializing in this field has supported and deepened my work, as have independent study and personal psychoanalysis.

The young people with whom I have worked in music therapy have been affected by a range of *traumatic* experiences: traumatic events preceding or surrounding a child's birth; repeated and prolonged separations in the first 3 years from a nonempathic mother; sexual abuse and neglect in early childhood; drug- and alcohol-abusing parents; witnessing violence between parents in the home; and/or successive and/or traumatic foster care and adoption processes. Persistent trauma in early childhood, where there have been overwhelming threats to basic safety and survival, may lead to developmental trauma disorder (van der Kolk, 2005). These children often present as pale and remote, yet hypervigilant; they are easily overaroused by ordinary movements, gestures, or sensory stimuli. The children may be so anxious that they will "shut down" their emotions or dissociate; become overly compliant; or become highly controlling and defensive, sometimes needing to withdraw physically from the situation (perhaps by hiding in a cupboard or a similar enclosed space). Their behavior and mood can change in a split second. In the occurrence of flashbacks of traumatic events, "the trauma is relived as isolated sensory, emotional and motoric imprints of the trauma, without a storyline" (van der Kolk, 2003, p. 183). Through its intrinsic sensory modalities and psychophysiological effects, music can be used in music therapy to help develop such children's continuity of self, capacity for sensory and symbolic play, and new narratives of being and being with others, untrammeled by trauma (Robarts, 2003, 2006, 2009).

Psychodynamic Music Therapy in the Field of Attachment Trauma

Psychodynamic music therapy has been well documented in collective and individually authored publications (Bruscia, 1998; Hadley, 2003; Wigram & De Backer, 1999). Music therapists specializing in trauma work are highly individual in their approaches or styles of working informed by a range of psychodynamic theories (Amir, 2004; Austin, 2008; Frank-Schwebel, 2002; Montello, 2003; Robarts, 2003, 2006, 2009; Scheiby, 2010; Schönfeld, 2003; Sutton, 2002). An essential aspect of all psychodynamically informed music therapy is receptivity to each client's internal world, particularly to musical and other aspects of transference and countertransference (nonverbal and verbal).

Musical and transference phenomena are complex visceral, emotional, and mental features of the therapeutic relationship. They are useful for understanding and working with a child's internal world and its constituent "object relations." They also present therapeutic challenges.

Holidays and any breaks in the children's therapy are prepared for, as is the ending of therapy. While children's confidentiality is strictly maintained except on a "need-to-know" basis, the music therapist works closely with parents and a multiagency team. This may include child protection, fostering, and adoption agencies.

In previous publications (Robarts, 2003, 2006, 2009), I have described some central aspects of music therapy that are particularly relevant to young people with unresolved early relational trauma and consequent developmental trauma disorder. In respect to attachment trauma, developmental psychology linked with affective neuroscience has emphasized the importance of the therapeutic attachment relationship in transforming interpersonal communicative relationships (Schore, 2001, 2003; Siegel, 2003; Stern, 2004; van der Kolk, 2003).

Issues and Challenges

Young people with unresolved attachment trauma present in music therapy with a wide range of issues that are challenging to both clients and therapists. This work requires heightened sensitivity; firm and highly adaptive therapeutic skills grounded in compassion; perceptive and creative use of mind and intuition; and a robust sense of reality. These young people present with the following, in various combinations: hypervigilance, hyperarousal, exaggerated startle response at the slightest trigger, disorganized or agitated behavior, withdrawal, a hardened or "hard-to-reach" demeanor, and emotional "tuning out." In such children, therapists are likely to meet a restricted range of feelings, impoverished capacity for play, and repetitive rituals in play (including self-harming or self-denigrating behavior or the reenactment of traumatic events). The more "acting-out" kind of behavior with poor capacity for play tends to be unsafe, because the children can easily become overexcited (and this may escalate into dangerous acts). It can be hard to maintain a vigilant stance while being open and receptive with such a child. To be firm yet relaxed requires a balance of skillful use of physical, verbal, musical, and spoken management in terms of boundaries to keep the child and the therapeutic relationship safe.

Added to these challenges is the scattered, fragmented, nonsequential nature of activity in the therapy room. Children may switch from screaming and kicking to remote, dissociative states. These switches are further complicated by the presentation of different stages of development in these children's behavior and their presymbolic and symbolic play. There is also the kind of "frozen" or "closed-down" child who presents with numbed responsiveness and a detached, avoidant style of relating and being. Often there is suicidal ideation or the exhibition of sexualized behavior in play. This may be accompanied by a controlling, intrusive style of relating, poor sense of physical interpersonal boundaries, physical and verbal abuse, and an unnaturally adult manner. In addition, there may be issues of shame and low self-esteem. Developmental delay and learning/attentional difficulties can all add to the attachment trauma and further affect the child's development.

All of these factors need careful understanding with regard to a child's feeling states and the symbolism in the child's play. The therapist needs to be able to understand where the child is developmentally at any given moment—and this may change from one moment to the next, with the child alternating between the coping strategies of a 6-year-old and those of the actual 14-year-old present in the room, all communicated either within the metaphors of symbolic play or more directly to the therapist. Features of the voice (such as volume and intonation), as well as the way in which the child is moving and generally behaving, inform the therapeutic process.

Avoiding Retraumatizing the Child

In working with children with PTSD and developmental trauma disorder in music therapy, the therapist needs to be aware of the impact that the sensory and interpersonal aspects of musical play and musical relationship may have, and the hyperarousal that even the slightest event may trigger. Frequently, the projections of an abused child's frightened and traumatized self make the therapist feel like one of the perpetrators of abuse. The therapist needs to develop a capacity to receive and then hold the intensity of transference feelings, along with any projections.

Mapping the Territory While Being Open to the New

Therapy processes are complex and multilayered, so that mapping the territory develops as part of one's craft (Robarts, 2000, 2003, 2009). Clinical experience is the most trustworthy route to theoretical understanding. My approach to music therapy sometimes embraces other art forms, such as drawing/painting, puppets, dance, and drama, in order to enrich the potential for children's symbolic play while affording a wide range of sensory experience. In my theory of symbolization, *poietic processes*, I elaborate the two-way channel between the preverbal and verbal self that allows integration to be nurtured in the therapy relationship (Robarts, 2003, 2009). The use of other expressive arts in music therapy sessions generally arises out of a child's spontaneous imaginative responses, and is developed within or alongside the music therapeutic process. Although I sometimes work solely in music (i.e., sound, instruments, voice), my clients constantly present all kinds of art forms, more accurately described by the Greek word for music, "mousike."

From a psychobiological perspective, the source of music and musicality has been described as "the intrinsic motive pulse" or "audible gesture" (Trevarthen, 1999, p. 175). "The essence of spontaneous musical expression is that it directly engages and activates the core of rhythmic and sympathetic impulses from which all human communication comes" (Robarts, 1998, p. 172). From the beginnings of life, music affects us. From 23 weeks of gestation, the fetus hears the intonation and timbre of its mother's voice, and recognizes this as its own mother's voice after birth (DeCasper & Carstens, 1981); this is the basis of prenatal attachment through sound. Parent–infant communication research shows our early intuitive emotional communication to be musical in all its dynamic forms—shaping and organizing the infant's developing brain, mind, and body through the parent's attuning to the infant in *protoconversational* forms, and thus building meaning and cultivating knowledge in relationships (Trevarthen, 1993). More recently, this process has been termed *communicative musicality*. It is a central, constructive feature of human relations and human development from the beginning of life and throughout the lifespan, and when it goes well, it lays the foundations of psychological health and well-being (Malloch & Trevarthen, 2009).

Conversely, if there are impairments or deficits in *intersubjectivity*, these will have a negative impact on the infant's core of rhythmic and sympathetic impulses, and thus on its developing brain connectivity and its self-regulatory and attachment capacities (Trevarthen, Aitken, Vandekerckhove, Delafield-Butt, & Nagy, 2006). In his descriptions of *affect attunement* in the infant–parent relationship, Stern (1985, 2004, 2010) has also described in musical terms the dynamic forms of vitality in early communication as a basis of attachment and emotional regulation in human psychosocial development. In music therapy, the regulating and shaping of musical–emotional communication are consistent with the constructs of communicative musicality and affect attunement.

Processes of Containment and Transformation in the Transference Relationship

I have found the psychoanalyst Wilfred Bion's concept of *containment* (Bion, 1962a, 1962b) very useful in music therapy. Bion developed this concept from Melanie Klein's original ideas of *transference* and the related intrapsychic processes of *projection*, *introjection*, and *projective and introjective identification*. To this, he added the idea of *transformation* to describe what happens when the mother/therapist receives the projections of infant/client, understands and thinks about them, and then gives them back in a useful form that can be felt with less anxiety and perhaps, at the right time, thought about—leading to his concept of the *container/ contained*. This has many parallels with the function of aesthetic form in the music therapy process described in this chapter. Bion emphasized not only the mother's receptivity to the infant's anxiety, but also her capacity to understand and give expression to the baby's unbearable feelings transforming them in ways that the baby can take in. If the baby's experiences are intolerable to its immature system, it then projects these feelings psychically into the mother, who then, identifying with the infant's emotional state and able to hold this state in her mind/feelings and understand it, gives the baby's feelings back transformed by her *understanding* response. In this way, Bion's explanation illuminates the processes of fragmentation and integration that take place in therapy as a client works toward creativity and well-being. This is helpful in considering the dynamic forms of the music therapy relationship.

Early object relations in terms of musical introjects and symbolization are also important (Robarts, 1994, p. 234). Regulatory processes in music involve the aesthetic creation of a space to think, and as such constitute a form of containment and transformation. Musical aspects of containment and transformation reside in the way the child is heard, listened to, and understood as much as being musically accompanied. This kind of "listening landscape" is the starting point and the point to which more active episodes in therapy return: The therapist remains open and receptive to what is arising in the moment, without expectation. Silence can enable a child to hear his or her own breathing, bringing the child a vital sense of being alive and present. A single tone, a sustained simple background of alternating harmonies (Austin, 2008), or a simple rhythm can be offered in a way that invites the child to respond if he or she wants to. Being with a traumatized child musically and affectively may center at first on letting the child explore the room and the instruments. It is important to let the child feel that he or she is in control and can check out everything, including the therapist!

While maintaining the boundaries of the therapeutic relationship, a therapist needs to respond sensitively and resourcefully to engage with a child's presenting developmental level(s). As explained earlier in this chapter, music is not necessarily the only form of engagement in music therapy; some children prefer to draw or play with toys, or roll on the mat. In music it is vital to create experiences of stability, often in the background of their other play preoccupations—such as a repeating melodic motive, an *ostinato* pattern, a shift in mood, a well-placed chord, a thickening or thinning of the harmonic texture, or a speeding or slowing of pace or tempo. All of these may offer some sense of connection, even without the child's response. Here the therapist's musical countertransference is akin to Bion's (1962a) maternal "reverie." Tuning into the *unsounded* music of the child's internal world is as important a process in music therapy as engaging in more overt modes of musical communication and play.

In a musical therapeutic relationship, children reveal their patterns of relating, motivations, and defenses, and often do so at varied developmental levels within a single therapy session. Augmenting positive and tolerable experiences of intersubjectivity through music is a primary concern, as is the assisting of emotional awakening and internalizing of experience when children's emotions are numbed or frozen. One only has to think of the physical pain of frozen limbs warming up to gain some appreciation of the pain of frozen emotions melting and beginning to flow. This is necessarily a slow and careful process. Music can engage children (and adults) at very early developmental levels when these are present in the therapy room. In adapting to the character and style that is likely to engage or respond to a particular client, simple musical form using musical techniques such as these can be used in infinitely flexible ways—from nursery songs to hip-hop, from blues to baroque.

In working with very disturbed children who have a fragile core sense of self, the therapist needs to be able to hold onto projected primitive anxieties for much longer than with clients whose ego function is stronger (Alvarez, 1992, 2010). Alvarez (1992) also describes the therapist's role in enlivening and engaging a child with significant developmental disorder and ego deficit. These facets of therapeutic work have importance in working with abused and traumatized children, whose self-protective defenses must be worked with sensitively by the therapist in order to build the children's capacity to trust, reflect on, and process experience. Working within the metaphors of children's songs, for instance, can enable maintaining much-needed defenses, while at the same time delicately bypassing these same defenses to address anxieties and nurture creative capacities.

Containing/Transforming Function of Improvised Songs: From Procedural Memory to Autobiographical Narrative

Song can bring forth emotions and images as autobiographical narratives from preverbal and visceral levels, from the procedural memory; this often integrates the dissociated, traumatized self-experiences in a freshly evolving here-and-now, supported by the music therapist. Developed in the early intimacy of infant–parent relating, the preverbal self is a social construction of implicit relational knowing (Siegel, 2012; Stern, 2004). When the preverbal self is traumatized in early development, the neural *template* of the intersubjective self is shattered, with lasting consequences. In music therapy, the underpinning of rhythm, pulse, or groove of the music increases the child's capacity for self-regulation, whereby a more secure and cohesive sense of self is experienced in musical coactivity. From this feeling of security and self-involvement, children with intelligence and language may begin singing their stories: autobiographical narratives or songs of self, often entirely in metaphor but clearly relating to themselves in a kind of borderland of half-conscious, half-unconscious.

One such child who improvised songs in music therapy was Lena (Robarts, 2003), whose case is described below. For the person who has suffered early trauma that has become embodied as part of the body–mind self, and is often beyond verbal recall, the power of music and singing can be a healing process (Austin, 2008). The preverbal, implicit, or procedural domain of the self is thought to function in quite a different way from the verbal self and declarative memory—the storehouse of our experiences that we can search and recollect consciously (Siegel, 2012). However, in my clinical experience, these two forms of memory or self-experiencing, implicit and explicit, can be bridged by art forms that *speak the language of the preverbal self.* In such cases, music can be used creatively not only in accessing the procedural domain of experience, but also in forging new relational experiences at that level, in musical interplay. These experiences are generally unplanned and arise spontaneously. The following case illustrations show how music therapy can bring new experiences of self into play, addressing unresolved trauma as well as developing normal healthy foundations of self.

Case Vignettes

The names of the children and the identifying features of their histories and therapy material have been changed to preserve confidentiality. For the same reason, songs and other material have been slightly altered, while retaining the salient therapeutic components.

Lena

Lena was an unwanted child who suffered severe neglect by her parents, and at the age of 2 years, during a traumatic separation from her mother, she was sexually abused by her grandfather. Throughout her early years, she was aggressive and provocative; as a result, she was excluded from nursery school. She then reported that she was being sexually abused by her brother and his friend. Lena felt she was "rubbish," a "throw-out," ugly, and unlovable. She was unable to learn effectively in school, and her bizarre behavior eventually raised sufficient concerns for her to be referred, at 9 years of age, to a child and adolescent mental health inpatient setting. There she stayed for 14 months. The unit staff was very conscious that she was being stigmatized by inpatient admission and made every effort to involve the whole family in regular therapy. Lena was also referred for music therapy once weekly (increasing to twice weekly after the first month), each session lasting 45 minutes.

Lena's music therapy fell roughly into three phases. The excerpts below (all described in the present tense, for greater immediacy) are drawn from Phase 1 and the very end of Phase 2. Phase 1 was characterized by listening; songs developing relationship and trust; idealization and self-protective defense; and symbolic use of musical instruments. In Phase 2, her defenses lowered: Her anxieties were expressed in song poems, later giving way to chaotic and eroticized play; flashbacks to early abuse; metaphors of the borderland between the unconscious and conscious in her improvised songs; and symbolic use of instruments. Phase 3 showed the beginnings of integration; expressions of sorrow at parting; and songs (again with powerful metaphors arising from her unconscious) showing hope for the future in images of transformation.

Session 3 illustrates the use of nursery songs, as well as the defensive yet incipiently creative nature of her symbolic play and use of the instruments. Session 4 then shows my introduction of spontaneous, co-active song improvisation that helped reach beyond her "happy" mask to work with her defenses against sadness, and later her much more disturbed, chaotic feelings connected with early abuse. A much later session (Session 37) demonstrates her use of an improvised song to reach a new level of integration.

Session 3: Nursery Songs; the "Music House"; Symbolic Use of the Instruments as Containers

Today Lena arrives in what I now recognize to be her habitual superficially happy mood. After briefly playing the piano, Lena then chooses to surround herself with musical instruments, creating a "music house" on the far side of the room. This symbolic use of the instruments is extended in later sessions, but in this session, the instruments are arranged to form a physical barrier as much as a container. She demands that I listen attentively to her playing without joining in myself. From within her barricade, however, she now begins to permit some musical interaction through familiar nursery songs. She requests "Pop Goes the Weasel," "Hickory Dickory Dock," and "Ring a Ring of Roses." Lena jumps up and down like a 3-year-old as she plays inside her music house, especially enjoying the dramatic moments in each song.

I improvise music matching Lena's movements and vocalize in response to her squeals of excitement, which I am concerned may overwhelm her. However, her physical responses to the music show how efficiently the music is regulating her tendency toward overexcitement in shared play. By improvising clear phrase structures in music that matches her mood, I can not only meet but also *hold* and steady her feelings, musically transforming them into excitement and pleasure that she can tolerate without becoming avoidant or emotionally disturbed. The nursery songs offer her a certain predictability in which she can begin to trust our relationship. Nevertheless, her use of the songs is also quite defensive and controlling.

I introduce altered diatonic (nonconventional) harmonies in my accompaniment of the nursery songs, bringing different emotional qualities into the music to resonate with Lena's overt and underlying feelings, which I pick up in my countertransference and from her musical expression. I sing about her feeling safe inside her music house. I also introduce a *rondo* form (a musical form with the structure ABACAD, etc.) that uses her familiar tunes as a secure basis, from which she then engages in free vocalizing and improvisational–conversational exchanges. This style of refrain and episodic improvisational play develops in subsequent sessions, building new creative self-expression while also allowing Lena to work through her feelings and past experiences.

Session 4: A Happy–Sad Song That Brings Lena in Touch with Her Real Feelings and Builds a More Trusting Working Relationship

Lena wanders around the room rather distractedly. I play the "Child's Tune" motif (sol-mi-la-sol-mi) in unison, interspersed with close-textured diatonic harmonies. Lena repeats a question from Session 1: "What's music therapy for, anyway?" I answer her musings about music therapy by leading into a gentle I-Ib-IV-V accompaniment—a repeating sequence of a four-chord harmonic progression—banal in its predictability, wherein lies its therapeutic value in this instance. It becomes a refrain, to which we return when the musical development of emotional expression is more than Lena can bear:

> We can sing a happy song. Cheer us up, cheer us up;
> We can sing a happy song to cheer us up today.

Lena plays a countermelody on the metallophone, stopping intuitively at each cadence. I repeat the first phrase of the song. Lena joins in, singing and beating a conga drum and a cymbal so chaotically that her singing is almost inaudible. I then offer a contrasting idea (verbally and musically, shifting to a minor key, including dissonances and added 7ths, 9ths, and slightly slowing the tempo). I make these minimal changes to steady her beating and to begin to get in touch with her sadness. I sing, "We can sing if we're sad . . ." (ending on an open cadence in the hope that she will take over with the next line). I deliberately use "we" as a way of indicating that there is someone to share the "not happy" feelings and to avoid referring too directly to her (which might trigger her defense against sadness). The melody, previously characterized by ascending intervals, now is inverted as a descending phrase, in a minor key and in a slightly slower tempo. Lena does not respond, so I sing another phrase: "We . . . can . . . sing, if we're sa-a-ad. . . ." This time Lena echoes: "We . . . can . . . sing, if we're sa-a-ad. . . ."

Lena's singing now enters fully into the music's sadder mood, adding her own inflection of the melody. I continue singing and accompanying, to sustain this mood: "Sometimes we're sad. . . ." Lena interjects quickly: " . . . or happy . . . ," continuing: "Sometimes we're full of sorrow; sometimes we laugh with joy, full of joy. The sky's nice and bright; there's happiness in the air." My music reflects this idea with rippling impressionistic sequences in the upper registers of the piano. I hear a gentle sadness in my music (still in a minor key) with slightly increased harmonic tension and dissonance, thereby holding the two contrasting moods that Lena has expressed. The sadness is too much for her to bear getting in touch with. She sings rather wanly: "We can be so happy . . ." She then stops singing and chatters at such speed that I can barely grasp any of it, except to understand that she wishes to "get back to the bit about being happy."

Her verbal, cognitive defense against any feelings that might overwhelm her is evident; her desperation about being happy rather than sharing her real feelings is particularly poignant. I concur with a "happy" phrase, hoping to reengage Lena's singing and feelings rather than her verbal defenses against her emotions. I sing: "Happy, happy day," but in a minor key, continuing to the minor-key "bridge" section of the song. Here I reintroduce the mood and feeling states that Lena has seemed to deflect and split off (by way of dissociating), and which I am now feeling strongly in my countertransference, as I sing: "Sometimes . . . we feel sad. . . ." This time Lena takes over the song again, expressing her feelings more authentically, with the image of a lonely, upset child:

> Sometimes we feel good;
> Sometimes we feel like we're small and the world's against us;
> Some days we feel joy, full of joy, and happiness in the air
> And lovely smiley faces . . .
> Children playing outside, happy and joy;
> Someone sitting on their own, being upset . . .

Lena beats the cymbal and drum *sforzando*. She stops just as suddenly as she has begun and returns to her singing, reverting to the idea of happiness. She continues singing with a touching lyricism, while I accompany her, marking the pulse and harmonically coloring some of the emotive phrases:

> Sometimes we're happy, sometimes we're sad,
> Sometimes we're glad, sometimes we're ungra . . . a . . . a . . . ateful,
> Sometimes we laugh, sometimes we sad
> Sometimes we laugh, sometimes we . . . cough (*she coughs*),
> Sometimes we laugh, sometimes we . . . grump,
> Sometimes we sulk, sometimes we're sad, sometimes we're full of sorrow . . .
>   again.

Holding on to the main issues of the narrative that pour from Lena in her songs and reflecting on them are central to this stage of therapy.

Session 37: A New Level of Integration

Lena's use of songs disappears almost entirely during a period when she presents highly disturbed behavior interspersed with dissociative states—remote, then chaotic and angry in turn. However, in Session 37 a new level of integration appears as she improvises a song about "The Haunted House." Many children imagine haunted houses, but this is a song poem that seems to be not just about any ghosts, but the ghosts in her life, in the home she grew up in. It contains powerful poetic images of resolution and integration, where good overcomes evil. All of this is communicated in metaphor, bringing experiences from the procedural realm to a half-consciousness—where I feel at this stage they should remain. Here is the hymn-like coda with its message of transformation in her song-poem, which Lena improvises while indicating to me (at the piano) what mood of accompaniment she wants, and encouraging me to repeat any motive or musical feature she finds *right* for her song as it evolves in the moment:

> As the world turns by, the house gets rottener and rottener;
> It gets uglier and creepier and ghostlier every day.
> And the people that spotted it have no desire
> And the people have noticed since it's been there.
> In a few years' time it's going to be knocked down
> Forever and ever and evermore.
> So one day a big bad windy storm—pshoo!—blows the house to bits . . .
> And the right notes (*Lena gestures to me to change the music*) make the next
>   day quiet . . .
> Nothing is left—just a chimney and half a door;
> The birds perch on what is left in there; the house is gone; no people in it.
> In a few years' time, the buildings there are shops and flats and houses,
> Forevermore . . . forevermore . . .

She then instructs me: "Ends! . . . End it!"

After a brief diversion, Lena continues singing, engaging easily with the new upbeat 5/4 meter or "groove" of my accompaniment:

> The house is forever gone; house is gone forevermore.
> Danger is nowhere in the world; bogey Martians have all gone.
> We have the joy of the sun; no badness on the earth.
> There is a goodbye today . . .
> There's a sun and come and wipe away evil.
> Evil has gone . . . when the house has been blown . . .
> The wind has gone . . .
> The evil has gone away from the derelict house. That's it, and it's gone.
> IT HAS GONE! (*Here Lena sings in an operatic style with great intensity.*)

Created in the moment with intensity of feeling coming from her soul, Lena's song-poems carried in metaphor aspects of autobiographical narrative, her past, the secrets in the family that haunted her and that were shaping her life. They represented the banishing of overwhelming evil, the transformation of shadowy ugliness with which she felt identified. Her music therapy drew to an end after 14 months when she moved to a residential school, before returning to live at home with family support from social services. Many years later I heard that she had married and had a child.

Laura

Laura presented as a pale, thin 7-year-old. Her clothes were old and dirty and hung on her bony body like rags. Intelligent but emotionally withdrawn, she presented as a "closed-down" and "frozen" child, with numbed feelings—unable to talk, much less smile. Laura seemed unreachable, just standing limply, then compliantly engaging in what she thought I expected of her. From babyhood and through the first 5 years of her life, Laura was repeatedly placed in foster care. During periods when her parents were living together (there were frequent separations), they were frequently unconscious from drug abuse; when conscious, they were arguing and attacking each other. By the time Laura was 6, she was used to looking after her parents and trying to survive in a highly stressful, unsafe home. She found safety in a cupboard beneath the stairs, or in her bedroom where she developed obsessive organizing and tidying types of play. At 7 years of age, she was taken permanently into foster care. Her new school then referred her to music therapy. For several years, I saw her twice weekly during school term time. The music therapy room was a space that Laura solemnly arranged to her liking. I noticed that she did not chatter to herself while she played; she was completely silent.

Initially, Laura engaged in some familiar, clearly patterned, improvised black-note piano duets. She seemed to be developing a sense of safety and trust in the clear phrasing and patterns of the music, and in the ways in which I accompanied her melodies. I noticed her body sometimes moving to the pulse of the music, enjoying its predictability and equally the very slight variations of the melodic and rhythmic patterns as she began to respond spontaneously. At the time I remembered Frances Tustin's account of "the rhythm of safety" in the infant–mother relationship as well as the therapeutic relationship, where new rhythmic experiences of self and other are created through the adapting of one to another in a shared, reciprocal experience (Tustin, 1986, pp. 268–275). However, I soon found that the piano duets became increasingly perfunctory, and that music making itself was being used by Laura as a defense against feeling—a means of blocking out unbearable feelings. I soon learned that it was her habit to switch off her spontaneous feelings to their safely numb state whenever they arose as she became engaged in her play.

In later sessions, it was encouraging to see this entrenched state shifting. Laura's play became fragmentary and disorganized, but more authentic; in many ways, it represented the patterns of her early experiences of frequent abandonment and uprooting from one foster home to another. I felt it was important to wait, attend, listen, and accept however she wished to use her sessions. Equally, it felt important to enliven and *lift* the mood of the sessions in some way by injecting some energy into the room. I am reminded of Alvarez's (1992) thoughts on the therapist's sometimes needing to alert and enliven the child. My offering her a sudden idea (with an intake of breath, raised eyebrows, and a sense of excitement) engaged her briefly, but was then rejected.

Rejecting me and music and controlling her world were central themes in Laura's therapy—just as, undoubtedly, she had been rejected and neglected as a child. Yet Laura came every week and, later, twice weekly. Laura found ever-inventive ways of disappearing and hiding during the sessions, much as she had evaded the violence between her parents. It also showed me how she erected barriers to provide physical safety. Inside her room at home, she had rearranged its contents almost daily, creating her own world over which she had control. She began to treat the therapy room in much the same way, except that she now used a large instrument cupboard in which to create her own private space, where she busily drew and labeled everything. (I had to preserve these labels from week to week—and in doing this I felt I was helping with the continuity of her play, which she had previously seemed incapable of maintaining.)

One day, from inside the cupboard, Laura began to tap. From the other side, I tapped back. An exchange of rhythmic patterns developed. This recurred in the following sessions; at last, there was some continuity of play that felt meaningful and spontaneous, coming from her own motivations. I wondered if my whistling instead of tapping in response might lead to Laura to use her voice expressively (she spoke barely audibly in the sessions). To my surprise, an exchange of whistled phrases ensued with dramatic melodic swoops up and down, in patterns and varying phrase lengths, questioning and answering each other. In her whistling, there were the first signs of spontaneous play and emotional expression, which were never heard in her speaking voice or instrumental play.

In this way, I encountered for the first time her sense of humor and playfulness. However, these musical exchanges lasted only briefly, returning to quiet tapping games and a guessing game she invented: I had to guess where her hand was on the other side of the wooden cupboard door. This felt like a very controlled game of hide-and-seek, where she definitely had the advantage. But it was also a game in which the purpose or goal was for me to *find/locate* the very spot where her hand was on the other side of the door. It grew to be a reciprocal game in which some real communication took place. Toward the end of one session, I heard her quietly singing a song to her parents: "I miss you, I'm sorry." From these tentative, simple musical exchanges, our therapeutic relationship grew in a more real way—working through the many painful experiences that had numbed her feelings, and bringing new experiences that opened the door to new possibilities in her life. This was a five-year-long therapeutic process.

Conclusion

This chapter presents an overview of music therapy with children with unresolved attachment trauma or developmental trauma disorder. I have described the nature of music and communicative musicality, and have linked these to early relational phenomena from developmental psychology and psychotherapy. Music therapy can provide a "listening landscape," as well as a "sounding of the self." Being musically and clinically resourceful, receptive, and open to the new, and serving as an actively responsive participant, are vital qualities in the music therapist. Working with children, especially those with developmental trauma disorder, I have learned much about the essence of what it is to be human, to be heard, to sound, to find one's voice, and to forge new experiences of self and well-being within and beyond the musical-therapeutic relationship.

ACKNOWLEDGMENTS

I would like to thank Dr. Barbara Wheeler for her helpful advice on this chapter. I would also like to thank Barcelona Publishers for their kind permission to include here in a revised form some excerpts from my chapter in *Psychodynamic Music Therapy: Case Studies* (Robarts, 2003).

REFERENCES

Alvarez, A. (1992). *Live company: Psychoanalytic psychotherapy with autistic, borderline, deprived and abused children.* New York: Routledge.

Alvarez, A. (2010). *The thinking heart: Three levels of psychoanalytic therapy with disturbed children.* New York: Routledge.

Amir, D. (2004). Giving trauma a voice: The role of improvisational music therapy in exposing, dealing with and healing a traumatic experience of sexual abuse. *Music Therapy Perspectives, 22*(2), 96–103.

Austin, D. (2008). *The theory and practice of vocal psychotherapy: Songs of the self.* London: Kingsley.

Bion, W. R. (1962a). A theory of thinking. *International Journal of Psycho-Analysis, 43*, 306–310.

Bion, W. R. (1962b). *Learning from experience.* London: Heinemann.

Bruscia, K. E. (1998). *The dynamics of music psychotherapy.* Gilsum, NH: Barcelona.

DeCasper, A. J., & Carstens, A. A. (1981). Contingencies of stimulation: Effects on learning and emotion in neonates. *Infant Behavior and Development, 4,* 19–35.

Frank-Schwebel, A. (2002). Developmental trauma and its relation to sound and music. In J. P. Sutton (Ed.), *Music, music therapy and trauma: International perspectives* (pp. 193–207). London: Kingsley.

Hadley, S. (Ed.). (2003). *Psychodynamic music therapy: Case studies.* Gilsum, NH: Barcelona.

Malloch, S. N., & Trevarthen, C. (Eds.). (2009). *Communicative musicality: Exploring the basis of human companionship.* Oxford: Oxford University Press.

Montello, L. (2003). Protect this child: Psychodynamic music therapy with a gifted musician. In S. Hadley (Ed.), *Psychodynamic music therapy: Case studies* (pp. 299–318). Gilsum, NH: Barcelona.

Robarts, J. Z. (1994). Towards autonomy and a sound sense of self. In D. Dokter (Ed.), *Arts therapies and clients with eating disorders* (pp. 229–246). London: Kingsley.

Robarts, J. Z. (1998). Music therapy and children with autism. In C. Trevarthen, K. Aitken, D. Papoudi, & J. Z. Robarts (Eds.), *Children with autism: Diagnoses and interventions to meet their needs* (pp. 172–202). London: Kingsley.

Robarts, J. Z. (2000). Music therapy and adolescents with anorexia nervosa. *Nordic Journal of Music Therapy, 9*(1), 3–12.

Robarts, J. Z. (2003). The healing function of improvised songs in music therapy with a child survivor of early trauma and sexual abuse. In S. Hadley (Ed.), *Psychodynamic music therapy: Case studies* (pp. 141–182). Gilsum, NH: Barcelona.

Robarts, J. Z. (2006). Music therapy with sexually abused children. *Clinical Child Psychology and Psychiatry, 11*(2), 249–269.

Robarts, J. Z. (2009). Supporting the development of mindfulness and meaning: Clinical pathways in music therapy with a sexually abused child. In S. N. Malloch & C. Trevarthen (Eds.), *Communicative musicality: Exploring the basis of human companionship* (pp. 377–400). Oxford: Oxford University Press.

Scheiby, B. B. (2010). Analytical music therapy and integrative medicine: The impact of medical trauma on the psyche. In K. Stewart (Ed.), *Music therapy and trauma: Bridging theory and clinical practice* (pp. 74–87). New York: Satchnote.

Schönfeld, V. (2003). "Promise to take good care of it!": Therapy with Ira. In S. Hadley (Ed.), *Psychodynamic music therapy: Case studies* (pp. 207–224). Gilsum, NH: Barcelona.

Schore, A. N. (2001). The effects of early relational trauma on right brain development, affect regulation, and infant mental health. *Infant Mental Health Journal, 22,* 201–269.

Schore, A. N. (2003). Early relational trauma, disorganized attachment, and the development of a predisposition to violence. In M. F. Solomon & D. J. Siegel (Eds.), *Healing trauma: Attachment, mind, body, and brain* (pp. 107–167). New York: Norton.

Siegel, D. J. (2003). An interpersonal neurobiology of psychotherapy: The development mind and the resolution of trauma. In M. F. Solomon & D. J. Siegel (Eds.), *Healing trauma: Attachment, mind, body, and brain* (pp. 1–56). New York: Norton.

Siegel, D. J. (2012). *The developing mind: How relationships and the brain interact to shape who we are* (2nd ed.). New York: Guilford Press.

Stern, D. N. (1985). *The interpersonal world of the infant: A view from psychoanalysis and developmental psychology.* New York: Basic Books.

Stern, D. N. (2004). *The present moment in psychotherapy and everyday life.* New York: Norton.

Stern, D. N. (2010). *Forms of vitality: Exploring dynamic experience in psychology, the arts, psychotherapy, and development.* Oxford: Oxford University Press.

Sutton, J. P. (Ed.). (2002). *Music, music therapy and trauma: International perspectives.* London: Kingsley.

Trevarthen, C. (1993). The self born in intersubjectivity: The psychology of an infant communicating. In U. Neisser (Ed.), *The perceived self: Ecological and interpersonal sources of self-knowledge* (pp. 121–173). New York: Cambridge University Press.

Trevarthen, C. (1999). Musicality and the intrinsic motive pulse: Evidence from human psychobiology and infant communication. *Musicae Scientiae* (Special Issue 1999–2000), 155–215.

Trevarthen, C., Aitken, K. A., Vandekerckhove, M., Delafield-Butt, J., & Nagy, E. (2006). Collaborative regulations of vitality in early childhood: Stress in intimate relationship and postnatal psychopathology. In D. Cicchetti & D. J. Cohen (Eds.), *Developmental psychopathology: Vol. 2. Developmental neuroscience* (2nd ed., pp. 65–127). Hoboken, NJ: Wiley.

Trevarthen, C., & Malloch, S. N. (2000). The dance of wellbeing: Defining the musical therapeutic effect. *Nordic Journal of Music Therapy, 9*(2), 3–17.

Tustin, F. (1986). *Autistic barriers in neurotic patients.* London: Karnac.

van der Kolk, B. A. (2003). Posttraumatic stress disorder and the nature of trauma. In M. F. Solomon & D. J. Siegel (Eds.), *Healing trauma: Attachment, mind, body, and brain* (pp. 168–196). New York: Norton.

van der Kolk, B. A. (2005). Developmental trauma disorder: Towards a rational diagnosis for children with complex trauma histories. *Psychiatric Annals, 35*(5), 401–408.

Wigram, T., & De Backer, J. (Eds.). (1999). *Clinical applications of music therapy in psychiatry.* London: Kingsley.

CHAPTER 6

Moving with the Space between Us

The Dance of Attachment Security

Christina Devereaux

Significant research findings have underscored nonverbal parent–child interaction as an important collaborative exchange that supports healthy development and enhances positive social relationships (Ainsworth & Bell, 1970; Beebe & Lachmann, 1998; Bowlby, 1969, 1988; Schore, 2001; Siegel, 2012; Tronick, 2003, 2007; Tronick & Beeghly, 2011). *Attuned* interactions between parent and child are nonverbal communications that assist individuals in building empathy/understanding and developing healthy attachment relationships. This attunement involves all of the physical senses and also depends on the awareness of sound, tone of voice, and nonverbal rhythms of communication. However, when there is consistent disengagement or disruption in this dance of interaction, both parent and child can be affected, influencing the security of the attachment relationship.

Attachment theory, an approach emphasizing parent–child interaction (Ainsworth, Blehar, Waters, & Wall, 1978; Bowlby, 1969, 1988), has been incorporated into a variety of theories providing many implications for clinical application and developmental research. Its core construct is a biologically based predisposition for physical proximity and connection between mother (or other primary caregiver) and child (Bowlby, 1988); the security of this attachment predicts later functioning. These theoretical constructs are widely applicable in assessment and intervention for individuals, groups, and families, especially within nonverbal psychotherapeutic disciplines such as dance/movement therapy (DMT).

This chapter first discusses how attachment, viewed as a metaphorical dance, can be enhanced through nonverbal attunement and body-based intervention. A more in-depth look into the discipline of DMT through the theoretical lens of attachment theory follows. Examples from DMT interventions with individuals with attachment needs support this discussion.

Theoretical Foundations: Attachment Theory and the Body

Bowlby (1969) emphasized the importance of a behavioral system that equips a child with body-based signal behaviors (i.e., smiling, crying) designed to keep the primary caregiver in reach. These signal behaviors are complemented by an exploratory system that allows the child to crawl away from the primary caregiver and explore the world, once a "secure base" (Bowlby, 1988) is established. In times of distress (e.g., separation from the primary caregiver or other stress), a child tries to resort to comfort by moving into closer proximity to the caregiver, resulting in the deactivation of the exploratory behavior. This emphasis on both the biological drive for proximity seeking when distressed, and the drive to explore out into the world when internalized security is established, highlights the importance of attending to nonverbal, body-based, interactive cues when one is examining attachment relationships.

Attachment research has proposed that a primary caregiver and infant have a goal to achieve a state of reciprocity, consisting of connectedness, intimacy, oneness, synchrony, and mutual delight, and that "to attain it they jointly regulate the interaction with interactive behaviors" (Tronick, 2007, p. 178). This is demonstrated in research (Brazelton, 1982; Tronick, 1980, 2007; Tronick & Beeghly, 2011) highlighting how infants, when faced with interactive ruptures, activate a number of predictable strategies designed to repair the mismatch or to cope with the failure via self-soothing or withdrawal. For example, Tronick's "still-face" research and subsequent studies (Tronick, 1980, 2003, 2007) obtained significant findings suggesting that when a caregiver disengages from the interactive cycle with an infant, the infant responds by attempting to reengage the connection through various strategies. Tronick and Beeghly (2011) discuss how an infant's capacity to make meaning out of the interaction with a primary caregiver occurs primarily through nonverbal cues, such as affect and movements. This strongly indicates that attachment security develops as a result of body-based nonverbal communication. They also suggest that the dyadic attachment relationship is a mutually regulating system of communication.

Tronick's research is highly significant to DMT, as it stresses the value and importance of the infant–caregiver relationship for the infant's socioemotional behavior, and shows how disruptions in the interactive exchange activate the attachment behavioral system. Schore and Schore (2008) have discussed how these attachment relationships are formed through nonverbal, body-based attunement (i.e., eye gaze, vocal tone, and facial expressions). Therefore, therapists can rely on nonverbal communication to form attachment relationships within the therapeutic alliance, since such communication acts as a mechanism to support interactive regulation with clients. These constructs are some of the core principles of the discipline of DMT.

Assumptions and Principles of DMT

Dance/movement therapists view movement of the body as both expressive and communicative, and utilize it both as a method of assessing individuals and as the mode for clinical intervention. DMT is based upon the belief that there is a fundamental interconnection between the mind and body; it is assumed that whatever is having an impact on the body will have a reciprocal impact on the mind. Therefore, a core principle of DMT is that healthy overall functioning relies upon the integration of mind and body (Levy, 2005). When there is a lack of mind–body integration, individuals may suffer from a variety of psychological disorders. Similarly, there is a foundational belief that examining one's movement vocabulary or range "opens a door to the study of patterns of early development, coping strategies, and personality configurations" (Kestenberg Amighi, Loman, Lewis, & Sossin, 1999, p. 2). An increased integration of a person's body parts and. awareness of others expands the individual's movement vocabulary, thus increasing his or her ability to communicate needs and desires.

DMT focuses directly on movement behavior as it emerges out of the developed therapeutic relationship. A DMT pioneer, Marian Chace, emphasized that "the therapeutic relationship is core to the meaning of movement structures that evolve between the dance therapist and those with whom he/she works and it is the interactive process that enables change" (Fischer & Chaiklin, 1993, p. 138). Furthermore, because "movement is a universal means of communication" (Erfer, 1995, p. 196), it is an especially useful therapeutic approach that can both provide a direct link to feelings and build a connection or relationship with others. Finally, because people's early attachment influences affect their later development of healthy relationships (Ginot, 2012; Schore, 2003; Schore & Schore, 2008; Siegel, 2012; Stern, 1985; van der Kolk, 2006), movement can serve as the common language for building communication and establishing secure attachment relationships.

DMT and Attachment Theory

Behrends, Müller, and Dziobek (2012) have discussed the evolving connections between different disciplines such as neuroscience and DMT. They suggest that it is "cructial to integrate the bodily dimension of perceptive and expressive processes as part of social interactions in diagnostic procedures and treatment plans for patients with problems with . . . social relationships" (p. 114), such as those with attachment difficulties. van der Kolk (2006) also emphasizes that effective treatment of developmental trauma must involve the traumatized individual's "learning to tolerate feelings and sensations . . . [and] learning to modulate arousal" (p. 277). Subramaniam's (2010) qualitative study examined how attachment theory and work within the attachment and relational framework informs the work of dance/movement therapists. The results of her interviews with attachment-oriented dance/movement therapists "demonstrated linking what the field of attachment-oriented psychotherapy has been calling for—an integration of more body-based and nonverbal interventions" (p. ii). Her results also suggested that approaches in DMT can "provide significant benefit for clients with disrupted attachment experiences . . . [by] working with the preverbal experiences of the self, which are in turn influenced by our early attachment relationships" (p. ii).

Other literature has highlighted the use of DMT to support, develop, enhance, or "rechoreograph" areas important to attachment relationships, such as emotional regulation (Betty, 2013; Hervey & Kornblum, 2006; Kornblum, 2002, 2008; Koshland & Wittaker, 2004), socioemotional development (Thom, 2010), body awareness (Moore, 2006), the bonding between infants and caregivers (Loman, 1998; Tortora, 2006), and attachment relationships within the family structure (Devereaux, 2008). However, a firmer scientific foundation and further research are needed to support and strengthen this evidence-base.

DMT does have a unique set of processes for promoting the emergence of bodily experience within the therapeutic movement relationship. The development of kinesthetically attuned interactions will support a client in establishing emotional regulation and a healthy attachment relationship. It is particularly important that clinical interventions include a "rechoreography" of new embodied patterns, so that "repair work" of insecure attachment relationships can occur through the body and become integrated on a bodily level.

The following sections address some concepts used in clinical intervention to support this focus, such as mirroring, attunement, mutual regulation, spatial exploration, and the use of connective tools. A case vignette follows this discussion.

Mirroring, Attunement, and Empathy

The DMT relationship begins with the process of *attunement* or "matching" (Tortora, 2006, p. 259), in which the dance/movement therapist experiences the qualitative aspects of a client's movement through reflecting back and conveying understanding of the client's communicative gestures.

In DMT, this is accomplished through relational dances and movement interactions such as trying on various body shapes, exaggerating or exploring various movement dynamics, and engaging in heightened moments of rhythmic synchrony. Indeed, the interactive movement relationship is essential in the dance/movement therapy treatment process (Berrol, 2006).

Through the use of the traditional DMT technique called *mirroring* or *empathic reflection* (Chaiklin & Schmais, 1993), the therapist reflects an individual's body rhythms, movement patterns, and/or vocalizations to begin the process of relationship formation. The goal is to attune to the client where he or she is, both physically and emotionally, and to establish a trusting therapeutic movement relationship that builds an awareness of the self and other. Because most of these attuned interactions occur on a nonverbal level, DMT can be an ideal treatment intervention in supporting the development of a safe therapeutic relationship emphasizing consistency, trust, and empathy—an experience that clients who exhibit severe attachment needs may not have had (Bowlby, 1988, Devereaux, 2008; Schore, 2003; Siegel, 2012). Because of these clients' challenges, establishing a therapeutic relationship can be extremely difficult. According to Chaiklin and Schmais (1993),

> There is a fine line between empathy on a movement level and mimicry. Mimicry involves duplicating the external shape of the movement without the emotional content that exists in the dynamics and in the subtle organization of the movement. . . . Empathy meant sharing the essence of all nonverbal expression resulting in . . . direct communication. (p. 86)

Therapeutic interactions that include imitation or reflection of a client's movements or actions and attunement to the individual's emotional state send the nonverbal message "I hear you, I understand you, and it's OK." Trust is established through nonverbal recognition and response to the client. Therefore, DMT can support healthier attachment relationships through the therapist's and client's participating in shared movement experiences and engaging in shared focus. These joint experiences can assist a client in feeling seen and joined with, and in reexperiencing attuned nonverbal interactions—all of which are imperative to establish a secure attachment.

The process of moving with someone through the art of dance empathically connects the therapist with the attachment-disordered individual, so that the experience of attunement can begin (Berrol, 2006; Fischman, 2009; Devereaux, 2012). "Knowing [the child's] rhythm, affect, and experience by metaphorically being in its skin . . . goes beyond empathy to create a two-person experience of connectedness by providing a reciprocal affect and/or resonating response" (Erskine, 1998, p. 236). In DMT, attunement is communicated not just by what is said, but also by facial or body movements; these signal to the child that his or her affect and needs are perceived, are significant, and make an impact on another (Devereaux, 2008, 2012). Schore (2003) asserts that to enter into this communication, one must be psychobiologically attuned not so much to the child's overt behavior as to the reflections of the rhythms of the child's internal state. These affective attunements, which are both spontaneous and nonverbal, are "the moment-to-moment expressions of [one's] regulatory functions occur[ing] at levels beneath awareness" (Schore, 2001, p. 14).

In DMT, once an initial attuned relationship is established, the therapist then serves as "a catalyst, gradually assisting in the expansion and elaboration of the patient's movements until they reach full expressivity— yet always watching the patient's emotional and kinesthetic reactions to this change and adjusting their empathic movements accordingly" (Merna, 2010, p. 111).

Mutual Influences in the Attachment Relationship

Another purpose of attachment lies in the experience of psychological containment of difficult and threatening affective states. Such containment is required for the development of a coherent self (Siegel, 2012). Fuertes, Lopes-dos-Santos, Beeghly, and Tronick (2009) emphasize that coping with strong affect (affect regulation) and caregiver behavior both seem to influence the formation of the attachment relationship, suggesting that attachment interactions have the capacity to be mutually regulating. These mutual influences, called *interactive/mutual regulation*, occur during times of shared affective moments where caregiver and child can become attuned in a synchronistic nonverbal exchange (Stern, 1985). According to Beebe and Lachmann (1998), during these shared experiences "contingencies flow in both directions between partners. That is, the behavior of each partner is contingent upon (influenced by) that of the other" (p. 485). Studies in infant mental health clarify the importance of mutuality and interactive movement relationship between the dance/movement therapist and the individual with an attachment disorder. Fischer and Chaiklin (1993) state:

> The dance therapist in the role of participant observer must have a clear realization and responsibility for his or her own dance in relation to the other individual. Just as the tension of any existing anxiety present in the mother induces anxiety within the infant, such tension in the therapist will affect the interaction. The meeting in movement of the therapist and the client assumes that both are part of the dialogue, even though one is identified as helper and the other as needing help. (p. 139)

As previously discussed, attunement and mirroring are of prime importance in order to establish a safe therapeutic relationship for clients in DMT, especially for clients who exhibit severe attachment needs and have not had feelings of security in past relationships (Baudino, 2010; Betty,

2013; Devereaux, 2008; Tortora, 2006). The therapist must also attend to his or her own embodied responses (i.e. countertransference) to serve as guideposts in the development of empathy (Subramaniam, 2010).

Spatial Exploration as Metaphor

Kossak (2009) has emphasized that attunement is a dynamic relationship where "the [client] begins to learn about relational space and safety" (p. 14). Spatial exploration as a metaphor for this safety of the relational space is an essential tool for therapists to utilize in DMT interventions. Dance/movement therapists give important attention to the full range of spatial exploration—such as moving on different levels (moving from the floor to standing) and maintaining physical distance between self and other—that occurs when they are moving with clients. This active exploration of the physical holding environment also allows a client to physically experience moving out and away into the movement space (widening the distance between therapist and client) or moving toward another (narrowing the distance between therapist and client). Interventions that emphasize the actual physical distance between self and other parallel the healthy development of the exploratory system (Bowlby, 1988). Other body-level interventions also provide opportunities for a client to reexperience a healthy sequence of movement development (Kestenberg Amighi, Loman, Lewis, & Sossin, 1999). For example, moving in the *horizontal* plane surrounding one's body involves spreading to open and reveal the body and reach to the furthest rim of ones's *kinesphere*, or personal space. This way of moving can be an expansive opening movement, while the opposite way of moving in the horizontal plane is generally enclosing or gathering oneself together, as if closing oneself off from the outside world. Ascending to the upright stance of the *vertical* plane provides a client with possibilities of rising and falling. Movement along this vertical plane is one of display: "Here I am!" Movements that explore advancing forward or moving backward through space, on what is referred to as the *sagittal* plane, directly highlight the exploratory system that Bowlby (1988) discusses. Therefore, when the therapist assists the client in using explorations that support the physical awareness of the kinesphere, or the awareness and expansion of multidimensional uses of the client's own body space, this can "facilitate the formation of complex relationships" (Kestenberg Amighi et al., 1999, p. 175).

When a client begins to internalize a secure base within the therapeutic alliance, the client has a safe opportunity to reexperience moving away out into space in the sagittal plane from the attachment figure, and then coming back in closer proximity in a new spatial configuration. The therapist can continue to attune to these relational dynamics by narrating the movement patterns as they are literally occurring. For example, "I noticed that when I came closer, you moved your body away. I wonder, how far do I need to go for you to feel comfortable? I am all the way in the corner, and

I'm still too close." Or, conversely, "You seem to be almost on top of me, and it's still not feeling close enough for you." When the therapist reflects back to the client the active, in-the-present-moment processes occurring within the attachment relationship, together the client and the therapist (through the movement metaphor) can make sense of and rechoreograph the attachment dynamics.

Bridging the Space with Connection Tools

Dance/movement therapists also emphasize the exploration of the physical space via the use of props (e.g., stretch fabrics, scarves, balls, and music) during sessions. These props serve as connective and communicative tools. They can provide a less threatening way to make various connections: from a client to others in a group, from one client to another, from therapist to client, from client to therapist, or from client to imagination and exploration. In particular, these connection tools can assist in providing a bridge of contact between therapist and client, and can also serve as a means "to express feelings and thoughts, which [create] an outlet for imagination and exploration" (Baudino, 2010, p. 126). For example, if the therapist initiates connection and joining to a client through the use of a scarf or a flexible piece of stretch fabric, the prop can create connection and provide a visual representation for the attachment relationship. The client can experience pulling against the therapist, joining in a less threatening way, or feeling the self as separate by carving out his or her own kinesphere or personal space bubble. The use of connective tools provides opportunities to play with the flexibility of distance, to experience resistance to or desire for closeness, and to dance and move the attachment relationship through an active and metaphorical process (Devereaux, 2012).

The use of music as an auditory external holding environment can support the sense of connection through rhythm to support and attune the individual to the energetic tone of the session. As therapist and client dance together to same rhythm with music, there is an embodied sense of connection. In addition, Erfer (1995) notes that "rhythm is a meaningful organizer of impulses" (p. 201).

In summary, a client who has experienced insecurity in the space around him or her may benefit through actual movement explorations that involve establishing a physical therapeutic container, defining a personal kinesphere, and bridging the relational or intermediate area of space between client and therapist. Such interventions can support the establishment of a relationship in a less intimate way than the use of touch, direct movement matching, or even verbalization can do.

In the following section, I describe a case in which the concepts described above are integrated with a clinical example. Specifically, I discuss how the DMT process came to assist an individual child client with rechoreographing his attachment insecurity and internalizing the capacity to regulate strong affect, healthy coping strategies, and experience an attuned secure base via the therapeutic alliance.

Case Vignette: Joey

Joey, an 8-year-old child, worked with me in once-a-week 50-minute DMT sessions in an outpatient clinic. His mother referred Joey to treatment after becoming severely concerned about his acting-out behavior at school (refusing to complete homework, angry outbursts, aggression with other peers, increasing fear of trying new things, and disrupting class) and his escalating behavior at home (verbal and physical aggression toward his older sibling and his mother).

Joey witnessed consistent verbal and physical abuse from his father toward his mother. His father was now inconsistently present in his life, and was involved in a new relationship where there was a baby on the way. Joey would come to DMT sessions and both verbally and nonverbally express his own underlying feelings of low self-worth. He appeared to be ambivalent about his relationship with his father, and this ambivalence seemed to be carried over into his patterns of interactions with his mother, sibling, and peers. His mother reported that at times, he would become clingy, sleep with her in her bed, and refuse to leave the house. At other times, when he would get angry, it appeared as if nothing could soothe him. He also began to be less comfortable with taking risks and exploring new things at school. His exploratory system was often deactivated, as he was often under stress, and his capacity for self-regulation was limited. My approach with him in DMT sessions was first to establish a trusting therapeutic alliance through attuned reflective relational experiences, where his nervous system could become regulated and he could internalize healthier coping strategies for expressing his underlying feelings, especially during times of heightened affect. Through this approach, Joey could begin to rechoreograph his coping strategies when under stress by internalizing a sense of embodied security.

In the beginning of our work together, Joey would often project his own insecurities onto me, both verbally (e.g., "You never do anything right") and nonverbally (e.g., when I would attempt to mirror his movements, he would reject these connections by moving away or placing an object between us to create more spatial distance). At the same time, he appeared to crave connection with me as his therapist. His mother reported that he would become anxious if they might be late to a session, and would request phone sessions if his mother could not bring him to therapy. Through the use of a connection tool, he began to use his sessions to explore his ambivalent feelings more deeply. The active and metaphorical processes of DMT allowed a secure attachment relationship to form, develop, and serve as a reparative experience.

Fairly early in the treatment process, Joey became invested in engaging me in a ritual game through the use of a soft foam ball. Rather than using the ball to connect directly with me, he would actively throw the ball against the wall and explore various ways to make it difficult for me to catch it. This initial stage of relating allowed me to see metaphorically how strong his defenses were in direct attuned-movement relationships. Instead of trying to change this spatial position of relating, I joined with him, moving in parallel, and narrated out loud verbally the challenges that he set forth for me. I attuned to his movement dynamics by matching his intensity with sound. He would not tolerate any direct movement mirroring or matching, but he did allow me to reflect his movements through the tone of my voice. Slowly, he also began to experiment with moving at varied intensity levels, and would attend carefully to how I would adjust my sound so that he could match and attune to the change in intensity. If I didn't "do it right," he would tell me. He was clearly telling me through his movement presentations that he wanted a relationship with me, but that it needed to developed at his own pace and in his own way. Furthermore, it was important that I tell him both verbally and nonverbally, through my own interactions, that I could accept all intensities of him, regardless of his ambivalence. This was the start of our relational dance.

As our sessions continued, I assisted Joey in movement involving different spatial relationships with me (i.e., beside each other, back to back, and eventually facing each other directly). We also engaged in dance explorations through imagery, where we would move at varied intensity levels and work on the acceleration and deceleration of these intensities (i.e., moving in "slow motion"; having an "instant replay" and starting again; speeding up to "hyper speed"; and finding a "relaxed place, like being on a desert island and just chilling"). At times, Joey would take charge of the speed and intensity at which we would move, but slowly he allowed me to have some ideas, and invited cues to help his body adjust to a different intensity. At other times, we engaged in a sort of "freeze dance," where we took turns being in charge of creating the music to make one person move and the other person freeze into a creative shape. Joey took joy in experimenting with different ways to keep his body in control even in a still position. His increasing capacity to share the leadership with me indicated increasing trust that I would follow his pace, and that I could be with him in all his affective states. In addition, his movements, regardless of their intensity, were accepted and attuned to. He began to take more and more risks with his body, while taking pride that he could stay in control when required to on a given cue. He was beginning to feel less ambivalent in the therapeutic relationship.

On one particular day, during the middle phase of treatment, Joey came into session very angry, but was not verbalizing any feelings. His body appeared tense, and his posture was enclosed. He was emotionally shut down and unresponsive to my attempts to engage him in verbal dialogue, yet I had a strong sense that he was craving some connection with me. It was clear that he needed to discharge and release his feelings; therefore, I engaged him solely through the body. I invited him to be the leader in a dance and to move his body as it needed to move. My intention was to observe closely to see whether he wanted me either to move with him or to watch him. To my surprise, he quickly started his dance. His movements were strong and direct, with high intensity. His body was showing his emotional state, but his rejections of my joining with him were heightened. I attempted several ways to find a way in to attune to him (verbally, nonverbally, and through sound), but most of these attempts were rejected. He continued to intensify his dance, but became emotionally dysregulated and began to become physically destructive in the therapy room (throwing objects, tearing things from the walls). It appeared as if what he needed to do at that moment in our attachment relationship was to actively test the boundaries of our secure relationship. I reflected back to him the safety guidelines of the therapy room, but also that I could see that he was "needing to make a mess." He watched me intensely as this occurred as if to see whether I could accept and contain the strong affective experience that he was holding. In this moment, I felt that he needed me to see physically how "messy" he felt inside. As I inquired about this physical representation of his emotional feeling, I watched his body relax, as if he felt me understanding him in a new way. He was able to leave the "mess" in the therapy room for me to "hold." In the following weeks, this was somewhat of a ritual ending for each session where he would decide how to "leave a mess," but slowly we began to collaborate during the closure. He would watch me assist him in cleaning up parts of the "mess," and he would care for other parts. Week after week, he left the therapy room in less of a "mess." It appeared as if he started to internalize that all intensities of his feelings (all of his "messiness") could be accepted, and that there was a container to express it. Most importantly, the rechoreography of his patterns of expression (aggression and outbursts) was starting to become embodied, and he was starting to develop emotional regulation.

After several more months, Joey was able to put feeling words to his emotion dances and make some insightful connections about his family situation and his underlying feelings. He appeared to have internalized the therapeutic alliance as a secure relationship that could hold all parts of him.

During our final session, Joey was drawn to a small, smooth, grayish stone that was in a bowl in the dance/movement therapy room. He picked up the stone and began to tap it on a table, in a clear rhythm. In order to attune to him, I picked up another stone and joined with his rhythm, engaging with him in a little "stone dance." At one point during this synchronistic nonverbal exchange, Joey's stone broke open, revealing the stone's "insides." Ironically, the inside of this stone was crystal-like. In awe and amazement, Joey examined the insides with intrigue. It was a perfect symbolic reflection of his own therapeutic process that I chose to reflect directly to him, "Isn't it amazing that on the outside it appeared so gray, dull, and ugly, but now that we can see the inside it has revealed all of its beauty?"

Discussion

Over the course of therapy, as I used Joey's movements to attune with his body state, a co-created, improvised dance of relationship emerged through the nonverbal exchanges in the movement process. This dance assisted Joey in modulating his own impulses and empowered him to activate his own regulatory capacities. As I engaged Joey in an attuned-movement communicative dialogue, our formerly insecure relationship developed into a dance of listening and reflecting back, allowing Joey to take full mastery over his own movement impulses. I would constantly look at my own countertransference, and would attune to him and to myself simultaneously. I focused on being mindful of Joey's pace and readiness to make connections between his movement presentations that were occurring through our relationship and his own underlying struggles. I could not say, "You're so angry because your father is inconsistently in your life, and hence you are creating messes." He was not ready—he did not have the internal working models, so to speak—to be able to internalize this. Over time, however, through the consistency, trust, and nonverbal attunement we developed, he was able to take in more and more and allow an attachment relationship to feel nourishing. The expansion of his movement vocabulary through his experiments with movement modulation assisted him in being able to translate this into affect regulation. His outbursts decreased. He was able to be more verbal about his feeling states, rather than holding them in until he exploded. He used healthier outlets to channel his underlying feelings and used his body as a resource to discharge and release tension.

The quality of the therapeutic relationship with Joey focused first on the need for me as the therapist to provide a consistent and uninterrupted psychological containment for the affective experiences that he could not verbally express. After this secure base was established and internalized, it allowed Joey to express the intensity of the affective experiences that he was holding inside. These were reflected in his movement presentations. His readiness to allow for regulation and connection with me as a secure base became evident when he began to explore a different spatial relationship with me: He was now moving with, facing, and in collaboration with me. This also informed me that he was tolerating the stronger affect that was being stimulated by his family situation, and that he felt he had an adequate emotional container to discharge and process these feelings.

Conclusion

As discussed in this chapter, the embodied experiences of individuals are essential to examining attachment behavior. Specifically, because movement is communication, it can provide information about a client's emotional state. In the context of the DMT relationship between client and therapist, intervention takes place in a relational and moving context that opens opportunities for attunement and reparative attachment relationships to happen.

The therapeutic process requires careful pacing, adequate holding, and accurate mirrored reflection within a trusting therapeutic relationship in order to allow for repair of ruptured attachment relationships. Once consistent and secure attachment is reexperienced within the therapeutic alliance and internalized, it can become a blueprint for new behaviors. Therefore, the new internalized relational dance can serve as a rechoreography of past attachment relationships, and the client can be influenced by the newly developing relationship with the therapist.

Repeated experiences of attuned and empathically reflected movement through the therapeutic movement relationship during the DMT sessions can provide a reparative secure base to assist clients in developing healthier attachment relationships with others. According to Siegel (2012),

> When attuned communication is disrupted, as it inevitably is, repair of the rupture can be an important part of reestablishing the connection. Repair is healing as well as important in helping to teach the child that life is filled with inevitable moments of misunderstandings and missed connections that can be identified and connection created again. (p. 51)

Therapeutic approaches such as DMT that work directly with the body provide new avenues for assisting clients with attachment needs through simultaneous physical and metaphorical processes. Dance/movement therapists have a unique capacity to approach and rechoreograph these clients' interactive struggles into healthier attachment relationships.

REFERENCES

Ainsworth, M. D. S., & Bell, S. M. (1970). Attachment, exploration, and separation: Individual differences in strange-situation behavior of one-year-olds. *Child Development, 41,* 49–67.

Ainsworth, M. D. S., Blehar, M. C., Waters, E., & Wall, S. (1978). *Patterns of attachment.* Hillsdale, NJ: Erlbaum.

Baudino, L. (2010). Autism spectrum disorder: A case of misdiagnosis. *American Journal of Dance Therapy, 32,* 113–129.

Beebe, B., & Lachmann, F. M. (1998). Co-constructing inner and relational processes. Self and mutual regulation in infant research and adult treatment. *Psychoanalytic Psychology, 15*(4), 480–516.

Behrends, A., Müller, S., & Dziobek, I. (2012). Moving in and out of synchrony: A concept for a new intervention fostering empathy through interactional movement and dance. *The Arts in Psychotherapy, 39*(2), 107–116.

Berrol, C. F. (2006). Neuroscience meets dance/movement therapy: Mirror neurons, the therapeutic process and empathy. *The Arts in Psychotherapy, 33*(4), 302–315.

Betty, A. (2013). Taming tidal waves: A dance/movement therapy approach to supporting emotion regulation in maltreated children. *American Journal of Dance Therapy, 35*(1), 39–59.

Bowlby, J. (1969). *Attachment and loss: Vol. 1. Attachment.* New York: Basic Books.

Bowlby, J. (1988). *A secure base: Parent–child attachment and healthy human development.* New York: Basic Books.

Brazelton, T. B. (1982). Joint regulation of neonate–parent behavior. In E. Tronick (Ed.), *Social interchanges in infancy: Effect, cognition, and communication* (pp. 7–22). Baltimore, MD: University Park Press.

Chaiklin, S., & Schmais, C. (1993). The Chace approach to dance therapy. In S. Sandel, S. Chaiklin, & A. Lohn (Eds.), *Foundations of dance/movement therapy: The life and work of Marian Chace* (pp. 75–97). Columbia, MD: Marian Chace Memorial Fund of the American Dance Therapy Association.

Devereaux, C. (2008). Untying the knots: Dance/movement therapy with a family exposed to domestic violence. *American Journal of Dance Therapy, 30*(2), 58–70.

Devereaux, C. (2012). Moving into relationship: Dance/movement therapy with children with autism. In L. Gallo-Lopez & L. Rubin (Eds.), *Play-based interventions for children and adolescents with autism spectrum disorders* (pp. 333–351). New York: Routledge.

Erfer, T. (1995). Treating children with autism in a public school system. In F. Levy (Ed.), *Dance and other expressive arts therapies* (pp. 191–211). New York: Routledge.

Erskine, R. (1998). Attunement and involvement: Therapeutic responses to relational needs. *International Journal of Psychotherapy, 3*(3), 235–244.

Fischer, J., & Chaiklin, S. (1993). Meeting in movement: The work of therapist and client. In S. Sandel, S. Chaiklin, & A. Lohn (Eds.), *Foundations of dance/movement therapy: The life and work of Marian Chace* (pp. 136–153). Columbia, MD: Marian Chace Memorial Fund of the American Dance Therapy Association.

Fischman, D. (2009). Therapeutic relationships and kinesthetic empathy. In S. Chaiklin & H. Wengrower (Eds.), *The art and science of dance/movement therapy* (pp. 33–53). New York: Routledge.

Fuertes, M., Lopes-dos-Santos, P., Beeghly, M., & Tronick, E. (2009). Infant coping and maternal interactive behavior predict attachment in a Portuguese sample of healthy preterm infants. *European Psychologist, 14*(4), 320–331.

Ginot, E. (2012). Self-narratives and dysregulated affective states: The neuropsychological links between self-narratives, attachment, affect, and cognition. *Psychoanalytic Psychology, 29*(1), 59–80.

Hervey, L., & Kornblum, R. (2006). An evaluation of Kornblum's body-based violence prevention curriculum for children. *The Arts in Psychotherapy, 33*, 113–129.

Kestenberg Amighi, J., Loman, S., Lewis, P., & Sossin, K. (1999). *The meaning of movement*. New York: Brunner-Routledge.

Kornblum, R. (2002). *Disarming the playground: Violence prevention through movement and pro-social skills training manual and activity book*. Oklahoma City, OK: Wood'N'Barnes.

Kornblum, R. (2008). Dance/movement therapy with children. In D. McCarthy (Ed.), *Speaking about the unspeakable: Non-verbal methods and experiences in therapy with children* (pp. 100–114). Philadelphia: Kingsley.

Koshland, L., & Wittaker, J. W. B. (2004). PEACE through dance/movement: Evaluating a violence prevention program. *American Journal of Dance Therapy, 26*(2), 69–90.

Kossak, M. S. (2009). Therapeutic attunement: A transpersonal view of expressive arts therapy. *The Arts in Psychotherapy, 36*, 13–18.

Levy, F. (2005). *Dance movement therapy: A healing art*. Reston, VA: American Alliance for Health, Physical Education, Recreation, and Dance.

Loman, S. (1998). Employing a developmental model of movement patterns in dance/movement therapy with young children and their families. *American Journal of Dance Therapy, 20*(2), 101–115.

Merna, M. (2010). *Compiling the evidence for dance/movement therapy with children with autism spectrum disorders: A systematic literature review*. Unpublished master's thesis, Drexel University.

Moore, C. (2006). Dance/movement therapy in the light of trauma: Research findings of a multidisciplinary project. In S. C. Koch & I. Bräuninger (Eds.), *Advances in dance/movement therapy: Theoretical perspectives and empirical findings* (pp. 104–115). Berlin: Logos Verlag.

Schore, A. N. (2001). Effects of a secure attachment relationship on right brain development, affect regulation, and infant mental health. *Infant Mental Health Journal, 22*, 7–66.

Schore, A. N. (2003). *Affect regulation and the repair of the self*. New York: Norton.

Schore, J. R., & Schore, A. N. (2008). Modern attachment theory: The central role of affect regulation in development and treatment. *Clinical Social Work Journal, 36*, 9–20.

Siegel, D. (2012). *The developing mind: How relationships and the brain interact to shape who we are* (2nd ed.). New York: Guilford Press.

Stern, D. (1985). *The interpersonal world of the infant*. New York: Basic Books.

Subramaniam, A. (2010). *Moving towards a secure base: The role of attachment theory in clinical dance movement therapy*. Unpublished master's thesis, Lesley University.

Thom, L. (2010). From a simple line to expressive movement: The use of creative movement to enhance social emotional development in preschool curriculum. *American Journal of Dance Therapy, 32*(2), 100–112.

Tortora, S. (2006). *The dancing dialogue*. Baltimore, MD: Brookes.

Tronick, E. (1980). On the primacy of social skills. In D. B. Sawin, L. O. Walker, & J. H. Penticuff (Eds.), *The exceptional infant: Psychosocial risks in infant environmental transactions* (pp. 144–158). New York: Brunner/Mazel.

Tronick, E. (2003). Things still to be done on the still-face effect. *Infancy, 4*(4), 475–482.

Tronick, E. (2007). *The neurobehavioral and social-emotional development of infants and children.* New York: Norton.

Tronick, E., & Beeghly, M. (2011). Infants' meaning-making and the development of mental health problems. *American Psychologist, 66*(2), 107–119.

van der Kolk, B. (2006). Clinical implications of neuroscience and PTSD. *Annals of the New York Academy of Sciences, 1071*(1), 277–293.

CHAPTER 7

The Integration of Drama Therapy and Play Therapy in Attachment Work with Traumatized Children

Eliana Gil
Teresa Dias

This chapter focuses on the application of drama and play therapies to advance therapeutic goals involving attachment issues in traumatized children. In particular, this chapter addresses work with children who have suffered complex interpersonal trauma during early development, and whose social, physical, emotional, and psychological functioning may have become disturbed or compromised. Contemporary wisdom about the treatment of childhood trauma is ample (D'Andrea, Ford, Stolbach, Spinazzola, & van der Kolk, 2012; Osofsky, 2011; Shaw, 2010) and provides a blueprint for clinical interventions for attachment issues associated with such trauma. Specifically, we (1) present a brief overview of the interface between drama and play therapies; (2) discuss the relevance of doing attachment work with traumatized children; and (3) describe drama and play therapy approaches that indirectly or directly address attachment issues with such children.

Drama Therapy and Play Therapy

Play therapy theories, techniques, and approaches are varied and unique (O'Connor & Braverman, 1997, 2009) and have shown to be effective in helping resolve a variety of psychosocial difficulties (Bratton, Ray, & Rhyne, 2005). Drama therapy likewise has diverse methodology, particularly in its clinical applications and clinical impact (Jones, 2010; Weber

& Haen, 2005). Drama therapy utilizes various aspects of dramatic performance and physical movements in order to encourage affective expression and its therapeutic benefits. Drama therapy and its companion discipline, psychodrama, emphasize spontaneity, creative expression, and affect enhancement. In general, drama therapists may begin as "theater people" with theatrical training and then receive specialized drama therapy and psychotherapy training. Psychodramatists tend to be psychotherapists first, who then train intensely in J. L. Moreno's psychodramatic method. Moreno (1934) defined *psychodrama* as "the science which explores the 'truth' by dramatic methods. It deals with interpersonal relations and private worlds" (p. 13).

Jones (1996) describes core processes of drama therapy similar to Schaefer's (1993, 1994) curative factors. These include dramatic projection; drama therapeutic empathy and distancing; role playing and personification; interactive audience and witnessing; embodiment (dramatizing the body); playing; life–drama connection; and transformation. Drama therapy has the potential to access constricted energy and cause release, to oxygenate the body, and to allow for self-initiated personal momentum to lead the way into discovery of internal concerns. As Jones (1996) states, "play enables the client in drama therapy to create within the session a playful relationship with reality" (p. 93). As suggested by Irwin (1983), there are developmental levels of play. Similarly, Jones (1996) conceptualizes a continuum, which includes the following key aspects: "sensory motor play, imitative play, pretend play, dramatic play, and drama" (p. 177).

It is difficult to take the play out of drama therapy or the dramatic component out of play therapy. Thus the merging of play and drama therapies is a natural and easy partnership, one that equips practitioners with a much richer repertoire for work with attachment and trauma. Drama and play therapies have several factors in common—specifically, playing, dramatic projection and distancing, and empathy building. In addition, many children naturally use embodiment as they "try on" and "act out" characters as they role-play and pretend, using their creative imaginations. Both play and drama therapies encourage expression through varied holistic activities that elicit physical, emotional, sensory, spiritual, and cognitive engagement, thereby evoking introspection, reflection, and change. In brief, play and drama therapy are *whole-brain activities*, which, according to Siegel and Bryson (2011),

> help our children become better integrated so they can use their whole brain in a coordinated way. For example, we want them to be horizontally integrated, so that their left-brain logic can work well with their right-brain emotion. We also want them to be vertically integrated, so that the physically higher parts of their brain, which let them thoughtfully consider their actions, work well with the lower parts, which are more concerned with instinct, gut reactions, and survival. (p. 7)

When utilizing therapeutic play in an environment of specially selected therapeutic toys, children make internal associations, project thoughts and perceptions, and attribute and delegate affective specificity to their toys and their stories. These projected externalizations, embedded with personal meaning, are kept at a safe enough distance for children to view them from afar, in order to permit gradual approaches to feared thoughts or emotions. In cognitive-behavioral terminology, children organically use their own projections to achieve *gradual exposure*—a way to desensitize themselves to or inoculate themselves against specific, intolerable sensations, cognitions, or feelings (Cohen, Mannarino, & Deblinger, 2006).

Children, Complex Trauma, and Attachment

The term *complex trauma* suggests a layering of difficulty that can have a major impact on general functioning, especially with more vulnerable populations such as children. Complex psychological trauma is defined by Courtois and Ford (2009) as "including traumatic stressors that (1) are repetitive or prolonged; (2) involve direct harm and/or neglect and abandonment by caregivers or ostensibly responsible adults; (3) occur at developmentally vulnerable times in the victim's life, such as early childhood; and (4) have great potential to compromise severely a child's development" (p. 1). The most significant aspect of complex trauma is that it is often caused by those who are most important in children's lives and who are supposed to meet their early needs for nurturing and survival. Probably the most insidious lesson of abuse is that "people who love you hurt you," and this early association can have a negative impact on a child's view of the world from that point forward. As Herman (2009) notes, the trauma is occurring within a *relational matrix* in which "the strong do as they please, the weak submit, caretakers seem willfully blind, and there is no one to turn to for protection" (p. xiv). She goes on to state that children may then develop self-loathing, as well as pervasive distrust of the abusive caregivers and others. In fact, abused children have myriad responses, including fierce loyalty to their abusive caregivers, anxious or insecure attachments to them, or fear or avoidance of them. But most importantly, since their primary caregiving relationships serve as their templates for future relationships and expectations (internal working models), complex trauma has huge implications for children's relational experiences with others. In addition, when abuse continues uninterrupted, children will develop more refined coping mechanisms and defenses that can keep them emotionally shut down, disconnected from others, and unable to negotiate their important needs.

Cook et al. (2005) describe six core components of treatment for complex trauma: safety, self-regulation, self-reflective information processing, integration of traumatic experiences, relational engagement, and enhancement of positive affect. Although these consensus-based areas provide a uniform direction to help children (and their families) recover from early trauma, clinical approaches by definition must remain relationally based, developmentally sensitive, evocative, trauma-informed, "brain-based," and engaging.

There has been consistent advocacy in the last decade for incorporating evidence-based practices into all clinical settings; this trend challenges clinicians to remain attentive to research studies that provide effective treatment outcomes. In the forefront of evidence-based treatment models for working with traumatized children is trauma-focused cognitive-behavioral therapy (TF-CBT). TF-CBT provides a structured and well-articulated model that emphasizes critical areas of care and provides guidance about the treatment trajectory with abused children and their families. Recently, TF-CBT's developers have emphasized the potential use of play activities to advance trauma-focused goals in ways that might engage younger children and their families in fuller participation (Cohen, Mannarino, & Deblinger, 2012). There are several other evidence-based models for working with childhood trauma (domestic violence, physical abuse) that include play-based interventions based on psychoanalytic principles of play therapy (see, e.g., van Horn & Lieberman, 2009, and Eyberg, 1988). Other evidence-based practices in working with children and families are emerging (Ford & Cloitre, 2009).

This past decade has also been one of innovation, technological advances, and great excitement as the field of neuroscience has gained great relevance in clinical work. Several threads of valuable and critical neuroscientific data now provide support for the theoretical foundation that has been laid since the 1970s. Leaders in the field of neuroscience have repeatedly noted the impact of trauma on the development of children's brains, pointed to the plasticity of the brain, and emphasized the fact that the brain repairs itself best in the context of relational health (Ludy-Dobson & Perry, 2010; Siegel, 2012).

Treatment of Complex Trauma in Children

When children enter treatment as a result of complex trauma, several key issues need immediate attention, particularly the pivotal concern of establishing safety and trust. Because children have by definition been hurt in the context of trusted relationships, their attachments to primary caregivers have been severely compromised, disrupted, or damaged. This happens when the predictable, repetitive patterns of caregiving and responding to children's basic needs are not consistently provided. Such children are never fully soothed, may associate caregiving with disappointment or anxiety, and have difficulty in developing self-regulation. When children cannot trust that their needs will be met, they develop anxiety and mistrust, and attempt to adjust their needs in a variety of ways. Children may learn to avoid eye contact; they may even learn to cry weakly or stay quiet; or they may exhibit a range of symptoms associated with stress, such as an acute or delayed startle response. Given an impaired caregiver–child attachment system, a child remains vulnerable and may develop anxious, avoidant, or disorganized interactions with caregivers.

In a therapy context, when therapists make themselves available for personal interactions, the therapist–child relationship can provoke anxiety; children may manifest that anxiety by exhibiting either overly compliant (fear-based) behaviors, or emotional or behavioral dysregulation (nervousness and hyperactivity). Moreover, children may become anxious when asked to "talk" to therapists about traumatic events. Decreasing and managing young clients' anxiety, and establishing a safe therapeutic environment, are therefore critical to meaningful progress.

A beginning therapeutic goal is to attend to child clients in a conscientious and reflective way, which will give these children the experience of collaborative communication. Alert observation can be learned and practiced in individual or group therapy settings through various drama and play therapy activities.

A Selection of Integrative Drama and Play Therapy Exercises

As noted earlier, the integration of drama and play therapy is one of the most natural, refreshing, and logical mergers that can occur. Play therapy already includes an appreciation for children's natural physicality; their mimicking through pretend play; their exaggerated emotional expression at times; and their availability for and engagement with fantasy, creative imagination, and enactments through story and play. Applying principles of drama therapy is good common sense and is inherently a good fit: Pretend play often spontaneously occurs within drama therapy. The following sections illustrate how specific treatment goals in work with traumatized children can capitalize on the blending of play and drama interventions. These individual and group exercises have two central therapeutic elements: focused attention and mirroring, which are the primary ways children learn and explore their worlds in the early years.

Individual Exercises

Synchronized Water Breaths

Synchronized water breaths are slow full-body breaths done side by side or face to face; the therapist can move from a side-to-side position to a face-to-face position over several sessions as the client's comfort grows. On the in-breath, arms go out to sides and then scoop down to ground (as if scooping water) and lifting over the head. During the out-breath, the overhead hands flow back down to the body and cross in front. Together, the therapist and child bring a subsequent breath in and bring arms out to sides again (the synchronization is more important than the choreography of arms).

This activity provides a co-regulating metaphor in which a therapist and a child client work in tandem, while at the same time the child is encouraged to oxygenate the body, is helped to decrease his or her anxiety, and is taught the breathing skills so necessary to self-regulation. This exercise can be even more engaging when child and therapist choose animal masks to wear; the mask provides the child with a buffer against feeling too exposed. Also, the movement itself suggests picking up water and gently allowing it to spill and wash over the body. The therapist can use a variation on the idea of "picking up water" and collaborate with the client at the beginning or end of a session to intentionally "pick up" a feeling, color, or attribute, and allow this to wash over the pair. For example, anxious children may benefit from scooping and pouring a feeling of "calm" over themselves, or the "love" of a favorite person. This exercise can become an opening or ending ritual that establishes predictability and delineates boundaries in the session.

Mirroring

As an exercise, mirroring has its roots in theater and is used in training actors to hone observation skills and character development (Boal, 1992; Spolin, 1986). It must be kept in mind that clients can experience face-to-face activities as intimate and intense, so in order to respect initial boundaries, clinicians are encouraged to use peripheral mirroring to establish therapeutic trust gradually. Recent research in neurobiology (e.g., Iacoboni, 2008) shows that mirror neurons may be critical neural elements in the evolution of language.

The classic, face-to-face mirroring exercise (Boal, 1992; Spolin, 1986) has value for building attunement, trust, and shared leadership. Therapists who are face to face with child clients without touching them can begin to move their bodies slowly, making faces and moving their arms while maintaining loose eye contact. Therapists encourage clients to follow their movements exactly, and then give the children the opportunity to lead while the therapists copy the clients' movements. As children engage in this exercise, they learn to regulate their physical and emotional states, and they have the opportunity to develop attunement by sharing resonating neurons in which physical states are mirrored and emotional states are conveyed.

"Healer" or "Wise Person"

Another drama therapy exercise can follow mirroring and is particularly useful in introspection and exploring inner strengths and self-empathy. In this exercise, the therapist facilitates the creation of a real or imagined character by asking the client to think of a "healer," or a "wise person," or "a person who knows a lot," or "a person who knows a lot about helping others." The child imagines a person with full detail, standing in front of the child or sitting in an empty chair. The child is encouraged to look over the imagined character from head to toe, noticing everything about how he or she looks, smells, and seems. Once the image is clear, the client can sit in the chair or stand in the place of the wise person (the moment of changing places or sitting in the empty chair is an important point, because the client literally and figuratively steps into the role of the other). The therapist suggests that the client take a minute to become the character, asking questions like "How does the wise person stand?" Once it is clear that the client is ready, the therapist interviews the "wise one." The following vignette illustrates the use of this exercise.

Case Vignette: Carla

Carla was 16 years old and had disclosed her brother's sexual abuse of her when she was 10 or so. For whatever reasons, this disclosure was met with minimization by her parents, and even a school guidance counselor had questioned whether she had imagined the abuse. Her mother's response, in particular, had made her skeptical about therapy in general and whether anyone would really believe her or be capable of helping her. The abuse had apparently continued for a while, until she was able to ask for and get a lock on her bedroom door; her brother also became more socially active and started spending much of his time away from home. Carla felt lonely in her home and spent most of her time in her room. She became depressed in her junior year of high school; she had been unable to make close friends, stating that she felt different from others her age. In the last few months prior to the referral, Carla's grades had also begun to plummet, partly due to her lack of motivation and disinterest in her current classes, teachers, and homework. Her parents opted to bring her to therapy at the point when her grades became a problem to them, and Carla was somewhat reluctant to invest much of herself in therapy.

Carla and I (Eliana Gil) had just moved into the end of the initial phase of treatment, and therapeutic trust had been established. Carla was now feeling happy to come see me and prioritized her appointment time, often insisting that her parents bring her even when their schedule was problematic. We had developed a fairly good therapy relationship, and I had worked hard to be viewed as trustworthy. I had told her that if I had seen her when she was 10, the whole family would have been asked to come to therapy, and everyone would have had to acknowledge how painful and confusing her brother's alleged abuse had been to her. She smiled when I told her that he would have been court-ordered into therapy right away, because what he was doing was not "normal"; in fact, it was abusive. (I had stated precisely the same to the parents when they came in to see me.)

Carla was hesitant to talk about the abuse or her brother, although she was agreeable to doing some focused work on what had happened, since it often "haunted her" and "came into her mind." I had assessed that she was having intrusive flashbacks, which are not unusual for individuals with unresolved complex trauma. I opted to use the "wise person" technique to begin to connect Carla with the part of herself that had been wise enough to report what she knew to be wrong, and wise enough to know that her parents had not done all they could to help her at that time. In addition, I thought it important to strengthen her coping strategies and inner resources prior to doing more specific trauma work. Without assigning blame, we proceeded with the "wise person" interview. Carla had established her receptivity to symbol work, metaphorical language, guided imagery, and role playing by using miniatures in our early sessions, so she easily went into the role of "wise person."

THERAPIST: What is your name?

CARLA: (*as the wise person*) Clementine.

THERAPIST: How do you feel about your name, Clementine?

CARLA: (*as Clementine*) It suits me perfectly.

THERAPIST: How so?

CARLA: (*continuing as Clementine*) I am small, I am sweet, and people are surprised at what a good fruit I am, even when they are looking for an orange and picked me by mistake.

THERAPIST: How old are you?

CARLA: I am without an age. I can look different ways, but where I live, there are no young or old—only beings who float in time.

THERAPIST: What are you wearing?

CARLA: Just robes, lavender robes, that don't pull or push anywhere. They just float with me as I go.

THERAPIST: How do you know Carla?

CARLA: Oh, I've been knowing her since she was about 5 years old.

THERAPIST: Five years old! You've known her 11 years. That's a long time!

CARLA: Yes, indeed, she and I are old friends—old souls, I mean, connected and bonded and very close.

THERAPIST: What can you tell me about your friend as a little girl?

CARLA: She was wise beyond her years, quiet, spent a lot of time in her room. She is very kind, kind-hearted, and spirited, like a wild horse galloping through a leafy forest.

THERAPIST: Kind and spirited. I see. How else would you describe her as a little girl?

CARLA: Loving, very loving—looking to be loved, really. She was always wanting hugs and kisses, but her parents were always busy, and her dad traveled a lot.

THERAPIST: So she wanted hugs and kisses, like most little girls do, but her parents seemed busy a lot of the time. So what did she do?

CARLA: Well, that's when she first started talking to me. She loved her brother a lot and he was only a few years older, and they spent a lot of time alone together. But he started hugging her too tight, and she didn't like it and told him so. But he just kept pushing and started doing other stuff she didn't like.

THERAPIST: So she turned to you for advice with this problem? What a smart girl to turn to you for help!

CARLA: Yes, she could see that this was not OK, that her brother seemed mean and angry some of the time, and that he wasn't being nice to her. So I asked her to tell her mother what was going on.

THERAPIST: Oh, so you were wise enough to give this important advice?

CARLA: Yes, and she listened right away, and tried two or three times to tell her mother.

THERAPIST: This is a very hard thing to do, to keep trying when her mother was not able to hear.

CARLA: Yes, but she managed it because she has a lot of "stick-to-it-veness"!

THERAPIST: And it sounds like she got support from you the whole way, even when her mother and father thought she was making a mountain out of a molehill.

CARLA: She knew she was right. She was there. She could see that something was wrong with her brother, especially when he kept trying to do more and more bad things to her.

THERAPIST: She was lucky to have you when it sounds like she was feeling very alone.

CARLA: Oh, yes, she was very alone, and that's when she started feeling that no one understood her—except for myself, of course. We had many, many long conversations, and she understood that parents sometimes do the best they can with difficult situations. She even thought, when she got a little older, that her parents were worried about him and wanted to hope and pray that she was exaggerating so that they wouldn't need to worry so much.

THERAPIST: Wow, she really is very kind . . . she tried hard to understand why her parents would want to think of this as normal. She surely was kind to them, but I wonder, wise one, how you felt about her being so lonely and not having anyone in her family believe her.

CARLA: She is truly amazing. She found a way to keep herself safe, and she kept telling other people outside the home, which I also thought was the right thing to do.

THERAPIST: How do you think she got through all this on her own and with your help?

CARLA: She is a very special, kind, and strong girl. She has lost her way a little now, but she knows deep down that what doesn't kill you makes you stronger.

THERAPIST: So she has gotten "strong at the broken places?"

CARLA: Yeah, that's right. She's tougher than she looks, and as I said, she's forgotten a little about all she went through to come out on the other side, but I think she'll remember a little. I know that I do.

THERAPIST: So what would you most like her to know from you today?

CARLA: I'd tell her, "Carla, you've been through rough times. You've had good times too. You need to find your compass again, like I've seen you put in the sandtray pictures over and over. You can do it. There are lots of important paths for you in the future."

THERAPIST: What's the one thing you think would help her the most right now?

CARLA: To know that her mother still loves her and doesn't blame her for what happened.

THERAPIST: That sounds like an important thing for her to know. All kids like to know that their parents love them and don't blame them. And, by the way, what is it that she thinks she's blamed for?

CARLA: She thinks they blame her for her brother's drinking problem and his getting into trouble after she told.

THERAPIST: Oh, I think it might be important to check that out with her parents and find out what they think instead of guessing.

CARLA: (*as Clementine*) That might be good. (*as herself*) I think I want to stop now.

THERAPIST: OK, wise one, just one last question: What surprises or delights you most about Carla?

CARLA: (*as Clementine again*) That she remains kind and expects the best from others.

THERAPIST: That sounds great. How did you get to be so wise?

CARLA: I talk to a lot of kids who need my help. I listen to them and learn from them too.

THERAPIST: Sounds great. OK, I'd like for you to begin to imagine your friend Carla and begin to step back into her shoes, so that Carla can come back into the room.

When Carla was reoriented to time and place, we debriefed a little by talking about the experience of her wise person and what she had learned from her today. She told me that she had not "seen her" in a long time and had forgotten how calm she felt when she talked with her. I told Carla that I was impressed by how much the two of them had in common. "I know," she said quietly. Subsequent sessions were guided by some of what had been disclosed in this conversation and included family therapy sessions.

This dramatic role play was quite revealing, showing when Carla's attachment disruption began. It was clear that at the age of 5, she had turned to her mother and father, who were unable or unwilling to hear her disclosure. In an effort to protect themselves from the truth, they minimized what Carla said, and turned away from her obvious need to be heard and believed. They did not do this maliciously; they were simply unequipped to know how to be of help to their daughter. But in turning away from Carla's disclosure and spoken need for protection, the mother in particular had also turned away from her emotional connection to her daughter, and from that point on functioned to avoid what was before her. Carla became a reminder of what the mother considered her failure, and this perception led to years of loneliness for them both. Now, 11 years later, it was not only relevant but crucial to bring them together to attempt an attachment reparation, a foundation that was necessary if more growth was possible for them in the future.

So I gingerly approached Carla about having joint family sessions with her parents, in an attempt to have them respond more appropriately to her initial disclosure. Although Carla thought it was too late (and not necessary) to have these sessions, we consulted with the wise one, Clementine, who agreed it was worth making the effort. We talked to Clementine often, and in so doing allowed Carla to tap into her own impressive internal resources and access the wisdom or advice she already possessed. Wisdom and knowing are elusive for many young clients. Many have suffered physical or emotional blows, and their positive identity formation has been compromised. This exercise can be changed to create someone who is a fan, cheerleader, or champion of a child and thinks positively of him or her. It may be the family dog, a teacher, or a favorite aunt. In using role reversal with these characters, children are able to see themselves more positively through the eyes of a trusted other. They are able to stand within the love that is available to them, and perhaps feel it more fully—embodied self-love is very powerful.

Group Exercises

Stop–Walk–Run

Groups can work toward group awareness and cohesion through Stop–Walk–Run (Zapora, 1995), which allows children to be anonymous leaders from within a group. While the group is instructed to mill around (to walk in a designated space, zigzagging in an unpredictable pattern, without touching), someone can initiate a "freeze" by simply stopping. The other children must follow the lead of any child who freezes first and must freeze until the whole group has stopped. Next, a new member initiates movement, which cues the group to resume. Without planning, the group members are invited to take the leadership role and are challenged to respond to the group as a whole. As the group has opportunities to practice moving together, members develop their ability to use peripheral vision while strengthening their sense of cohesion. Through this activity, children learn to be attuned and sensitive to each other and to behave in respectful ways. They also learn to be both leaders and followers, and can experiment with being in and out of control without fear. This exercise also builds group cohesion, because it allows children to feel a part of something larger than themselves, and is safe and mutually created.

Mirroring within a Group

Mirroring can also encourage acceptance in a group, in that it gives children the sense of being seen and accepted by others. Mirroring exercises may be expanded as groups become more cohesive. For example, as a circle group game, an embodied check-in can be mirrored back. Older kids can be given a prompt such as "How are you feeling about being in group?" or "How was your day before group?" In a circle, children take turns choosing a sound and movement to reflect their check-in—for example, a frustrated body shake accompanied by a growl if they are feeling annoyed or irritated. Then the whole group is encouraged to mirror back the check-in as a validating experience. The person who has demonstrated an embodied feeling is usually pleased to have been heard, and the group has made way for each member to be the focus of brief attention.

Emotional Statues

In a group setting, children are asked to mill around, and the therapist calls out the name of an emotion such as "Sadness." The children are asked to walk while embodying that emotion (embedding the emotion physically), and the therapist then notices and highlights the physical attributes in the children. For example, the therapist can say, "I see many heads are hung down, and shoulders are slumped," or "People are walking slowly and sighing a lot." Then on the count of 3, the therapist calls a "freeze," and children are asked to create a statue of the emotion. For some children, holding still is already addressing their issues of impulse control. Once children have created their affective statues, the therapist introduces the idea of "turning up the volume" as on a radio. With each clap, children are encouraged to exaggerate the sadness (or other emotion) into a new sculpture.

Therapists determine how much to turn the intensity up or down, depending on children's reactions to the exercise and their ability to stay in control and involved with the exercise. On a scale of 1–10, the emotional intensity can be escalated from a 3 to a 5, back down again, then up to 10, then back down to 3. As closure for this activity, children are asked to mill around again and shake off their feelings, restoring their bodies to a normal walk. The therapist can bring attention to common physical signs of emotions, such as fist clenching or holding breaths, so that children learn to associate their somatic experience and their affective states. One of the interesting outcomes to this exercise is that children begin to develop an understanding of affective scaling (i.e., the concept that their feelings can be smaller or larger) and that they have some degree of control over increasing or decreasing their emotions. (The clinical use of affective scaling has become quite popular—e.g., the Subjective Units of Distress Scale.)

Another variation of this exercise is family sculpting, popularized by Papp, Silverstein, and Carter (1973) and originated by Virginia Satir. One family member is asked to "sculpt" family members to represent his or her perceptions of family relationships—how close or distant they feel, or how they view others on an emotional level. For example, family members can be shaped into positions that manifest affect, such as crossed arms and pursed lips for anger, or open arms and smiles for welcoming. Clearly, this exercise can quickly identify attachment concerns and give family members a chance to identify them in a graphic and physical way—not only as they currently exist, but as they might be imagined or desired. Drama therapists consider sculpting a pivotal way for clients to activate their bodies and physically *try on* the positive attributes that they seek.

Big–Bigger–Biggest

Big–Bigger–Biggest is adapted from a Playback Theater exercise by Salas (1993). The therapist selects three group members to be the "actors" on stage. The other group members become audience members, and the roles are rotated throughout the group therapy session. The three actors stand side by side. A group member calls out an emotion, and each actor steps forward to show the emotion in a sculpture, with increasing intensity. After the third actor has finished, the audience claps for all three of them enthusiastically. Each actor has had a chance to express embodied emotion in a unique way; to amplify the intensity of each emotion; to watch two other group members do their renditions; to be visible to the audience; and to be acceptable to and accepted by the audience.

In drama therapy, the goal is to expand every client's repertoire of affect identification, modulation, and expression. Therefore, children participating in this exercise are challenged to try on a muted or more expressive affect in order to expand their own emotional repertoire. A "de-role" (which can be as simple as a physical brush-off) can be built into this and other more emotionally intense exercises, to allow the children to disengage from acting out troubling emotions and to attain regulatory closure. The creation of the "stage" can be as simple as asking the audience to sit in one area as the actors come onstage in another area; using this language sets the tone without fuss.

Specific Activities for Addressing Attachment Issues in Complex Trauma

There is a general consensus that childhood trauma is best addressed directly, in order to give clients the opportunity to integrate the experience in a healthy way; however, *processing* is a term that means different things to different people. As mentioned previously, Cook et al. (2005) provide guidance about specific aspects of processing trauma, including self-reflective information processing and the integration of traumatic experiences. What becomes clear is that the intended goals include some type of self-reflection, opportunities to correct cognitive distortions, affective release, and eventual restoration of personal power through controlled recall. All of these will eventually allow the person to integrate the experience as one of many—one that does not hold undue power and influence over future choices and options. Central to future choices and options are the selection and management of interpersonal relationships, which can be compromised by a lack of trust and by negative expectations of relationships as harmful rather than potentially rewarding.

It is also considered crucial to help clients create accurate trauma narratives. Memories of the trauma become less intensely felt as clients have repetitive exposure to and reevaluation of such narratives. One of the questions in work with young children is whether their narratives have to rise to the experience of full consciousness, or whether their narratives can be conducted through play, art, or other means of self-expression (Gil, 2010). This debate is likely to continue.

Drama and play therapies provide many mechanisms for reflection that can help with the goals of trauma processing (which we suggest will include reflection, improved management, and transformation of some type, as well as the capacity to regard past events with decreasing emotional intensity). Below, we describe some activities that have the potential to help accomplish goals associated with trauma processing within an increasingly trusted therapeutic relationship.

Integrating the Social Atom and the Play Genogram

J. L. Moreno, the founding father of psychodrama, originated the activity known as the *social atom* in the 1930s (Moreno, 1934). The social atom is similar to a *genogram* (McGoldrick & Gershon, 1986), in that it serves as a graphic representation of a relational map that can be drawn on paper. The major difference between a genogram and a social atom is the emphasis on the subjective world of the client. With a social atom, the client maps out connections to those people or institutions that have an impact on his or her life at the present time. Moreover, proximity and distance are used to indicate the sense of closeness or distance in each relationship. Because this activity focuses primarily on a client's subjective perceptions of important relationships, and particularly on whether these relationships are viewed as sources of emotional nurturance and support, it is relevant to the work of resolving traumas occurring in an interpersonal context.

Gil (2003) has developed a *play genogram* that uses miniatures to enliven the paper-and-pencil genogram (McGoldrick, Gerson, & Petry, 2008). We suggest these adaptations: (1) a paper-and-pencil social atom, animated with miniatures; and (2) a social atom with brightly colored circles and squares of different sizes. Both of these approaches help elicit children's fuller participation in these therapeutic strategies, and decrease their resistance to following a path of self-contemplation. Children, in particular, may find it less threatening to miniaturize or play out their concerns or problems than to discuss them verbally. These processes can eventually lead to verbal conversations that might not have been available in other ways. In addition, the act of *choosing* miniatures is a projective technique that communicates rich metaphoric information to the therapist without words. Drama therapy adaptations may include an "interview" of the characters on the social atom, conducted in the same way that the director would interview the auxiliary characters in an enacted psychodrama (Dayton, 2005).

Social Atom with Miniatures

The therapist first provides the child with a large sheet of paper with several concentric circles drawn on it, and invites the client to draw him- or herself in the center, using a circle if the client is female or a square if the client is male. Next, the client adds images (shapes or colors) of the people, institutions, and pets that are important to him or her. The child is instructed to put the people and places that play a big role in his or her life closer to the symbol in the center representing the child. The purpose is to create a relational map from the client's point of view. Once the client seems to have added the significant people and institutions, he or she can then pick a miniature to represent each shape in the social atom, placing them directly on the page at proximities representing their actual closeness or distance to the child. (See Figure 7.1 for two different examples.)

Once the miniatures are selected and placed, and depending on the child's age and propensity for verbal communication, the therapist can initiate an exploratory dialogue by signaling the child to "say as much or as little about the things you have chosen and their closeness to your circle." These conversations should be explorative, and should stay within metaphorical language unless the child shifts to first person. For example, it may be better to ask, "The owl seems to be facing in this direction. What does it see?" than "I see the object you've chosen for your mother is looking away from you." The first question is explorative, and the second is interpretive; the latter can have the effect of causing the child to feel self-conscious or self-protective. Processing any metaphorical work must be carefully approached, in order to maximize the child's engagement rather than inadvertently cause defensive responses (Gil, 2010). The social atom map can be photographed and discussed at later times; or the child can be asked to embody one of the chosen miniatures to bring it more to life; or the child can be asked to take one miniature and give it a voice (dialogues between two or more miniatures can even be elicited).

As mentioned above, a drama therapy adaptation of this activity can include an interview with some of the characters chosen. For example, the therapist can ask specific miniatures an array of questions, such as these:

"Who are you?"
"How long have you known [the client]?"
"How did you first meet [the client]?"
"What did you first notice about [the client]?"
"What one thing have you learned about [the client] that you didn't know at first?"
"What kinds of things do you and [the client] like to do together?"
"What kind of things do you say to [the client]?"
"What's the best advice you have ever given [the client]?"

The questions can be designed to gain information, but can also serve as a warm-up for dramatic play. An important element to remember is always to guide the child to end the explorations in the role of him- or herself. Even when other characters are animated, the exercise needs to be finished with the client as him- or herself.

If a child spontaneously includes, or is asked for therapeutic purposes to include, the abuser in the atom, it is not advisable to have the child role-play that particular role. In the case of a known abuser, a conversation could occur about him or her from others' point of view. This is a subtle and important difference that the therapist controls for obvious reasons.

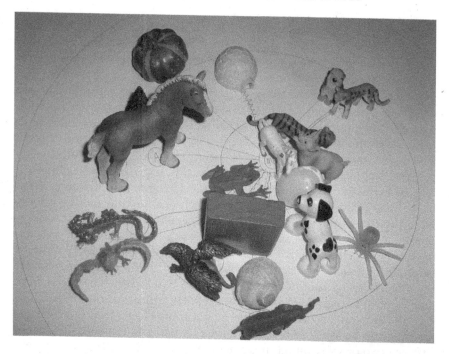

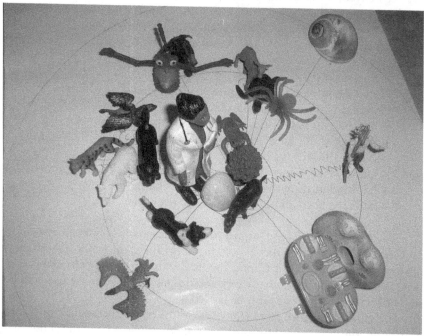

FIGURE 7.1. Two examples of a social atom with miniatures.

The social atom can also be enhanced and explored by using art materials or miniatures to represent the *types* of relationships that are drawn on the paper. For example, a child may choose to represent a rocky relationship between two characters in an atom by drawing a zigzagged line. The line may be blocked or broken in some relationships that have been discontinued. Once the line representing the connection is added, the line itself can be animated with art materials. Miniatures may provide additional information and metaphors to the relational line, such as a rock that blocks a connection or a snake that threatens a path.

Social Atom with Circles and Squares

Another adaptation of the social atom is to have a child draw a large circle on a large sheet of paper and place the sheet on the floor in an ample area. Then the child picks a circle or square to represent the self (as in the previous exercise, a circle if the child is female and a square if the child is male). The child next picks other sizes and colors of circles and squares for people in his or her life, and places them close to the central circle/square or far away (see Figure 7.2). Once this graphic social atom is created, the

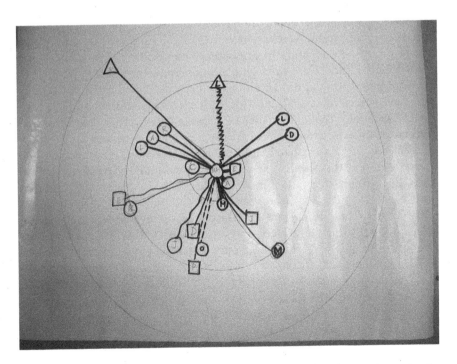

FIGURE 7.2. A re-created example of a social atom placed on concentric circles. The circle and square symbols represent females and males, while the triangles represent significant institutions.

child can step into the circles/squares of others, in order to be interviewed by the therapist. Each circle or square in and of itself carries important information—for example, how "big" or "small" this person is to the child, and in terms of color, how intense, muted, bright, and so on the energy that the child sees in this person is. A drama therapist is obviously interested in the actual embodying of the person that the child can portray as he or she takes the role of each person, while an art or play therapist may be more interested in the spaces between the circles/squares and how to interact playfully with those spaces, or how the colors convey their own meaning about the child's experience of each person.

Conclusion

Play and drama therapists have much in common: Both play and drama are free and natural phenomena that emerge spontaneously in childhood, and yet therapists who make use of both have struggled to establish their disciplines as credible mental health practices with legitimate potential to advance therapeutic goals. Both play and drama therapists believe that emotions can become unavailable for expression for a variety of reasons, and both provide ample opportunities for release that are not restricted to verbal communication. Much more holistic by definition, play and drama engage the mind and body in attempts to cause internal movement and transformative experience through reflection and expression.

Childhood trauma has traditionally been described as overwhelming a person's perceived capacity to cope with external stressors, and its treatment is generally thought to include expression of affect, cognitive and perceptual shifts, assimilation of fragmented memories, and sensory and physical release. Traumatized children can feel isolated, stigmatized, and compromised in their ability to establish or maintain important relationships. In addition, their attachment to others can feel frightening and necessary at the same time, causing them to feel dysregulated in the presence of caregivers. Trauma must be addressed directly or indirectly in order for these children to move forward and create new and more positive future options for themselves. Drama and play therapists are in a unique position to advance the goals of trauma resolution by providing clients with tools that give them the necessary combination of resources and safety to reflect, give voice, express affect, make shifts in perception and thinking, and eventually feel a greater sense of mastery and control.

REFERENCES

Boal, A. (1992). *Games for actors and non-actors.* New York: Routledge.
Bratton, S. C., Ray, D., & Rhine, T. (2005). The efficacy of play therapy with

children: A meta-analytic review of treatment outcomes. *Professional Psychology: Research and Practice, 36*(4), 376–390.

Cohen, J. A., Mannarino, A. P., & Deblinger, E. (2006). *Treating trauma and traumatic grief in children and adolescents.* New York: Guilford Press.

Cohen, J. A., Mannarino, A. P., & Deblinger, E. (Eds.). (2012). *Trauma-focused CBT for children and adolescents: Treatment applications.* New York: Guilford Press.

Cook, A., Spinazzola, J., Ford, J. D., Lanktree, C., Blaustein, M., Cloitre, M., . . . van der Kolk, B. (2005). Complex trauma in children and adolescents. *Psychiatric Annals, 35,* 390–398.

Courtois, C. A., & Ford, J. D. (2009). Defining and understanding complex trauma and complex traumatic stress disorders. In C. A. Courtois & J. D. Ford (Eds.), *Treating complex traumatic stress disorders: An evidence-based guide* (pp. 13–30). New York: Guilford Press.

D'Andrea, W., Ford, J., Stolbach, B., Spinazzola, J., & van der Kolk, B. (2012). Understanding interpersonal trauma in children: Why we need a developmentally appropriate trauma diagnosis. *American Journal of Orthopsychiatry, 82*(2), 187–200.

Dayton, T. (2005). *The living stage: A step-by-step guide to psychodrama, sociometry and experiential group therapy.* Deerfield Beach, FL: Health Communications.

Eyberg, S. (1988). PCIT: Integration of traditional and behavioral concerns. *Child and Family Behavior Therapy, 10,* 33–46.

Ford, J. D., & Cloitre, M. (2009). Best practices in psychotherapy for children and adolescents. In C. A. Courtois & J. D. Ford (Eds.), *Treating complex traumatic stress disorders: An evidence-based guide* (pp. 59–81). New York: Guilford Press.

Gil, E. (2003). Family play therapy: "The bear with short nails." In C. E. Schaefer (Ed.), *Foundations of play therapy* (pp. 192–218). New York: Wiley.

Gil, E. (2010). Children's self-initiated gradual exposure: The wonders of posttraumatic play and behavioral reenactments. In E. Gil (Ed.), *Working with children to heal interpersonal trauma: The power of play* (pp. 44–66). New York: Guilford Press.

Herman, J. (2009). Foreword. In C. A. Courtois & J. D. Ford (Eds.), *Treating complex traumatic stress disorders: An evidence-based guide* (pp. xiii–xvii). New York: Guilford Press.

Iacoboni, M. (2008). *Mirroring people: The new science of how we connect with others.* New York: Farrar, Straus & Giroux.

Irwin, E. C. (1983). The diagnostic and therapeutic use of pretend play. In C. E. Schaefer & K. J. O'Connor (Eds.), *The handbook of play therapy* (pp. 148–173). New York: Wiley.

Jones, P. (1996). *Drama as therapy: Vol. 1, Theory, practice and research.* New York: Routledge.

Ludy-Dobson, C. R., & Perry, B. (2010). The role of healthy relational interactions in buffering the impact of childhood trauma. In E. Gil (Ed.), *Working with children to heal interpersonal trauma: The power of play* (pp. 26–43). New York: Guilford Press.

McGoldrick, M., & Gerson, R. (1986). *Genograms in family assessment.* New York: Norton.

McGoldrick, M., Gerson, R., & Petry, S. (2008). *Genograms: Assessment and intervention* (3rd ed.). New York: Norton.

Moreno, J. L. (1934). *Who shall survive?: A new approach to the problem of human interrelations.* Washington, DC: Nervous and Mental Disease Publishing.

O'Connor, K. J., & Braverman, L. M. (1997). *Play therapy theory and practice: A comparative presentation.* New York: Wiley.

O'Connor, K. J., & Braverman, L. M. (2009). *Play therapy theory and practice: Comparing theories and techniques* (2nd ed.). Hoboken, NJ: Wiley.

Osofsky, J. D. (2011). *Clinical work with traumatized young children.* New York: Guilford Press.

Papp, P., Silverstein, O., & Carter, E. (1973). Family sculpting in preventive work with "well families." *Family Process, 12*(2), 197–212.

Salas, J. (1993). *Improvising real life: Personal story in Playback Theater.* Dubuque, IA: Kendall/Hunt.

Schaefer, C. E. (Ed.). (1993). *The therapeutic powers of play.* Northvale, NJ: Aronson.

Schaefer, C. E. (1994). Play therapy for psychic trauma in children. In K. J. O'Connor & C. E. Schaefer (Eds.), *Handbook of play therapy: Vol. 2. Advances and innovations* (pp. 297–318). New York: Wiley.

Shaw, J. A. (2010). A review of current research on the incidence and prevalence of interpersonal childhood trauma. In E. Gil (Ed.), *Working with children to heal interpersonal trauma: The power of play* (pp. 12–25). New York: Guilford Press.

Siegel, D. (2012). *The developing mind: How relationships and the brain interact to shape who we are* (2nd ed.). New York: Guilford Press.

Siegel, D., & Bryson, T. P. (2011). *The whole-brain child: Revolutionary strategies to nurture your child's developing mind.* New York: Delacorte Press.

Spolin, V. (1986). *Theater games for the classroom: A teacher's handbook.* Evanston, IL: Northwestern University Press.

van Horn, P., & Lieberman, A. F. (2009). Using dyadic therapies to treat traumatized young children. In D. Brom, R. Pat-Horenczyk, & J. Ford (Eds.), *Treating traumatized children: Risk, resilience, and recovery* (pp. 210–224). New York: Routledge.

Weber, A. M., & Haen, C. (Eds.). (2005). *Clinical applications of drama therapy in child and adolescent treatment.* New York: Brunner-Routledge.

Zapora, R. (1995). *Action theater: The improvisation of presence.* Berkeley, CA: North Atlantic Books.

CHAPTER 8

Overcoming Complex Trauma
with Filial Therapy

Glade L. Topham
Risë VanFleet
Cynthia C. Sniscak

Children experiencing complex trauma offer significant challenges to their parents or other caregivers, as well as to the therapeutic process. Their histories are interwoven with maltreatment and attachment disruptions, leaving these children with serious emotional, behavioral, and social difficulties, further complicated by a decreased ability to trust the adults in their lives. Because their behaviors can be extreme and sometimes destructive, children with complex trauma can become a source of significant frustration to those who care for them. A negative interaction pattern can exacerbate the problems, yielding even greater stress and exasperation for all involved.

Filial Therapy (FT) has been used successfully with many children with attachment trauma—within the care system (foster care, kinship care), with adoptive families, and during the reunification process with their own biological parents (VanFleet, 2006b; VanFleet & Sniscak, 2003; VanFleet & Topham, 2011). There are a number of reasons why FT is an extremely valuable treatment for these children, and these are discussed in this chapter, along with case illustrations of how the FT process works to resolve emotional, behavioral, and relational problems while resolving the trauma and attachment issues that fuel children's maladaptive behaviors.

This chapter begins with a description of FT and some of its variations, followed by a discussion of the relevance of FT in meeting the needs of these children and the families that care for them. A section that highlights the research evidence for the efficacy of FT is followed by case vignettes illustrating its use with child victims of interpersonal trauma and attachment disruption.

Filial Therapy

FT was the brainchild of Drs. Bernard and Louise Guerney in the late 1950s, and they have guided its research and development as a powerful family therapy intervention from the beginning, nearly 50 years ago (B. G. Guerney, 1964; L. F. Guerney, 2003; L. F. Guerney & Ryan, 2013; VanFleet, 2013). It is a deceptively simple approach that fully integrates play therapy and family therapy, with a foundation and methods that draw from all the major schools of psychological thought (Ginsberg, 2003; L. F. Guerney & Ryan, 2013; VanFleet, 2011a, 2011b, 2011c, 2013). FT engages parents or caregivers as the primary change agents for their children; this was a novel idea when FT was created, and it remains so today. Therapists who are fully trained in FT's psychoeducational framework teach parents to conduct special 30-minute nondirective play therapy sessions with their own children. The therapists directly supervise the early parent/caregiver–child play sessions until the parents master the necessary skills, after which the therapists provide continuing support as the family members hold the play sessions at home unsupervised (or are supervised indirectly by video).

Overview

To avoid cumbersome language, the term *caregivers* is used from here on to refer to whichever parents, grandparents, kinship caregivers, foster parents, or adoptive parents are involved with a child during the FT process.

FT was developed for children ages 2½ to 12—the ages at which children use imaginary play the most to express their feelings, wishes, and dilemmas—but we have extended its use to children with complex trauma as old as 16. Because of their developmental disruptions, children who have experienced trauma and attachment disruptions often function socially and emotionally as if they were younger, thereby making it possible to apply FT with some adolescents with little variation.

In FT, a therapist teaches caregivers four basic skills for use within the caregiver–child play sessions. These play sessions are nondirective in nature, following the principles and practices of child-centered play therapy (CCPT) (Axline, 1969; Cochran, Nordling, & Cochran, 2010; Landreth, 2012; VanFleet, Sywulak, & Sniscak, 2010; Wilson & Ryan, 2005). The caregivers conduct a 30-minute play session with the child each week, and in cases where there are other children in the family, it is desirable that they each have a 30-minute play session with the caregivers as well. This prevents a singling-out effect on the target child, while facilitating the development of healthy attachment relationships within all of the dyads in the family (VanFleet, 2013). Furthermore, all adult caregivers in the household are strongly encouraged to participate.

In FT, the therapist first demonstrates one or more CCPT sessions for the caregivers (usually one with each child in the family), and discusses each session thoroughly with the caregivers. The therapist then takes approximately three 1-hour sessions to train the caregivers to conduct the play sessions. This is done using an empathic, positive, and playful approach, culminating in mock play sessions in which the therapist role-plays a child while a caregiver practices all of the skills. The therapist gives encouraging feedback to caregivers as they do this. After this, each caregiver conducts approximately four to six play sessions with the child that are directly supervised by the therapist. Each of these sessions includes a feedback segment, in which the therapist provides skill feedback and discusses play themes and daily concerns with the caregivers. Only after caregivers have mastered the skills of the play sessions and understand how to identify and understand play themes do they begin unsupervised play sessions at home. They continue to meet with the therapist to discuss the home play sessions and to begin generalizing the skills they've learned to daily life. When conducted with individual families, FT typically takes between 15 and 20 hourly sessions, although the number of sessions can easily be extended as needed for families dealing with serious trauma and attachment issues.

The Skills Taught to Caregivers

Therapists teach four basic play session skills to the caregivers: *structuring, empathic listening, child-centered imaginary play,* and *limit setting* (see VanFleet, 2006a, 2012, and 2013, for details). *Structuring* includes the messages given to a child to establish the relatively permissive climate of the playroom upon entry, as well as 5-minute and 1-minute warnings that the play session is ending. *Empathic listening* refers to brief descriptions of what the child is doing (tracking) and reflections of the child's feelings, as expressed either directly by the child or indirectly through the imaginary characters in the child's play. *Child-centered imaginary play* requires the caregiver to play out roles that are assigned by the child, and to play them in a manner that follows the child's lead. The child is viewed as both the director and an actor in the play, and the caregiver is an actor under the child's direction. *Limit setting* is used to establish safety and boundaries in the play; in FT, caregivers learn to state a limit, to give a warning, and to carry out the consequence if the child disregards the limit. In all cases, if a child breaks the same limit three times during a session, the session ends. This quickly reestablishes caregiver authority, since most children enjoy the play sessions and do not wish them to end. The skills of empathic listening and imaginary play foster a permissive environment in which the child can explore, express, and enjoy. This permissiveness is balanced by the skills of structuring and limit setting to ensure safety and establish ultimate caregiver authority.

Training Adjustments for Children with Complex Trauma

In work with children with complex trauma, adjustments are sometimes made to the usual FT process (VanFleet, 2006b; VanFleet & Sniscak, 2003). Caregivers need more information about trauma, attachment processes, and the relationships of these to child behaviors and well-being. For example, they need to understand how past trauma and attachment disruptions can result in extreme behaviors and emotional reactions over which children seem to have little control. A better understanding of the importance of secure attachment and how it is fostered provides a framework for the FT that the therapist is recommending. Furthermore, these children are more likely to play in aggressive or sexualized ways because of their histories, so it is sometimes advisable to add an extra mock play session to show the caregivers how to respond to emotionally difficult material during the play sessions.

Didactic and Dynamic Elements of FT

FT consists of a blend of didactic and dynamic elements that unite to create positive change for both children and caregivers. The didactic element involves the training process to prepare caregivers to conduct the play sessions and master the CCPT play session skills. The dynamic element includes the discussions that therapists hold with caregivers to help them recognize and understand children's play themes, as well as empathic explorations of the caregivers' own feelings and reactions to the play and the process. Play sessions frequently trigger caregiver reactions that can prevent the caregivers from being responsive to the child. The skilled FT practitioner processes these reactions in a manner that helps caregivers develop understanding and make their own changes as needed.

Formats and Variations

FT was initially developed as a family group intervention, which is an efficient and cost-effective format for FT. This approach is detailed in L. F. Guerney and Ryan (2013); the 20-week group model described there can be shortened or lengthened as needed. VanFleet (2006a, 2013) has described the use of FT with individual families in detail, as well as a number of other group formats and resources. VanFleet, Sniscak, and Faa-Thompson (in press) describe a 14- to 18-week group FT format for use specifically with foster parents and adoptive parents. When therapists are properly trained and adhere to the values, principles, and process of FT, the method has great flexibility for effectively meeting the complex needs of families of children with serious trauma and attachment problems. The section that follows discusses an integrated model for treating attachment trauma, and provides the rationale for using FT with these children and their caregivers.

Targets of Treatment for Attachment Trauma

Attachment and trauma are intertwined for children. When children experience trauma, it threatens the attachment relationship, as well as children's trust that they are safe and that attachment figures will protect them. Furthermore, children with insecure attachments may have more trouble recovering from the effects of trauma and may also be more vulnerable to the effects of future trauma, because they may lack both the internal and external resources and supports to deal with overwhelming experiences. Therefore, the treatment of child trauma and of attachment disruption needs to be informed by both attachment and trauma theories (Busch & Lieberman, 2007).

A useful framework for guiding treatment of chronic interpersonal trauma or complex trauma in children that integrates attachment and trauma theories is the *attachment, self-regulation, and competency* (ARC) treatment framework (Blaustein & Kinniburgh, 2010; Kinniburgh, Blaustein, Spinazzola, & van der Kolk, 2005). The ARC model is not a treatment protocol, but rather a framework that highlights key areas and targets of treatment for child complex trauma, based on the existing body of research on the effects of child trauma. Below we list the three areas and 10 components or targets of the ARC model, as well as the associated challenges commonly seen in children who have experienced complex trauma. Then we use the ARC framework to describe how FT addresses the key caregiver and child targets of effective treatment for complex trauma.

Attachment

The four target areas of *attachment* in the ARC framework are *caregiver management of affect*; *attunement*; *consistency of response*; and *routines and rituals*. In the case of complex trauma, caregivers, who in the past have failed to provide proper protection and care for their child, frequently have poor emotional awareness and poor emotion regulation skills; these deficits significantly impairing their ability to be responsive and available to their child. Furthermore, even in cases where there is no history of maltreatment or neglect with current caregivers, it is frequently difficult for caregivers to manage their emotional experiences in response to the sometimes volatile behavior and emotions of a child who has experienced complex trauma. Furthermore, children who have experienced complex trauma are frequently accustomed to chaos in their family systems, leaving little sense for consistency, predictability, and safety (Arvidson et al., 2011).

Self-Regulation

The three target areas of child *self-regulation* in the ARC framework are *affect identification, affect modulation,* and *affect expression.* Children who have experienced trauma often experience overwhelming negative emotions, with limited awareness of these emotions or their origins; have few strategies for modulating their inner experience; and are frequently unable to communicate effectively with others about their inner experience (Kinniburgh et al., 2005).

Competency

The two target areas of developmental *competency* in the ARC framework are *executive functions,* and *self-development and identity.* Children who have experienced trauma often feel little sense of influence over their environments and have difficulty with problem solving and persevering with challenging tasks. They also commonly experience an internalized negative self-concept as a result of traumatic experiences and inconsistent care from attachment figures. Furthermore, trauma commonly interferes with children's development and may result in a delay in developmental competencies. The final building block of the ARC model is *trauma experience integration.* Children who have experienced trauma frequently have a fragmented internal experience that is overwhelming, leaving the children with little ability to make sense out of the internal experience and the associated events (Arvidson et al., 2011).

FT and Treatment of Complex Trauma

FT is well suited for the treatment of complex trauma in children because a child is treated within the context of the caregiver–child relationship; treatment focuses simultaneously on improvement in the child, the caregiver, and the caregiver–child relationship; treatment attends to all of the key targets of treatment as specified in the ARC model; treatment can be flexibly applied with biological, foster, or adoptive parents; treatment is structured and time-limited; the nondirective nature of the caregiver–child sessions allows FT to be utilized to treat a wide range of child symptoms and caregiver–child relationship problems; and treatment is positive and strength-based. Below we describe how FT addresses the targets of the ARC model in the areas of attachment, self-regulation, and competency.

Attachment

Caregiver Management of Affect

While developing and refining the four FT skills, caregivers learn to manage their own internal experiences in interaction with their child. The empathic listening and child-centered imaginary play skills challenge caregivers to set aside (i.e., regulate) their own personal needs, fears, and reactions in order to be fully present for their child. In setting limits, caregivers learn to manage their reactions in order to stay emotionally present and avoid shaming or rejecting their child. An important component of the work in helping caregivers improve self-regulation happens in the feedback sessions that follow play sessions. There the therapist helps caregivers identify points of emotional reactivity during the play session, helps caregivers identify and talk through possible reasons for their reaction from their own backgrounds, and helps caregivers understand the child's behaviors from trauma and attachment perspectives. Through these discussions, caregivers become more self-aware and more intentional about self-regulation.

Attunement

At the core of the empathic listening and child-centered imaginary play skills is caregiver attunement. A focus on these skills pushes caregivers to attune to and reflect the child's inner experience, including feelings, desires, and intentions. Child-centered imaginary play causes caregivers to flex their attunement "muscles" as they strive to play in the ways they sense the child wants or needs them to play. During the postplay feedback sessions, the therapist fosters caregiver attunement by engaging caregivers in reflective discussions regarding the meaning of the child's play and what might be going on for the child (as viewed through developmental and trauma lenses). Furthermore, the therapist models attunement in interaction with caregivers by attending to the caregivers' internal experience.

Consistency of Response, and Routines and Rituals

Utilizing the structuring skill, caregivers learn to create consistency and predictability during play sessions by providing the same introduction and concluding statement to play sessions and by providing a 5-minute and a 1-minute warning before concluding the session. Furthermore, the playroom is set up in the same way with the same toys for each play session. Caregivers are taught to generalize the structuring skills outside of play sessions by creating consistency and predictability in the child's schedule and environment, and to be particularly attentive to trauma triggers for the child when doing so. For example, children who have experienced complex trauma frequently become anxious and fearful at bedtime. In addition to common bedtime rituals, caregivers might do a bedroom check with a child to be sure the room is "safe," turn on extra night lights, leave the door open a crack, and give the child a stuffed animal to watch over him or her (Arvidson et al., 2011).

Self-Regulation

Affect Identification

Using the empathic listening skill, caregivers verbally reflect a child's feelings, intentions, and desires throughout play sessions, helping the child become attuned to and accepting of his or her own internal experience.

Affect Modulation

In play sessions, children are provided with various toys that tend to lead to up-regulation of arousal (e.g., bop bags, swords, aggressive animals) and various toys that tend to lead to down-regulation of arousal (e.g., a sandtray, baby dolls, bottles). In the safety of the play session, children who may initially be fearful of particular states of arousal are able to experiment gradually with different arousal states, and to experience an increasing sense of mastery over those states. Caregiver-imposed limits provide children with opportunities to regulate behavior and emotion; caregiver reflections reinforce the children's emerging regulation abilities (e.g., "You are really mad that you can't color on the wall, but you figured out something that you could color on").

Affect Expression

As children become increasingly aware of and accepting of their emotional experience as a result of caregiver reflections, it becomes easier for children to express their feelings. In many cases, as children become accustomed to caregiver reflections, they begin to provide their own narrations of thoughts and feelings in later stages of FT. In generalizing the empathic listening skill, caregivers are taught how to continue to assist their children in understanding, modulating, and expressing emotions in conjunction with everyday experience.

Competency

Executive Functions

The nondirective play sessions in FT provide a fertile context for children to develop problem-solving skills. In this context, children experience control over their environment and can take on simple problems at first (e.g., building a basic tower), then increasingly difficult problems (e.g., putting a dart correctly in a dart gun) as they gain confidence. Large barriers to problem solving for children who have experienced trauma are poor frustration tolerance and a limited ability to persist in the face of challenge. In FT, caregivers' reflections help scaffold children's problem solving, helping the children regulate frustration and sustain focus and effort. Furthermore, esteem-building reflections by caregivers (e.g., "It was so hard to figure out how to get the dart to go into the gun, but you turned it until you figured it out, and now you got it to work!") help children consolidate their emerging skills and develop confidence.

Self-Development and Identity

Caregivers' reflections about children's internal experience help children develop a sense of being unique, as well as an internal acceptance of their uniqueness. A positive sense of self is also fostered as children gain mastery over their environment, reinforced by caregiver reflections of their positive feelings (e.g., "You are really proud you were able to make that tower so high").

Trauma Experience Integration

A central objective of FT is to create a context in which children can "play through" past traumatic and distressing experiences. Within the context of the caregiver–child play sessions, a child is able to play through and gain mastery over previously overwhelming memories, experiences, and emotions, and by so doing to integrate fragmented internal experience.

Supportive Research

A number of positive child outcomes have been demonstrated in FT treatment programs, including increased emotional expression, decreased depression and anxiety, increased self-confidence, and decreased behavioral problems. Additional positive outcomes include increased caregiver sensitivity, empathy, and acceptance; decreased caregiver stress; and improved caregiver–child relationships (see VanFleet, Ryan, & Smith, 2005, for a review). A recent study (Topham, Wampler, Titus, & Rolling, 2010) examining the predictors of treatment success in FT found that higher levels of caregiver distress and poorer child emotion regulation at pretest were predictive of significant reductions in child behavior problems across treatment. Similarly, poor caregiver emotion regulation at pretest was predictive of significant increases in caregiver acceptance across treatment. Although research has not yet examined whether FT leads to improvement in caregiver and child emotion regulation, this study indicates that caregivers and children with poorer emotion regulation (as is commonly the case with children who have experienced complex trauma) are likely to experience positive gains in FT, leading to speculation that the positive changes are a function of improving emotion regulation.

Case Vignettes

The identifying information in the case illustrations that follow has been changed, and the illustrations may represent composites of several families. All of them represent realistic depictions of the FT process at work, however.

Tory

Tory was 3 years old when she was removed from the care of her biological mother. She had been burned on the bottom half of her body by a hot bath, and had been in a major medical facility for many months healing from the effects of this abusive experience. Tory was referred for play therapy due to the trauma of sustaining her injuries, the numerous painful medical procedures related to those injuries, her lengthy hospital stays, and the loss of her primary caregiver. More surgeries were expected in her future. In addition to the abuse, Tory's primary caregiver, who had cared for her since she was an infant, died of a heart attack when Tory was alone with her. Furthermore, her dependency placement took her away from her two siblings.

Tory met her new foster family when she was still in the hospital. When she presented for treatment, she was a shy, introverted, and withdrawn child who had considerable developmental delays in most areas of functioning. She had significant communication problems and was very difficult to understand when she attempted to speak. The treatment plan focused on three goals: (1) assisting the family with developing a secure attachment, (2) helping Tory to heal from the past trauma, and (3) helping her with her developmental issues. At the time the family presented for outpatient psychotherapy, Tory was fitting into the foster family quite well. There were no significant behavioral problems, except that she seemed to have nightmares related to her prior trauma, and she often cried with frustration if she could not master things. Tory was described by her foster mother as lovable, persistent, resilient, and independent. It was mutually decided that FT would be the primary intervention to promote a healthy relationship and attachment, while working on developmental and trauma issues. After the FT process was well established, a number of additional directive play therapy interventions were woven into the treatment to work on some of her more specific issues.

Tory's play was delayed for her age, most likely as a result of her history. She moved from toy to toy without any consistent themes or sequence. She did not engage her foster mother or father during play sessions with them, but kept her back to them. The therapist encouraged the foster parents, during their respective play sessions with her, to move to a position at her side where they were better able to see her play and make eye contact with Tory as they empathically listened.

Trauma themes emerged early in the parent–child play sessions. Without talking, Tory played very roughly with the baby dolls. She shook the babies repeatedly and hit them. She held them down and pressed on them. She threw them across the room and piled them on top of each other. She then hit the bop bag and aggressively pushed everything away from her. Themes seemed to be related to power, control, aggression, and prior trauma.

As FT play sessions with her foster parents continued, Tory's play became less chaotic and more focused on developmental and trauma mastery and on relationship building. As the play expanded, Tory showed patterns and themes related to exploration, trust building, mastery, problem solving, developmental play, relationship, nurturance, and self-identity. She became interested in making sure the doll babies always had enough food and were well cared for. She then moved to water play, pouring water into different containers and spilling it. Although this play often represents developmental mastery, it was especially significant for Tory, because she had initially been afraid of the sounds of water being poured. This fear may have been related to her traumatic experience.

As Tory expanded her interest in the toys in the playroom, she put on many masks, trying to trick her foster parents. She then removed them to show her parents that it was really her underneath, saying, "It's *me!*" Hiding behind and trying on different identities constitute a common theme among children who are working on developing a secure attachment. At first, Tory had been afraid of all the masks in the playroom, but her tolerance of them and other "scary" toys grew as her anxiety decreased within the relationships with her foster mom and dad.

Tory eventually found the emergency vehicles and the hospital set. She began putting figures inside the ambulances. After the play sessions switched to the home setting, she began playing with the medical kit. At first she played with these items by herself, giving herself shots. After a couple of sessions like this, she hesitantly began treating her foster mom.

As the play sessions continued and Tory worked through her traumatic experiences, the attachment with her foster parents grew, and Tory's play resembled what one would expect of a child at her developmental level. She was then able to attend preschool, and was adopted by her foster parents. Later, the family also adopted her two siblings, and the parents held regular one-to-one filial play sessions with all three children. The mother called 9 months after discharge to report that everyone in the family looked forward to their continuing weekly play sessions. The play sessions, coupled with the parents' use of their now-generalized skills in daily life, were still yielding excellent results.

Lilly

Lilly was removed from her young mother's care for neglect and was placed in the foster care system. This first placement was found to be abusive, and the child was removed and then placed in kinship care with her grandmother. Most unfortunately, for a second time, Lilly had been placed in an abusive home; this time, she received such severe injuries that she had to be hospitalized for several months. Lilly suffered brain injury so severe that part of her brain had to be removed to allow for swelling. When she was well enough to be released, she was unable to walk and had lost the use of one of her arms and a hand. The grandmother who had perpetrated the abuse was found guilty and sentenced to many years in prison.

Given Lilly's history of attachment disruption, severe abuse, inconsistent care, and medical trauma, it was not surprising that she had become a child with challenging behaviors. She was introduced to her new foster mothers while still in the hospital. One of her new parents had to be out of town for the first several months of her placement, further interfering with the development of a secure attachment. Moreover, Lilly's medical treatment continued, with numerous additional hospital stays and difficult treatments.

When Lilly presented for therapy, she had already been adopted by the foster mothers, who reported concerns relating to anxiety, temper tantrums, fearfulness, oppositional behaviors, and defiance. Lilly constantly tested limits and tried to triangulate her parents. Her well-intentioned adoptive parents invited her birth mother, her other grandmother (not the perpetrator of the abuse), and her half-brother to share vacations with them once a year. After these visits, Lilly became especially dysregulated and difficult to manage. The adoptive family asked for help to assist Lilly in resolving her trauma-related issues, regulating her emotional reactions, and controlling her maladaptive behaviors. They also requested assistance with attachment issues. FT was the primary intervention used with this family, although other play interventions were used as well to facilitate progress.

Both parents attended every training and therapy session. It took Lilly several weeks of parent–child play before she trusted that she could actually do "almost anything you want." Her early play involved frequent checking to make sure the parent playing with her was happy with what she was doing—a common theme in children who have anxious attachments. Soon Lilly started to take risks related to aggressive play, such as shooting guns and trying some disrespectful words.

Once Lilly began to trust that her mothers meant what they said and were accepting of her play, she expanded her play themes. She began to play aggressively with the bop bag, beating it and then pretending to shoot one or the other of her moms repeatedly, telling her she was a bad person. Within just a couple of play sessions, she began asking her moms to join her in fighting the "bad people" together. There was soon evidence of behavioral improvement, and the parents developed confidence in generalizing some of the play session skills to daily life.

Just as the significant improvements seemed to be consolidating, Lilly had to attend a rehabilitation program that seemed to trigger her sensory memory of her traumatic experiences, resulting in a huge escalation of her problematic behaviors. The therapist helped the parents, who were confused by the escalation, understand Lilly's extreme reactions and behavioral regression in the context of her trauma. Together, they developed strategies for showing understanding of Lilly's triggered emotions while managing her behaviors.

During this period, Lilly had a particularly difficult week. She had numerous outbursts and tantrums, was oppositional much of the time, and showed great fear at bedtime. The parents, with the clear understanding of trauma gained from FT, discovered that the time of year coincided with Lilly's initial traumatic hospitalization and her entry into her new family. They suspected that another powerful sensory memory had been awakened.

The therapist suggested a more directive play therapy activity to assist Lilly with discharging some of the distress she felt about her frequently mentioned abusive grandmother. In this family play intervention, Lilly drew a large picture of the perpetrator. Lilly, her mothers, and the therapist threw wet wads of toilet paper at the perpetrator, simultaneously shouting at the symbolic perpetrator that she could no longer hurt children and that she would be in jail for a long time. Lilly's parents also let Lilly know that they would never let the perpetrator near her again. Lilly started yelling at the symbolic perpetrator she had drawn, telling the paper representation of her grandmother what she would no longer tolerate from her, and at the same time talking about what her grandmother had done to her. Lilly exclaimed loudly, "She almost killed me!" As her moms joined in, she got bolder and more intense, using three complete rolls of toilet paper.

After this 20-minute activity, Lilly had an FT session with one of her mothers. Interesting themes after the directive play emerged. She asked this mom to help her build a double-thick wall of large cardboard blocks, indicating that they would be safe in there. She said that there was only one way in and one way out. Lilly proclaimed that she was the boss of that place and no one was welcome except her two moms. Her mother accurately reflected that it was a safe place; they were all together; and nothing bad could happen to them within those double walls. When Lilly left the playroom, after giving her mom a hug, she seemed relaxed and calm. The parents reported seeing a huge improvement in her affect and behavior after this session. Lilly's play became less intense, and she focused on mastery, problem solving, and her relationship with her mothers. She seemed happy, laughing frequently both during her play sessions and in daily life. The gains were maintained for the duration of her therapy and thereafter.

Joshua

At age 4, Joshua was removed from his mother's home for neglect and placed in the custody of child protective services. When he was referred to therapy 6 months later, Joshua had been removed from several foster homes due to behavioral problems. There was a possibility that he had been exposed to drug and alcohol abuse by adults in the mother's home. It was definitely known that Joshua had been exposed to pornographic material and had witnessed parental sexual activity, including incest: He told the therapist that he had tried to stop his grandfather from having sex with his mother, but he had been unable to stop it. He also described being sexually abused by two men who frequently visited his home. Joshua told his therapist that he "was kicked out of school for being 'bad.' "

Joshua had been diagnosed with attention-deficit/hyperactivity disorder, oppositional defiant disorder, and reactive attachment disorder; his diagnosis also included a notation for "neglect of child." His first foster mother had identified issues related to impulsivity, aggressiveness, oppositional behavior, and destructive behaviors. She reported that Joshua seemed to exhibit a lack of conscience and cause-and-effect thinking, and that he had been cruel to animals in their home.

The school had reported that Joshua was urinating on things and exhibiting inappropriate sexualized behaviors. At home, he played with dolls and stuffed animals in a sexualized way, and his caseworker reported that he inappropriately touched other children. He wet his pants and masturbated frequently.

Initially, the therapist attempted to involve Joshua's foster parents in FT, but his placements were too unstable; his behavior was so dysregulated that the first few foster families would not keep him in their homes. The therapist used individual CCPT until there was more stability in his placements and relationships. From the start, Joshua's play was extremely trauma-based, including lots of aggression and sexualized play, especially after visits with his biological mother and grandfather. His play was chaotic and intense. He was often very agitated as he played. Joshua's play themes related to sex, protection, danger, anxiety, safety, rescue, power, control, aggression, good versus evil, limit testing, exploration, relationship, and loss. Limit setting was frequently needed during the play sessions to keep Joshua safe and regulated.

After 6 months of weekly CCPT sessions and disrupted placements, Joshua was placed in an appropriate foster home. His newest foster mother was eager to learn and conduct FT play sessions with him. During the training phase, the therapist added an additional mock training session to assist her with the expectation and management of traumatic play. Two FT play sessions were conducted on a weekly basis—one at home and the other in the playroom under the therapist's supervision, because Joshua's play was very trauma-based, intense, and disturbing to the mom. She needed the therapist's support and feedback to help her understand the play themes and their relationship to his traumatic experience and behavioral issues.

Joshua's play sessions often focused on a bad or dangerous situation, like a robbery or catastrophe of giant proportions. Often his foster mother was the victim in the imaginary play. He played the role of the strong and powerful "good guy" who dispatched the villain or put him in jail. For several sessions at the beginning of the parent–child play sessions, Joshua shifted between the roles of victim and victimizer. This is a frequent theme for children who have been traumatized, as they try to work out and make sense of their experience. For several sessions, Joshua tied up the "bad guy" (bop bag) with a rope and pretended to cut off his private parts, asking him, "Now how do you like that?" He then covered the bop bag's wounds with many Band-Aids. After this he put the bad person in "jail" and asked his foster mother to help him get "bad people." Together they made sure the world was a safe place.

FT was very beneficial for this child. There were positive changes in behavioral self-regulation, attention, focus, peer relationships, and general well-being. Joshua became closer and more trusting as his attachment with his foster mother grew.

Joshua's play themes greatly expanded as his trust grew. At the beginning of his therapeutic work, his play was chaotic, disorganized, and non-sequential. Sexual themes were a frequent focus in his behaviors and his play. Almost immediately after beginning FT, there was a reduction in sexual acting out and sexual play themes, as well as a reduction in sexually inappropriate language both in and out of the playroom.

As Joshua's play in the playroom became less hyperactive, impulsive, and chaotic, and more organized, so did his general functioning, with a few exceptions. He was now capable of playing out themes that were intentional and focused. His play themes became more sequential and healthier.

As FT sessions continued, Joshua's play themes focused on relationship, attachment, mastery, and self-esteem. Some play themes that are common to children with histories of trauma and attachment disruption were still evident; however, they were now accompanied by positive themes, including nurturance, healing, family and problem solving. For example, Joshua often asked his mother to become the mother of the doll babies, and together they cared for them—giving them bottles and food, and making sure they were tucked in for naptime. He also prepared food for his mom, asking her what she would like and making sure that she had everything that she needed.

As FT play sessions continued at home, more directive play therapy sessions were conducted in the office. These focused on safe and appropriate touch; understanding what to do when touch is not safe; peer relationship issues; impulse control and self-regulation; attention and focus; understanding foster placement and the loss of his mother and extended family; feelings identification; and sharing feelings appropriately. There was also work on stress management, relaxation techniques, and relationship and attachment issues. Several sessions of canine-assisted play therapy focused on creating relationships and treating animals kindly. In one of their last office sessions, Joshua and his foster mom painted each other's faces with face paint, looking into each other's eyes, smiling, laughing, and asking the therapist to take a picture. Shortly afterward, Joshua's foster mom became Joshua's adoptive mom. FT sessions continued at home, with ongoing benefits for the mom, the child, and the relationship.

Conclusion

Children whose lives have been marred by maltreatment and attachment disruptions struggle with a variety of maladaptive emotional reactions, behaviors, and relationship patterns. Their caregivers face significant challenges as they try to create a safe environment in which to overcome trauma and build secure attachments. FT offers an ideal intervention to address the complex needs of both children and their caregivers. Under the supervision of an appropriately trained FT practitioner, caregivers learn to conduct special nondirective play sessions with children, creating the safety and understanding needed for children to process and overcome prior trauma and gradually develop healthy attachments with caregiving adults.

In this chapter, we have provided a brief description of FT, which integrates family therapy with play therapy. We have shown how FT fits within the ARC treatment framework for complex trauma by addressing caregiver management of affect, attunement, consistency of response, and routines and rituals. After an overview of the relevant research, we have concluded with case vignettes of FT in action. Because FT addresses both child and family needs so thoroughly and effectively, it should be considered a leading therapeutic modality for children with complex trauma and their caregivers.

REFERENCES

Arvidson, J., Kinniburgh, K., Howard, K., Spinazzola, J., Strothers, H., Evans, M., . . . Blaustein, M. (2011). Treatment of complex trauma in young children: Developmental and cultural considerations in application of the ARC intervention model. *Journal of Child and Adolescent Trauma, 4,* 34–51.

Axline, V. M. (1969). *Play therapy* (rev. ed.). New York: Ballantine Books.

Blaustein, M. E., & Kinniburgh, K. M. (2010). *Treating traumatic stress in children and adolescents: How to foster resilience through attachment, self-regulation, and competency.* New York: Guilford Press.

Busch, A. L., & Lieberman, A. F. (2007). Attachment and trauma: An integrated approach to treating young children exposed to family violence. In D. Oppenheim & D. F. Goldsmith (Eds.), *Attachment theory in clinical work with children: Bridging the gap between research and practice* (pp. 139–171). New York: Guilford Press.

Cochran, N. H., Nordling, W. J., & Cochran, J. L. (2010). *Child-centered play therapy: A practical guide to developing therapeutic relationships with children.* Hoboken, NJ: Wiley.

Ginsberg, B. G. (2003). An integrated holistic model of child-centered family therapy. In R. VanFleet & L. F. Guerney (Eds.), *Casebook of Filial Therapy* (pp. 21–47). Boiling Springs, PA: Play Therapy Press.

Guerney, B. G., Jr. (1964). Filial Therapy: Description and rationale. *Journal of Consulting Psychology, 28,* 303–310.

Guerney, L. F. (2003). The history, principles, and empirical basis of Filial Therapy. In R. VanFleet & L. F. Guerney (Eds.), *Casebook of Filial Therapy* (pp. 1–19). Boiling Springs, PA: Play Therapy Press.

Guerney, L. F., & Ryan, V. M. (2013). *Group Filial Therapy: A complete guide to teaching parents to play therapeutically with their children.* Philadelphia: Kingsley.

Kinniburgh, K., Blaustein, M., Spinazzola, J., & van der Kolk, B. A. (2005). Attachment, self-regulation, and competency. *Psychiatric Annals, 35*(5), 424–430.

Landreth, G. L. (2012). *Play therapy: The art of the relationship* (3rd ed.). New York: Routledge.

Topham, G. L., Wampler, K. S., Titus, G., & Rolling, E. (2011). Predicting parent and child outcomes of a Filial Therapy program. *International Journal of Play Therapy, 20,* 79–93.

VanFleet, R. (2006a). *Introduction to Filial Therapy* [DVD]. Boiling Springs, PA: Play Therapy Press.

VanFleet, R. (2006b). Short-term play therapy for adoptive families: Facilitating adjustment and attachment with Filial Therapy. In H. G. Kaduson & C. E. Schaefer (Eds.), *Short-term play therapy interventions for children* (2nd ed., pp. 145–168). New York: Guilford Press.

VanFleet, R. (2011a). Filial Therapy: What every play therapist should know. Part One of a series. *Play Therapy: Magazine of the British Association of Play Therapists, 65,* 16–19.

VanFleet, R. (2011b). Filial Therapy: What every play therapist should know. Part Two of a series. *Play Therapy: Magazine of the British Association of Play Therapists, 66,* 7–10.

VanFleet, R. (2011c). Filial Therapy: What every play therapist should know. Part Three of a series. *Play Therapy: Magazine of the British Association of Play Therapists, 67,* 18–21.

VanFleet, R. (2012). *A parent's handbook of Filial Therapy: Building strong families with play* (2nd ed.). Boiling Springs, PA: Play Therapy Press.

VanFleet, R. (2013). *Filial Therapy: Strengthening parent–child relationships through play* (3rd ed.). Sarasota, FL: Professional Resource Press.

VanFleet, R., Ryan, S. D., & Smith, S. K. (2005). Filial Therapy: A critical review. In L. A. Reddy, T. M. Files-Hall, & C. E. Schaefer (Eds.), *Empirically based play interventions for children* (pp. 241–264). Washington, DC: American Psychological Association.

VanFleet, R., & Sniscak, C. C. (2003). Filial therapy for attachment-disrupted and disordered children. In R. VanFleet & L. F. Guerney (Eds.), *Casebook of Filial Therapy* (pp. 279–308). Boiling Springs, PA: Play Therapy Press.

VanFleet, R., Sniscak, C., & Faa-Thompson, T. (in press). *Filial Therapy group program for foster and adoptive families: A practitioner's manual* [working title]. Boiling Springs, PA: Play Therapy Press.

VanFleet, R., Sywulak, A. E., & Sniscak, C. C. (2010). *Child-centered play therapy*. New York: Guilford Press.

VanFleet, R., & Topham, G. (2011). Filial Therapy for maltreated and neglected children: Integration of family therapy and play therapy. In A. Drewes, S. C. Bratton, & C. E. Schaefer (Eds.), *Integrative play therapy* (pp. 153–175). Hoboken, NJ: Wiley.

Wilson, K., & Ryan, V. (2005). *Play therapy: A non-directive approach for children and adolescents* (2nd ed.). London: Elsevier.

CHAPTER 9

Theraplay in Reunification Following Relational Trauma

Phyllis B. Booth
Sandra Lindaman
Marlo L.-R. Winstead

Isaiah, a 6-year-old boy living in a low-income, chronically violent neighborhood, was found looking for food in the garbage. When the police took him home, they found his mother incoherent and high on crack. The child was immediately placed in foster care and had no contact with his mother. One month later, the foster mother contacted a therapist; she was concerned about Isaiah's aggression, defiance, unresponsiveness to affection, and extremely controlling behavior at home and school. Theraplay with Isaiah then began. Over the course of the next 6 months, the biological mother abstained from drugs, and her life became more stable. The court allowed supervised visits with the goal of reunification. Although Isaiah was calmer in his foster home, he fell back into patterns of aggression, defiance, opposition, and intense mood swings during visits with his mother. His mother was attempting to regain custody and to use the new strategies she was learning in parenting class, but could not seem to get control of the situation. The therapist started to include the biological mother in therapy, and discovered that she had been in foster care herself. In both her biological and her foster families, she had experienced attachment disruptions and severe abuse.

As therapists planning treatment for the relational trauma sustained by Isaiah's family, we asked ourselves:

- What impact had the lack of safety and responsive caregiving had in the lives of Isaiah and his mother?
- What would help this foster mother meet Isaiah's needs during placement?
- Would it be possible to support Isaiah's biological mother enough to make reunification feasible?
- What kinds of treatment would facilitate socioemotional health and healing for this mother and her son?

The Theraplay®[1] model would answer these questions in this way: Because the mother had not received responsive caregiving or felt safe as a child, she was unable to play her part in the healthy interaction that would have led to a secure attachment and long-term mental health for her son. Both she and Isaiah needed to share new experiences that would change their views and expectations, and to create relationships that would meet their needs for safety, intersubjectivity, regulation, mutual enjoyment, and ongoing healthy development. The first step would be to provide these experiences for Isaiah and his foster mother. The question of whether Isaiah's mother could achieve the stability and mental health needed to make reunification possible would depend on the quality of support she receives and on her own inner strength.

In this chapter, we describe the Theraplay approach to working with children and parents who have suffered relational trauma. We start by discussing the nature, impact, and treatment of relational trauma; we then present the Theraplay model, its history, its theoretical basis, and a typical treatment plan. An account of the Theraplay treatment with Isaiah, his foster mother, and his biological mother concludes the chapter. Theraplay was supplemented at crucial points by other modalities, but contributed in large part to the success of the family's treatment.

The Impact and Treatment of Relational Trauma

The mental health field has begun to look at the significant effect of trauma on the relationships and ongoing neuroaffective development of young children. Terms commonly used to describe this new view of trauma are: *developmental trauma*, referring to the interpersonal and developmentally adverse nature of child trauma (van der Kolk, 2005); *complex trauma*, describing seven domains of impairment of critical developmental experiences (Cook, Blaustein, Spinazzola, & van der Kolk, 2003); and *relational trauma*, acknowledging that the source of neglect or abuse is often the primary caregiver (Schore, 2001). In this chapter, we use *relational trauma* to

---

[1]Theraplay is a registered service mark of The Theraplay Institute, Evanston, Illinois.

describe the experience of Isaiah and his biological mother. In their childhoods, each of them was faced with the paralyzing dilemma that the very caregivers who should have been the source of comfort and protection were instead the source of neglect and pain.

Allan Schore (2003) describes how the preverbal emotional communication between parent (or other primary caregiver) and infant in a healthy attachment relationship shapes the maturation of the infant's right brain. The parent attends closely to the child and follows the minute facial, vocal, and gestural cues of the infant. As the parent attunes to the ups and downs of the infant's bodily arousal, the two gradually learn each other's rhythms and together create a new, specific shared rhythm. Through this moment-to-moment dance of attunement, they come to understand each other. Any misstep in this process creates a moment of stress, which the sensitive parent repairs with a return to synchrony. Through this process, the child becomes capable of regulating positive and negative emotions as he or she grows.

The emotional communication of the abusive and/or neglectful parent is less synchronized and less playful. Reactions to the infant's stressful emotions are minimal, unpredictable, inappropriate, or rejecting. Schore (2003) notes,

> Instead of modulating, she induces extreme levels of stimulation and arousal, and because she provides no interactive repair the infant's intense negative states last for long periods of time. Prolonged negative states are toxic for infants and although they possess some capacity to modulate low-intensity negative affect states, these states continue to escalate in intensity, frequency and duration. (p. 124)

When a caregiver does not connect with a child's active bid for attunement, the child experiences shame. When that shameful reaction is paired with a caregiver's sustained anger or lack of repair, the child experiences a humiliation that is damaging to the developing brain and to the regulation of emotion. This child enters a hyper- or hypoaroused physical and emotional state outside the autonomic nervous system's window of tolerance, resulting in reduced ability to function adaptively and flexibly (Siegel, 2012). In summary, when early trauma alters the development of the right brain the child's ability to process socioemotional information, regulate body states, and cope with emotional stress is impaired, leading to serious consequences for the development of the bodily and emotional self (Schore, 2003).

How should we treat such relational trauma? Schore and Schore (2008) advise that therapists must understand the importance of early dyadic regulation, right-hemisphere development, and the formation of implicit procedural memory. Effective intervention should focus on the preverbal, facial, vocal, and gestural communications that occur within the healthy attachment relationship. This focus will lead to optimal development of the limbic system and right-brain functions, and ultimately of the child's affect regulation (Schore, 2003).

Theraplay treatment, as described in this chapter, is a re-creation of the positive emotional communication of the securely attached parent and child through its emphasis on attuned, synchronous, and reciprocal right-brain-based interaction, appropriate up- and down-regulating to widen the window of tolerance, attention to bids for attunement, opportunities for repair in the here-and-now, and reflection with and guidance of the parent to move into a healthier relationship with the child. Appropriate modifications of Theraplay for trauma have been expanded in the third edition of the Theraplay text (Rubin, Lender, & Miller, 2010).

The Theraplay Model

Theraplay takes as its model the sensitive, responsive, playful give-and-take that occurs naturally between parents and their healthy young children—the kind of interaction that creates secure attachment, supports healthy brain development, and leads to long-term mental health. The goal is to develop regulation, social skills, positive internal working models for parents and child, and secure attachment through the emotional communication of reciprocal right-brain interaction.

History of Theraplay

Theraplay, developed in the early 1970s as a mental health treatment for preschoolers, has a history of meeting attachment needs before the term *attachment* was widely used and understood. In 1969, Ann Jernberg, a clinical psychologist, was awarded the contract to provide psychological services to the Head Start program in Chicago. In that first summer, our team identified a large number of children who needed help; we also found that there was little chance of meeting their needs within existing treatment centers. Jernberg came up with a simple solution for this problem: We would train lively young people to engage in one-on-one play with each troubled child. We had no toys, no games, and no play therapy tools. In each case, there was just an unhappy child and a lively adult who was prepared to pay full attention to the child and to entice him or her into interactive play.

We found that this kind of play worked magic. Soon, unhappy, withdrawn children become livelier, more outgoing, and more responsive; angry, aggressive, acting-out children settled down and began to interact appropriately with others. It was obvious that these children felt much better about themselves and were ready to engage with others in friendly interaction. They became lively, alert youngsters who did well in school (Jernberg, 1979; Jernberg & Booth, 1999).

John Bowlby's just-published theory of attachment (Bowlby, 1969/1982) offered us a partial explanation for our success: In his terms, we had changed the children's *internal working models*. Children learn about themselves and what they can expect from others in the repeated face-to-face experience of interaction with important adults in their world. The unhappy children we were working with came to us with negative views of themselves and fears that they couldn't count on a caring response from adults. By presenting such a child with a new experience of feeling safe and being responded to, admired, and enjoyed, a caring adult had created a new and more hopeful internal working model for that child.

Presently, mental health and education professionals in the United States and 37 other countries in a variety of settings practice Theraplay with children ranging in age from infancy to adolescence. Current best practice is described in the third edition of the Theraplay text (Booth & Jernberg, 2010). The Group Theraplay model was developed (Rubin & Tregay, 1989) and expanded and described in further publications (Munns, 2000, 2009). Sunshine Circles (Schieffer, 2012) is a classroom application for conveying the Theraplay principles of connection, cooperation, and socioemotional growth. Theraplay training and certification programs are administered by The Theraplay Institute (*www.theraplay.org*). In 2009, Theraplay was rated as demonstrating "promising research evidence" by the California Evidence-Based Clearinghouse for Child Welfare (2012). Its rating of 3 on a 5-point scale indicates that Theraplay meets the following standards: No empirical or theoretical evidence exists that Theraplay has a substantial risk of harming clients, as compared to its possible benefits; a manual is available; two peer-reviewed studies utilizing some form of control have been published (Siu, 2009; Wettig, Coleman, & Geider, 2011); and the outcome data support the benefits of Theraplay.

In addition, applications published since 2000 include Theraplay in residential care for youth with severe behavior problems (Robison, Lindaman, Clemmons, Doyle-Buckwalter, & Ryan, 2009), in a domestic violence shelter (Bennett, Shiner, & Ryan, 2006), in the Finnish SOS Village long-term fostering project (Mäkelä & Vierikko, 2004), with substance-abusing mothers (Salo, Lampi, & Lindaman, 2010), in adoption (Booth, 2000), and with children on the autism spectrum (Bundy-Myrow, 2012). The Theraplay model has been compared favorably to other parent–child interaction methods (Mäkelä & Salo, 2011). Combinations of Theraplay and other treatment modalities include Theraplay and dyadic developmental psychotherapy (DDP; Becker-Weidman & Schell, 2005), Theraplay and eye movement desensitization and reprocessing (EMDR; Gomez & Jernberg, 2013), and Theraplay and play therapy trauma treatment (Booth & Gil, 2011).

Dimensions of Theraplay

We turn now to describe the basic concepts of Theraplay and the research and theory that explain its effectiveness. We distinguish four basic dimensions of healthy parenting that we use to assess and to plan treatment, based on the specific needs of the parents and child: *structure, engagement, nurture*, and *challenge*.

Structure

Guidance and structure provide a sense of safety, organization, and regulation for both the child and the parents. We respond to the child's need for dyadic regulation of his or her experience, and for having an adult who can be counted on first to keep the child safe and later to set limits and provide a model for appropriate behavior. We structure simple, playful activities—such as blowing cotton balls back and forth, popping bubbles, and making a stack of hands together—using signals for when to start and variations in pacing and predictability to meet the child's need for regulation. We help parents (who may themselves be dysregulated) to experience the comfort of being guided in their interactions with their child, and in turn to learn to take the lead. In the case of neglect/trauma, establishing safety is particularly important. Many traumatized children exhibit controlling behavior, which comes from a need to be safe rather than from a need to be oppositional. We consider a young child's efforts to be prematurely autonomous and in charge of interactions to be a burden that the guided interaction of Theraplay can relieve.

SUPPORTING RESEARCH AND THEORY

The development of a healthy relationship requires the presence of a caring adult who can make the baby feel that this adult can provide safety, support, and guidance (Bowlby, 1988). Innate capacities exist in both parent and child to keep them close in order to be safe. If it were not so, babies could never survive (Bowlby, 1969/1982). During the first 2 years of life, repeated patterns of interaction create neural circuits and their corresponding internal working models of attachment relationships. As the child enters the second year of life, adult guidance and clear rules provide the foundation for self-regulation, resilience, and self-confidence (Baumrind, 1991; Grotberg, 1997). Rather than creating dependency, adult guidance and secure relationships are the foundation of self-reliance; "autonomy grows out of attachment" (Shahmoon-Shanok, 1997, p. 38).

In order to change the negative patterns of a child who has experienced relational trauma and to create mature neural circuits, it is necessary to provide a similarly direct, interactive, and sensitive emotional experience that challenges the old patterns and expectations (Hart, 2008; Schore, 2003).

New understanding of experience-dependent brain development and of the effects of neglect and trauma on the developing brain supports our focus on meeting the child's younger emotional needs, on finding ways to calm the dysregulated child, and on creating feelings of safety for the traumatized child (Perry, 2006; van der Kolk, 2005). Brain research places affect regulation at the center of healthy development (Schore, 1994).

Engagement

Engaging activities—such as peek-a-boo, clapping games, decorating each other with feathers, or "flying" the child on the adult's knees—create connection, optimal arousal, and shared joy. This playful, responsive interaction gives the child a new experience of his or her body and how to interact with others in a lively, coordinated manner. Theraplay treatment is geared to the child's current state of arousal and makes use of the nonverbal language of the right brain—facial expression, eye contact, movement, rhythm, and touch—to create the deep levels of neural integration that must be developed before it is possible to communicate on the mentalizing and narrative levels later on. We create "now moments" of intense connection and shared meaning, which lead to a major shift in internal organization and sense of self (Mäkelä, 2003; Tronick et al., 1998). We respond in an attuned and reflective manner to both the parent and child; in turn, we help the parent respond with synchrony and affective resonance to the child's readiness for interaction. If there has been relational trauma, the parent and child may never have experienced this joyful companionship. It is therefore particularly important that the therapist guide the parent in creating such experiences. In order to respond sensitively, parents must be able to reflect on their own and their children's internal states, and to understand the link between the children's behaviors and underlying mental states; parents who have little positive experience with emotional communication and connection in their own lives find this difficult to do (Fonagy, Gergely, Jurist, & Target, 2002; Slade, 2002).

SUPPORTING RESEARCH AND THEORY

When babies seek interaction and parents delight in the smiles and laughter they share with their children, a second innate capacity is demonstrated: the drive to share meaning and the joy of companionship. The process of *intersubjectivity* occurs in face-to-face human interaction resulting in a shared state of feelings and actions, making it possible for two people to synchronize their movements and to resonate with one another's feelings (Trevarthen & Aitken, 2001). In responding to a child, a sensitive parent attunes to the level and tone of the child's emotion, or "vitality affect" (Stern, 1985). An infant learns about his or her own feelings by seeing them mirrored in a parent's face (Winnicott, 1971). This sharing of emotional experience leads to empathy and a sense of connection (Stern, 1995). Mirror neurons also contribute to our understanding of the intentions of others (Iacoboni, 2008).

Stephen Porges's (2011) *polyvagal theory* provides insights into the way the human autonomic nervous system unconsciously mediates social engagement, trust, and intimacy. Well-defined neural circuits—particularly the vagal system, connecting facial, throat, heart, and stomach muscles involved in communication and emotional processing—support shared social engagement behaviors and the defensive strategies of fight, flight, or freeze. All of these capacities make it possible for babies and their responsive parents to establish an intimate, intersubjective experience in which they are present to each other and share meaning and companionship (Hughes, 2007; Siegel, 2006; Trevarthen & Aitken, 2001). Feeling safe, as discussed above in regard to the structure dimension, is essential to the activation of the social engagement system. Children who feel anxious and fearful do not readily enter into rhythm, resonance, and synchrony, and therefore find it difficult to understand the intentions of others and join in the interactive dance (Hart, 2008). Members of families who are not securely attached become hesitant to engage in intersubjective experience with one another because it does not feel safe or rewarding (Hughes, 2007).

Nurture

Nurturing experiences—such as caring for hurts, feeding, singing a lullaby, or making powder handprints—help calm and regulate the child and create feelings of self-worth. When adults respond empathically to a child's need for comfort and reassurance, they create a safe haven that is vital to the child's sense of being valued and protected. Touch is an essential ingredient in most nurturing experiences. We provide many opportunities for safe and appropriate therapist–child and parent–child physical contact and stimulation of all the senses. If a parent has difficulty touching a child gently, the therapist first demonstrates such touch with the child; next he or she practices with the parent; and finally the therapist guides the parent with the child. If a child or parent has experienced neglect or abuse, as Isaiah and his mother had, we introduce safe touch gradually and are very sensitive to both the parent's and the child's responses. Our goal is that they will be able to experience the benefits of healthy touch throughout their lives together.

SUPPORTING RESEARCH AND THEORY

Attachment research (Ainsworth, Blehar, Waters, & Wall, 1978) indicates that the sensitive, contingent responses of a caring parent are an important factor in the development of secure attachment. "Nurturing interactions form the basis of secure relationships" (Goldsmith, 2007, p. 211). Tender, comforting responses create an atmosphere of acceptance that helps the child feel that he or she has a safe haven to return to in times of stress. Touch is fundamental to human experience, first for survival and then for meaning (Brazelton, 1990). An infant requires the warmth of body contact to support the immature regulatory system. Touch and warmth raise the levels of the hormone oxytocin, which is calming to adult and child alike (Mäkelä, 2005). Human infants who are not touched and handled sufficiently at an early age may develop a distorted body image (Weiss, 1990). A large body of animal and human research supports the value of touch in stimulating development of premature infants (Field, 1995), creating the capacity to relate to others (Harlow, 1958), and reducing stress (Tronick, Ricks, & Cohn, 1982).

Challenge

Challenging activities—such as balancing on a stack of pillows, punching a newspaper, or keeping a balloon in the air—help a child experience feelings of competence, mastery, and playfulness. We choose the activities carefully so that the child can experience success. We also pay attention to the child's level of arousal, providing interludes of calm that regulate the experience. The child learns not only to expand his or her horizons, but to count on adults to be there when needed. Challenge activities are also used to respond to a child's resistance with acceptance and interest in the child's abilities. Attending to the appropriate level of challenge can help a parent who expects too much or too little from a child, or who finds it hard to focus on positive accomplishments. In working with a child who has experienced neglect or trauma, gentle, well-chosen challenge activities can help the child feel strong and free to act.

SUPPORTING RESEARCH AND THEORY

The lively, playful interaction between parents and their young children provides stimuli to all the senses. Tactile, vestibular, and proprioceptive systems are involved in the sense of self and the ability to interact in healthy ways with others (Williamson & Anzalone, 1997). The shared joy of interactive play creates a strong emotional bond and programs the brain to be fully social. Play episodes provide opportunities for affective synchrony and for co-regulation, which enhance the development of brain synapses (Hart, 2008). When the excitement of physically active play is co-regulated by an attuned caregiver, the child develops the capacity to regulate high states of arousal (Stern, 1974). As noted neuroscientist Jaak Panksepp (2009) suggests, "Any therapist who can capture the therapeutic moment in mutually shared play episodes will have brought the client to the gateway of happy living" (p. 17).

The Theraplay Treatment Process

The complexity of the family's needs in the case of Isaiah made the treatment process longer and involved more treatment segments than the typical Theraplay sequence. Over the course of treatment with this family, parts of the program described below were repeated with the different caregivers; other treatment modalities were added as needed. Theraplay treatment for children or parents with developmental problems may also be longer and involve other modalities.

Families experiencing mild to moderate difficulties in relationship and behavior typically participate in a series of 18–26 weekly sessions, with 2–4 follow-up sessions at quarterly intervals over the next year. The first session is an information-gathering interview with the parents. The second and third appointments are observation sessions using the Marschak Interaction Method (MIM; Theraplay Institute, 2011), in which the child and one parent perform a series of tasks together. The interactions are videorecorded and later analyzed by the therapist in preparation for a fourth session with the parents. In that session, the therapist and parents discuss their observations of the interaction and agree on a plan for treatment. In the fifth session, the therapist demonstrates Theraplay activities with the parent, and they discuss the purpose of the activities, the child's potential reactions, and the parent's reflections on the experience.

Sessions 6–25 involve direct Theraplay with the family, adapting to the child's developmental needs the kind of playful interactions that parents and young children naturally engage in together. The interaction includes structuring, engaging, nurturing, and challenging activities in combinations geared to the specific needs and problems of the individual child and family. The therapist and the parents meet after every third session without the child, to discuss progress and goals.

Parents observe all Theraplay sessions, and when they are ready, join in the activities with the therapist and child. The Theraplay model ideally involves two therapists—one who interacts with the child, and one who works with the parents. When two therapists are present, the parents' therapist observes with the parents and discusses the rationale for the activities (e.g., encouraging the development of trust and self-esteem, building a sense of self as lovable, developing confidence, permitting pleasurable experiences, encouraging intimacy, developing a positive body image, strengthening perceptual–motor coordination). This discussion includes ways in which the parents can implement these ideas at home. If only one therapist is involved, these discussions take place with the parents at the end of each session, by phone, or at a separately scheduled time.

The final treatment session ends with a goodbye party. The parent–child interaction assessment and any standardized tests are readministered and discussed with the parents to reflect on progress and make recommendations. Two to four follow-up sessions are scheduled with parents and child over the next 12 months.

Case Vignette: Theraplay in Isaiah's Journey Home

Additional Background

Child welfare first became involved with this family when Isaiah was 2 years old. The day care staff reported that they witnessed the mother repeatedly spanking Isaiah very hard on the bottom and aggressively flicking his mouth. The report was confirmed, and family preservation services were provided. For the next 4 years, the child welfare system received a number of reports related to the mother's behavior, but Isaiah stayed in the home until he was found looking for food in the garbage. At this point, the caseworker supported termination of parental rights and wrote that Isaiah had "no attachment" with his mother, Tonya. The case reports did not contain any reference to the biological mother's history in foster care as a victim of abuse and trauma.

Treatment with the Foster Family

The first step in Isaiah's journey was the Theraplay work with him and his foster parents.

Referral

The desperation in the voice of the foster mother, Cynthia, was clear as she described her struggles with Isaiah:

> "I have no idea what to do. I try to talk to him, and he covers his ears; I try to hug him, and he punches me; I give him gifts, and he breaks them on purpose; I ask him to be patient, and he pees all over my bed. He cries for his mama, so I let him call his mama; then he throws the phone on the floor and cusses at her, me, my husband, and anyone else around. I thought I could do this, but I'm not so sure. He acts the same way at school, and he has no friends. His teacher doesn't even like him. The caseworker says that this is normal, and it will stop, but I think Isaiah is in real trouble and I don't know how to help him. I don't know everything he's been through, but something has made him the way he is. Can you please, please, please help us?"

Assessment

I (Marlo Winstead) met with the foster parents, Cynthia and Kirk, for an intake interview. They were committed to doing their very best with Isaiah, but they felt completely unsupported by the child welfare system and very inadequate as caregivers. I administered a variety of child behavior scales and projective measures to learn about Isaiah. I also administered the MIM to learn more about Isaiah's healthy and unhealthy relational strategies.

He was easy to engage and enjoyed being playful. He exhibited anger and aggression during challenge and structure tasks, however, and he tried very hard both overtly and subtly to gain control of the tasks. During nurture tasks, he was ambivalent and fearful of receiving nurture, but wanted to care for his foster parents.

Theraplay with the Foster Mother and Child

Because the foster mother was the primary caregiver and the foster father was less available, I began Theraplay sessions with Isaiah and Cynthia in the foster home. The goals were to foster positive, relational, and experiential interactions that would result in shared joy and healing, while simultaneously targeting Isaiah's difficulty with adult direction (structure), his initial response of defeat when presented with a new activity (challenge), and his aversion to being cared for (nurture). I planned on incorporating Tonya, the biological mother, into treatment when she gained her visitation privileges.

As we see with many traumatized children, Isaiah was suspicious, easily dysregulated when touched, and hypervigilant. Similar to his presentation in the MIM, he was the most uncomfortable during tasks that focused on the dimensions of structure and nurture. Out of respect for his trauma history, I slowed down and made attunement my primary goal, reminding myself that I was seeking affective resonance, synchrony, and cooperation. I spoke in a clear, confident, and calm way and asked permission to make physical contact during our sessions. Cynthia was present during our first two sessions, observing and taking note of the successful and less successful techniques.

During Session 3, Cynthia watched as Isaiah bopped a balloon back and forth with me—first with his hands, and then, as I gradually increased the challenge, with his knees, feet, elbows, and head. Isaiah was initially reluctant, but my praise and encouragement helped him feel supported and confident in his ability to be the "best balloon bopper" ever. The success he experienced helped him to accept structure when Cynthia joined the session and decided which body part we would use to hit the balloon, and when the activity would start. Accepting Cynthia's direction and guidance during enjoyable activities increased the likelihood that Isaiah would accept her direction not only in sessions, but outside of sessions when they were not engaged in fun activities.

Little by little, Isaiah became more comfortable; he was less inhibited, he smiled a bit more, and he began to engage in playful ways. In Session 6, we had a "moment of meeting." Isaiah was feeling very confident after punching through three sheets of newspaper I was holding. Together we wadded the paper tightly into little balls to throw into the hoop I then made with my arms. I said, "When I say, 'Ready, set, go,' I want you to throw the ball into my arms. Ready . . . set . . . ," but before I said "go" he released the ball. In an accepting manner, I picked up the ball and said, "Wow, you have a great shot on 'set,' so let's see you throw the ball on 'set' this time.

Ready . . ." He threw the ball as hard as he could at my face, with a seeming intent for harm. I calmly picked up the ball, gently held his hand, and said, "We don't have any hurts when we're playing. I'm not for hurting, *and* I am not going to hurt you." Isaiah looked up and locked eyes with me. After intently scrutinizing me in a very no-nonsense, "I'm looking deep into your soul" kind of way, he said, "OK, then." It was as if we made a pact not to hurt one another. He seemed to absorb the fact that I was there to help him.

In Sessions 4–10, Cynthia started to participate actively in the Theraplay activities under my guidance and direction. She gradually moved from co-leading to leading activities like "blow me over, pull me up," copying each other's movements, and tracing shapes on Isaiah's back. My role became that of coach, teacher, and supporter, in order to focus the work on the relationship between Isaiah and Cynthia instead of me. Cautiously, Isaiah allowed himself to be vulnerable and accept Cynthia's structure and nurture. His maladaptive behaviors at home and school decreased, and positive behaviors (i.e., sharing and helping) took their place. Isaiah settled into the rituals of Theraplay, and looked forward to the sessions as well as to the Theraplay "homework" that Cynthia was doing with him between our sessions.

Sessions 10–14 proved to be difficult for Isaiah because of out-of-session changes in his life. Since his biological mother, Tonya, was getting stronger, completing her service plan, and maintaining sobriety, Isaiah began weekly 2-hour supervised visits with her. It seemed that Isaiah's tumultuous and traumatic early years with her made it difficult for him to believe that she was actually "better." Isaiah wanted to see his mother but was defiant, oppositional, and aggressive during the visits; she was very hurt and discouraged. In the sessions with the foster mother, I added DDP (Hughes, 2007) techniques into our Theraplay sessions, to provide a safe space to process the mixed emotions Isaiah was feeling toward his mother; he wanted to be with her and hoped for her to love him, but he was also distrustful, hurt, and angry because of her actions in the past. The foster mother continued to provide comfort and care in the difficult moments both in therapy and outside of sessions. With the biological mother's visitation granted, and the continued goal of reunification, it was time to transfer the work of strengthening relationships and increasing capacity for attachment to Tonya and Isaiah.

Theraplay with Both the Foster and Biological Mothers and the Child

An MIM between Isaiah and Tonya revealed Tonya's desire to be in relationship with Isaiah, and her commitment to using the new parenting skills she was learning. Isaiah engaged with Tonya for fleeting moments throughout the assessment, but he was very controlling and did not respond to her attempts to structure or nurture him. During the MIM feedback session with Tonya, she shared her own history of relational trauma, which included physical and sexual abuse, foster care, and numerous romantic relationships in which she was the victim of domestic violence. Before including Tonya in Theraplay sessions, I spent time connecting with her through providing education and support in regard to her history and how it was informing her parenting.

Sessions 15–18 included both Tonya and Cynthia, in order to help everyone make the transition and to generalize the growth, development, and acquisition of skills to Isaiah's "new" relationship with Tonya. Isaiah initially regressed to mild resistance, dysregulation, and hypersensitivity to touch. I attuned closely to his verbal and especially to his nonverbal signals, and worked hard to support everyone. It was both confusing and helpful for Isaiah to see his mother and foster mother endorse each other and work together. Over time, the content of the sessions implicitly gave him permission to love and care about both of them without feeling that he was betraying one or the other. The continued integration of DDP techniques gave Isaiah explicit permission to care about and to be cared for by both women.

The primary goal was attunement and affective resonance among all members of the session. At one point, Cynthia hid a dot of powder on Isaiah's elbow, and Tonya found and rubbed it in. This simple activity led to natural giggles and shared smiles that demonstrated cooperation among the three, trust as Isaiah's muscles relaxed when his eyes were closed, and progress with Isaiah's capacity for accepting nurture and Cynthia's provision of nurture in a healthy and safe way. It was a bittersweet session when Cynthia finally made the transition out of the therapeutic work. Isaiah and Tonya both missed Cynthia's presence, but after this, Tonya seemed to come out of her shell and was more confident in her participation.

Theraplay and Other Treatment with the Biological Mother and the Child

Over the next 8 months, treatment included Theraplay sessions as well as DDP (Hughes, 2007) techniques as described above, EMDR (Lovett, 2007), sandtray therapy (Homeyer & Sweeney, 2010), and projection through narrative work with puppets (Johnson & Clark, 2001). Outside of sessions, Tonya vacillated between her old methods of interaction (i.e., shouting, spanking, harsh discipline, unrealistic expectations, and rejecting behavior) and the new skills and strategies she was learning. She sometimes reported feeling hopeless because her "case" lingered on in the child welfare system, but she gradually became more powerful and competent to raise her child with new ideas and a fresh outlook.

Theraplay Session: Saying Goodbye to the Foster Parents

Seventeen months after placement and more than 65 therapy sessions later, Isaiah was going home, but not before experiencing a very healthy goodbye with his foster parents. Opportunities to honor the time spent with Cynthia and Kirk were maximized throughout the session. After measuring Isaiah's growth since coming into foster care by measuring his hands and feet with crepe paper strips, we made a "circle of love" out of a long strip of paper to provide a visual image of the relationship shared with his foster parents. I used a teddy bear as my foster son, "Ralph," who visited and shared his story (Johnson & Clark, 2001). This technique resonated on a very deep level, but also created sufficient psychological distance and safety for Isaiah. Questions such as "If you love me, why am I moving?", "Did I do something bad, and is that why I am moving?", and "Will you still love me?" were answered. At the close of a difficult session, Isaiah received lots of nurture, a shared snack, a story (*I Love You Through and Through*; Rossetti-Shustak, 2005), and a special song ("Twinkle Twinkle Little Star, what a special boy you are . . ."; Booth & Jernberg, 2010, p. 538). The message of a deep, warm, genuine, and sincere desire for relationship was conveyed through laughter, shared joy, acceptance, attuned and positive interactions—and tears. The foster parents allowed themselves to be vulnerable, which was not surprising, but Isaiah mirrored that vulnerability and did not use his unhealthy adaptive strategies to avoid or dismiss his feelings.

Outcome

Tonya was able to overcome innumerable hurdles from her past and her present in order to bring her child home; it took almost 2 years of hard work, which included a total of approximately 100 therapy sessions. There are still areas of growth for Tonya, but she has captured the essence of Theraplay within her parenting. She truly "sees" Isaiah for who he is, and her level of acceptance has significantly increased. Tonya no longer employs physical punishment; her capacity for providing nurture has improved; and as a result, she has more success in helping her son regulate his affective, emotional, and physical states. Isaiah's aggressive outbursts decreased significantly while his verbalization of feelings increased. He accepted structure and nurturing from his mother similar to other children his age, and he started taking risks, like trying out for a basketball team. For Isaiah, Theraplay provided an opportunity to experience the depth of love that his mother felt for him and to start to heal the deep wounds of neglect and abuse.

Conclusion

In this chapter, we have presented a vignette illustrating the use of Theraplay as a major part of the treatment for a young boy and his mother, both of whom had suffered relational trauma. The attachment-based approach provided a forum for relational repair and healing, as well as the necessary guidance and support to enter into the hard work of mending wounds and rebuilding trust.

The therapeutic journey with this family included the following steps:

- Helping the child form a safe connection with his foster parents, in order to reduce his violent behavior and prepare him to be open to a healing experience with his biological mother.
- Creating a safe and supportive experience for the biological mother, in which she could begin to reflect on her own feelings and those of her son.
- Giving the biological mother an opportunity to work together with the foster mother, so that she could benefit from her experience, use her support to understand her child's needs, and gain confidence in her own ability to respond appropriately.
- Collaboratively creating a well-planned transition for this child from the foster home back to living with his mother.

AUTHORS' NOTE

We dedicate this chapter to the case vignette families (foster and biological), all families in the child welfare system, all foster parents, and especially to our colleague Mary Pat Clemmons, LCSW, who died in 2012 while writing her doctoral dissertation about Theraplay and reunification. Her passion for her clients and for life continues to inspire us.

REFERENCES

Ainsworth, M. D. S., Blehar, M. C., Waters, E., & Wall, S. (1978). *Patterns of attachment: A psychological study of the Strange Situation.* Hillsdale, NJ: Erlbaum.

Baumrind, D. (1991). The influence of parenting style on adolescent competence and substance use. *Journal of Early Adolescence, 11*(1), 56–95.

Becker-Weidman, A., & Schell, D. (2005). *Creating capacity for attachment: Dyadic developmental psychotherapy in the treatment of trauma–attachment disorders.* Oklahoma City, OK: Wood'N'Barnes.

Bennett, L. R., Shiner, S. K., & Ryan, S. (2006). Using Theraplay in shelter settings with mothers and children who have experienced violence in the home. *Journal of Psychosocial Nursing and Mental Health Service, 44*(10), 38–47.

Booth, P. (2000). Forming an attachment with an adopted toddler using the Theraplay approach. *The Signal: Newsletter of the World Association for Infant Mental Health, 8*(3), 1–9.

Booth, P., & Gil, E. (2011). *Integrating Theraplay techniques into trauma treatment.* Paper presented at the 28th Annual International Play Therapy Conference, Sacramento, CA.

Booth, P., & Jernberg, A. (2010). *Theraplay: Helping parents and children build better relationships through attachment-based play* (3rd ed.). San Francisco: Jossey-Bass.

Bowlby, J. (1982). *Attachment and loss: Vol. 1. Attachment.* New York: Basic Books. (Original work published 1969)

Bowlby, J. (1988). *A secure base: Parent–child attachment and healthy human development.* New York: Basic Books.

Brazelton, T. B. (1990). Touch as a touchstone: Summary of the round table. In K. E. Barnard & T. B. Brazelton (Eds.), *Touch: The foundation of experience* (pp. 561–566). Madison, CT: International Universities Press.

Bundy-Myrow, S. (2012). Family Theraplay: Connecting with children on the autism spectrum. In L. Gallo-Lopez & L. C. Rubin (Eds.), *Play-based interventions for children and adolescents with autism spectrum disorders* (pp. 73–96). New York: Routledge.

California Evidence-Based Clearinghouse for Child Welfare. (2012). *Theraplay.* Retrieved from *www.cebc4cw.org/program/-2*

Cook, A., Blaustein, M., Spinazzola, J., & van der Kolk, B. (Eds.). (2003). *Complex trauma in children and adolescents: White paper from the National Child Traumatic Stress Network.* Retrieved from *www.nctsnet.org/nctsn_assets/ pdfs/edu_materials/ComplexTrauma_All.pdf*

Field, T. (1995). *Touch in early development.* Mahwah, NJ: Erlbaum.

Fonagy, P., Gergely, G., Jurist, E. L., & Target, M. (2002). *Affect regulation, mentalization, and the development of the self.* New York: Other Press.

Goldsmith, D. F. (2007). Challenging children's negative internal working models: Utilizing attachment-based treatment strategies in a therapeutic preschool. In D. Oppenheim & D. F. Goldsmith (Eds.), *Attachment theory in clinical work with children* (pp. 203–225). New York: Guilford Press.

Gomez, A. M., & Jernberg, E. (2013). Using EMDR therapy and Theraplay. In A. M. Gomez, *EMDR therapy and adjunct approaches with children* (pp. 273–297). New York: Springer.

Grotberg, E. H. (1997). The International Resilience Project: Findings from the research and the effectiveness of interventions. In B. Bain (Ed.), *Psychology and education in the 21st century: Proceedings of the 54th Annual Convention of the International Council of Psychologists* (pp. 118–128). Edmonton, Alberta, Canada: IC Press.

Harlow, H. F. (1958). The nature of love. *American Psychologist, 13,* 673–685.

Hart, S. (2008). *Brain, attachment, personality: An introduction to neuroaffective development.* London: Karnac Books.

Homeyer, L. E., & Sweeney, D. S. (2010). *Sandtray: A practical manual* (2nd ed.). New York: Routledge.

Hughes, D. A. (2007). *Attachment-focused family therapy.* New York: Norton.

Iacoboni, M. (2008). *Mirroring people: The science of empathy and how we connect with others.* New York: Farrar, Straus & Giroux.

Jernberg, A. (1979). *Theraplay: A new treatment using structured play for problem children and their families.* San Francisco: Jossey-Bass.

Jernberg, A., & Booth, P. (1999). *Theraplay: Helping parents and children build better relationships through attachment-based play* (2nd ed.). San Francisco: Jossey-Bass.

Johnson, S. P., & Clark, P. (2001). Play therapy with aggressive acting-out children.

In G. Landreth (Ed.), *Innovations in play therapy: Issues, process, and special populations* (pp. 239–256). Philadelphia: Brunner-Routledge.

Lovett, J. (2007). *Small wonders: Healing childhood trauma with EMDR*. New York: Free Press.

Mäkelä, J. (2003, Fall–Winter). What makes Theraplay effective: Insights from developmental sciences. *Theraplay Institute Newsletter*, pp. 9–11.

Mäkelä, J. (2005). Kosketuksen merkitys lapsen kehityksessä [The importance of touch in the development of children]. *Finnish Medical Journal, 60*, 1543–1549.

Mäkelä, J., & Salo, S. (2011). Theraplay—vanhemman ja lapsen välinen vuorovaikutushoito lasten mielenterveysongelmissa [Theraplay—Parent–child interaction treatment for children with mental health problems]. *Duodecim, 127*, 29–39.

Mäkelä, J., & Vierikko, I. (2004). *From heart to heart: Interactive therapy for children in care. Report on the Theraplay Project in SOS Children's Villages in Finland 2001–2004*. Espoo, Finland: SOS Villages Finland Association.

Munns, E. (Ed.). (2000). *Theraplay: Innovations in attachment-enhancing play therapy*. Northvale, NJ: Aronson.

Munns, E. (Ed.). (2009). *Applications of family and group Theraplay*. Lanham, MD: Aronson.

Panksepp, J. (2009). Brain emotional systems and qualities of mental life: From animal models of affect to implications for psychotherapeutics. In D. Fosha, D. J. Siegel, & M. F. Solomon (Eds.), *The healing power of emotion: Affective neuroscience, development & clinical practice* (pp. 1–26). New York: Norton.

Perry, B. D. (2006). Applying principles of neurodevelopment to clinical work with maltreated and traumatized children: The neurosequential model of therapeutics. In N. B. Webb (Ed.), *Working with traumatized youth in child welfare* (pp. 27–52). New York: Guilford Press.

Porges, S. W. (2011). *The polyvagal theory: Neuropsycholgical foundations of emotions, attachment, communication and self-regulation*. New York: Norton.

Robison, M., Lindaman, S., Clemmons, M. P., Doyle-Buckwalter, K., & Ryan, M. (2009). "I deserve a family": The evolution of an adolescent's behavior and beliefs about himself and others when treated with Theraplay in residential care. *Child and Adolescent Social Work Journal, 26*(4), 291–306.

Rossetti-Shustak, B. (2005). *I love you through and through*. New York: Cartwheel.

Rubin, P., Lender, D., & Miller, J. (2010). Theraplay for children with histories of complex trauma. In P. Booth & A. Jernberg, *Theraplay: Helping parents and children build better relationships through attachment-based play* (3rd ed., pp. 359–403). San Francisco: Jossey-Bass.

Rubin, P., & Tregay, J. (1989). *Play with them—Theraplay groups in the classroom: A technique for professionals who work with children*. Springfield, IL: Thomas.

Salo, S., Lampi, H., & Lindaman, S. (2010). Use of the Emotional Availability Scales to evaluate an attachment-based intervention—Theraplay—in substance abusing mother–infant dyads in Finland. *Infant Mental Health Journal (Supplement), 32*, 77.

Schieffer, K. (2012). *Sunshine Circles(r): Interactive playgroups for social skills development and classroom management.* Evanston, IL: Theraplay Institute.

Schore, A. N. (1994). *Affect regulation and the origin of the self: The neurobiology of emotional development.* Hillside, NJ: Erlbaum.

Schore, A. N. (2001). The effects of early relational trauma on right brain development, affect regulation, and infant mental health. *Infant Mental Health Journal, 22*(1–2), 201–269.

Schore, A. N. (2003). Early relational trauma, disorganized attachment, and the development of a predisposition to violence. In M. F. Solomon & D. J. Siegel (Eds.), *Healing trauma* (pp. 107–167). New York: Norton.

Schore, J. R., & Schore, A. N. (2008). Modern attachment theory: The central role of affect regulation in development and treatment. *Clinical Social Work Journal, 36,* 9–20.

Shahmoon-Shanok, R. (1997). Giving back future's promise: Working resourcefully with parents of children who have severe disorders of relating and communicating. *Zero to Three, 17*(5), 37–48.

Siegel, D. J. (2006). An interpersonal neurobiology approach to psychotherapy. *Psychiatric Annals, 36*(4), 248–256.

Siegel, D. J. (2012). *The developing mind: How relationships and the brain interact to shape who we are* (2nd ed.). New York: Guilford Press.

Siu, A. F. Y. (2009). Theraplay in the Chinese world: An intervention program for Hong Kong children with internalizing problems. *International Journal of Play Therapy, 18*(1), 1–12.

Slade, A. (2002). Keeping the baby in mind: A critical factor in perinatal mental health. *Zero to Three, 22*(6), 10–16.

Stern, D. N. (1974). The goal and structure of mother–infant play. *Journal of the American Academy of Child Psychiatry, 13*(3), 402–421.

Stern, D. N. (1985). *The interpersonal world of the infant: A view from psychoanalysis and developmental psychology.* New York: Basic Books.

Stern, D. N. (1995). *The motherhood constellation: A unified view of parent–infant psychotherapy.* New York: Basic Books.

Theraplay Institute. (2003). *Marschak Interaction Method (MIM): Manual and cards* (3rd ed.). Chicago: Author.

Trevarthen, C., & Aitken, K. J. (2001). Infant intersubjectivity: Research, theory, and clinical applications. *Journal of Child Psychology and Psychiatry, 42*(1), 3–48.

Tronick, E. Z., Bruschweiler-Stern, N., Harrison, A. M., Lyons-Ruth, K., Morgan, A. C., Nahum, J. P., . . . Stern, D. N. (1998). Dyadically expanded states of consciousness and the process of therapeutic change. *Infant Mental Health Journal, 19*(3), 290–299.

Tronick, E. Z., Ricks, M., & Cohn, J. F. (1982). Maternal and infant affective exchange: Patterns of adaptation. In T. Field & A. Fogel (Eds.), *Emotion and early interaction* (pp. 83–100). Hillside, NJ: Erlbaum.

van der Kolk, B. (2005). Developmental trauma disorder: Towards a rational diagnosis for children with complex trauma histories. *Psychiatric Annals, 35,* 401–408.

Weiss, S. J. (1990). Parental touching correlates of a child's body concept and body sentiment. In K. E. Barnard & T. B. Brazelton (Eds.), *Touch: The foundation of experience* (pp. 425–432). Madison, CT: International Universities Press.

Wettig, H. G., Coleman, A. R., & Geider, F. J. (2011). Evaluating the effectiveness of Theraplay in treating shy, socially withdrawn children. *International Journal of Play Therapy, 20*(1), 26–37.

Williamson, G. G., & Anzalone, M. (1997). Sensory integration: A key component of the evaluation and treatment of young children with severe difficulties in relating and communicating. *Zero to Three, 17*(5), 29–36.

Winnicott, D. W. (1971). *Playing and reality.* London: Tavistock.

CHAPTER 10

The Creative Use of Metaphor in Play and Art Therapy with Attachment Problems

Eliana Gil

Many practitioners have long regarded metaphor as a pivotal and central focal point in therapy. Specifically, clinical interest persists in the manner in which clinical metaphor takes center stage, and therapists listen for, invite, or explore metaphor in order to assist clients toward positive therapeutic gains. Play and art therapists consider metaphor work a natural part of their field of study. These expressive therapists have a profound recognition of the importance of clients' having the emotional distance and the inherent safety that they can enjoy as a result of having something stand in the place of something else. In addition, play and art therapists are taught to "stay with" the metaphors created, rather than making jarring verbal interpretations of similarities between the metaphors and real life.

This chapter discusses and presents various ways of working with metaphors—both inviting and responding to clinical material highlighted in metaphorical language or images. Metaphor work is likely to be helpful with any client, but I focus on the use of metaphor to enhance parent–child attachment in dyads where such attachment is confused, hurtful, or ambivalent. These situations can occur because of parental inability or unwillingness to provide consistent and empathic care or children's compromised receptivity.

Defining *Metaphor*

Metaphor is defined in different ways, but common ground exists among these definitions. It is usually considered something that is used to represent something else, a symbol. The word comes from the Greek word *metapherein*, which means "to carry over" or "to transfer." A symbol can be broadly understood as a representation, a mark, a pictogram, or a sign. Symbols can be toys, images in art, or physical signs such as a peace sign, but they can also be conveyed through language, and this happens often. Consider how often we hear terms such as "I'm running on half-empty," or "My cup runneth over," or "His boat hasn't docked yet." Our language is rich with metaphors that are used as shorthand for other, more complex concepts.

My adult client Doug started talking to me about what was going on in his life, and as he did so his affect became flat and his words sing-song and monotonous, to say nothing of vague. I felt disconnected from him, as if he were trying to "keep a lid" on what was really bothering him. At one point, he said, "The clearest way I can describe it is that I feel like I'm sinking in quicksand." Now I felt immediately connected, because his metaphor captured his sense of desolation, despair, and urgency completely. Metaphors often present the listener with a mental picture of something conceptual that resonates on a deeper level.

The clinical use of metaphor has been widely discussed. It probably gained its greatest visibility with the brilliant work of Milton Erickson (Erickson & Rossi, 1979), who is credited with inspiring hundreds of clinicians to place their trust in the innate value of metaphors, created by clients and clinicians alike. Erickson earned great reverence through his brilliant use of metaphors with clients, who, he felt, could create their own meaning. He felt that in this way, clients would learn lessons that might otherwise be too painful for their conscious minds to tolerate; he believed that the stories could get in "sideways," while more direct interventions might be denied entry. Erickson was truly a master at creating provocative, insightful, and powerful metaphors that his clients listened for intently and that are still remembered in the clinical community (Lankton, 2004). In the play therapy field, these traditions have been well continued by Joyce Mills (*www.drjoycemills.com*) and Nancy Davis (1990).

Esparza (2012) describes therapeutic metaphors as among the most elegant tools for assisting people in the process of personal transformation and growth. He further describes them as communicating from and with the subconscious mind, bypassing the critical faculties of the conscious mind. In therapy, a metaphor can represent a client's problem and often provides up a solution to the problem in an indirect way. My client Doug, for example, in presenting the "sinking in quicksand" metaphor, had to address whether to allow himself to "sink" or whether to gather resources for the fight to get out. Ricoeur (1967) states that metaphors work as an intermediary element between the languages of logic and of emotion, imagination, and affection.

Onnis et al. (2007) state that "The metaphor, because of its 'evocative' and not explicative power has the advantage [of] allud[ing] to the preverbal and unconscious level, without pretending to make it explicit; in this way on the one side it can elude some defensive mechanism, [and] on the other side it opens spaces for a more free and 'creative' translation by [whoever] receives it" (p. 2). Guiffrida, Jordan, Saiz, and Barnes (2007) encourage clinical use of metaphors because they can promote several therapeutic functions, including relationship building with clients, accessing and symbolizing emotions, uncovering and challenging clients' tacit assumptions, and introducing new frames of reference. Surely these functions greatly increase clients' receptivity to clinical interventions. Esparza (2012) finds therapeutic stories useful in that they can stimulate creativity (energy); they can illustrate points; they can open up possibilities; they can introduce doubt in the mind of a client who sees a position in only one way; and they can suggest options and possibilities.

Child Maltreatment and Attachment

The topics of child maltreatment and its effects on attachment are addressed throughout this book. For purposes of this chapter, it is important to emphasize that early disruptive, violent, or neglectful parental interactions will create internal working models that have far-reaching implications for young children. Specifically, children seem to learn the lesson that "people who love you will hurt you, reject you, or want sexual contact with you," and thus their efforts to get their needs met for affection, attention, protection, or nurturance are confused and compromised. These issues are exhibited whenever children interact with others—and given the intimate nature of the therapist–child relationship, they seem to be activated particularly strongly in the therapy process.

Case Vignette: Christine and Sarah

The case of Christine and her mother, Sarah, illustrates clinical work with metaphors.

Background

Christine was referred for treatment after having been placed in foster care a year earlier, at the age of 4. When she was removed from her mother, Sarah, 24, she had many signs of physical abuse at the hands of her aggressive father, Mike.

Christine was interviewed by a child protective services worker in tandem with a juvenile police officer, and she refused to respond to any questions. The officers had more luck with her mother, who, upon hearing the extent of Christine's injuries, told them about Mike's alcohol/drug abuse and what sounded like a classic history of domestic violence, including both physical and emotional abuse of Sarah and Christine. Sarah insisted that she had gone to great lengths to protect her daughter—locking her in the closet when Mike was drinking or using drugs, and telling her to run next door when Mike was beyond her control. She also talked about long hours of huddling together in the closet, waiting out Mike's explosive tirades. Sarah was under the impression that if Christine did not *see* her mother being beaten, she would be spared any emotional distress. Little did Sarah know that young children are seriously affected by a climate of fear and anxiety, by listening to their parents being beaten, and most definitely by being hidden or shoved out the door by their parents. In addition, Sarah was surprised to learn that children experience a unique type of distress at seeing their parents unable to protect themselves, and guilt at their own inability to help them.

When Christine was taken into the county's custody and was placed in foster care, Sarah fell into a deep depression and became homeless; without her daughter, she temporarily lost her will to live. But Sarah was a true survivor. In her shelter for the homeless, she was receptive to kind guidance from a social worker, and slowly but surely she revealed a predictable history of her own witnessing of violence and chaos when she was a child. She had run away from home after being sexually abused by one of her mother's boyfriends, and had never looked back.

Sarah met Mike at a dance club when she was 17, and she became pregnant almost immediately. She hinted that their first sexual encounter was not consensual and that he moved in immediately after meeting her. She noted that he acquired large quantities of money sporadically, and Sarah soon discovered that he sold drugs. Mike moved Sarah's roommate out quickly and was emotionally abusive from the start, but Sarah's first beating occurred when the baby was about 3 weeks old and she could not quiet her. Mike was intolerant of the child's screaming from the beginning, and he would take his anger out on Sarah. Sarah described her relationship to Mike as "weird," adding, "I don't think we ever liked each other."

After the unpredictable and violent environment with Mike, the shelter provided Sarah with a deep sense of relief. She would later tell me, "I woke up in the morning and knew it would be a good day. I would work hard to get back my daughter, and now I believed that it was possible for me to work for things I wanted. I felt like a fog was lifted and I could make decisions for myself." Her life had taken a wrong turn when she was young and vulnerable. Mike was 18 years older than she was, and he was obviously very self-involved, impulsive, and dangerous. He had held her captive for years, and once Sarah was born, she too was exposed to a chaotic and unsafe existence. Sarah consistently stated that she loved Christine and would do whatever it took to get her back. She had a lot of obstacles to overcome in order to achieve this goal: She had to get a job, find a place to live, and show some kind of stability in her life. Her motivation was palpable, however, and it was as if she was positioned to make a significant growth spurt in her emotional maturity. My job was to help Sarah and Christine establish a warm and safe attachment with each other, since their attachment had been so deeply disrupted from the outset.

Just as Sarah was thriving in a safe environment, Christine had made a positive attachment to her new foster parents, Dan and Gerttie. Although I was grateful that Christine was feeling secure, I recognized the challenges of divided loyalties for her, so I quickly asked Gerttie to encourage Christine to call her "Gerttie" rather than "Mom," and to remind Christine about her mom, Sarah, whenever she could. Gerttie had already tried to correct her foster child when Christine called her "Mom," and Christine's compromise was to call her "Grandma Gerttie," which several of Gerttie's grandchildren called her as well.

Dan and Gerttie were in their 50s; they were grandparents to a number of young children and excellent caregivers. They had been married during their first year in college. They were quiet and warm individuals, and they chose to be foster parents to give back some of their good fortune. Their children were either in college or married, and they had decided together that they could offer a good temporary home to a child in need. Christine was the third foster child they had taken into their home.

They described a frightened, shy, anxious child when Christine first arrived at their home. She still had some physical injuries that needed tending and rest. Gerttie settled Christine into her oldest daughter's room, which had a canopy bed, a small vanity table, pictures of puppies and kittens, and a beautiful night light that made stars on the ceiling and had soft music playing. Gerttie stayed with Christine all night the first few nights so that the child could rest. Christine kept asking for her mother and wondered whether Sarah had died. Gerttie reassured her and tried to make her comfortable. Once in the first week when Gerttie came to see her in the morning, Christine was under the bed and appeared cold and shaking. Her eyes were open, and she was sucking her fingers. Gerttie was concerned about Christine and made an investment of time and attention to ensure her adjustment to her new home. Gerttie didn't know that Christine had often slept in a closet, that she had never had a room of her own, and that her sleep was often interrupted by violent outbursts from Mike or Mike's friends. Sarah also volunteered that her own fears and worries caused her to be "nervous and worried" all the time, and thus she did not eat or sleep well herself.

It took Gerttie a full 2 months to get Christine settled into her new environment. After that, Christine followed her around the house, wanted to hold her hand, and called her "Mommy" despite Gerttie's encouragement to do otherwise. She still asked after her own mother, continually asking whether Sarah was dead. She was allowed to see her mother after 3 months, once Sarah was back on her feet emotionally. Sarah was anxious to see her daughter and was surprised to see Christine shy away from her and cling to Gerttie when she first saw her. This caused Sarah to cry and be sad, at which point Christine would no longer look at her. The social worker had tried to prepare Sarah for a wide array of possible responses in Christine, and although she had heard that sometimes children take a while to warm up, she was also shocked and disheartened by Christine's clinginess to her foster mother.

Christine Comes to Therapy

The presenting concerns of the social worker were Christine's anxiety, clinginess, and ambivalence toward her mother. In addition, Gerttie wanted guidance about how to prepare Christine for supervised visits, and how to help Christine when she became dysregulated after visiting with her mother. These visits had just begun, but they seemed to destabilize Christine.

When she arrived for her first therapy session, Christine sat in Gerttie's lap and looked away when I said hello. She seemed acutely anxious, but she appeared to relax a little when I told her that she and Gerttie could both come into my play therapy office. I told her there might be some things in my room that she would like. I showed Gerttie and Christine around, saying that I wasn't sure what she would like to play with, but she could look around and decide what to do. For the first four meetings, Christine stayed in Gerttie's lap while Gerttie and I sat together and played with different toys, hoping to interest Christine, who seemed a comfortable fixture in this warm foster parent's lap. I noticed a glimmer of interest in Christine as Gerttie and I played with a baby girl doll, fed her a baby bottle, and changed her diapers. At the end of this session, I decided to put the doll, diapers, and baby bottle in a bag; I told Christine that I wanted her to take the doll home this week, play with her, take good care of her, and bring her back the following session. Slowly but surely, this technique began to yield results as Christine became more and more comfortable in the play therapy office and with me. I asked Gerttie to begin to give Christine opportunities to tolerate more and more time without her, so Gerttie would take longer and longer bathroom breaks during the sessions. When she returned to the office, she would sit on a couch and be present while Christine and I played together. Eventually Christine began to enter the play therapy office easily by herself, although she would sometimes go to the door, open it, and make sure that Gerttie was still waiting for her in the waiting room.

Sandtray Scenario: **Up a Tree without a Ladder**

Christine had liked the feel of the sand in the sandtray from about the 10th session forward. She put her little fingers in the sand with great hesitation at first, but when Gerttie covered her own hand and asked Christine to find it, Christine finally smiled a little as she uncovered Gerttie's hand. This session (about 3 months into therapy) was the first time Christine put miniature objects in the tray. The metaphor she created became pivotal to our understanding of her perceptions of her life, and it also provided us with a way of helping her with her current ambivalence about her mother.

As shown in Figure 10.1, Christine placed a large, sturdy tree in the center of the tray. This tree had a cavity on the bottom, and she filled that cavity with a porcupine. She then placed a mother and a baby deer in the branches, high inside the tree. Behind the tree, she placed a very large and sturdy house on the right side. On the left side of the tray, she placed a structure that appeared to be a rock formation (the sort of thing that usually goes inside fish tanks) and had openings in several places. There was a dolphin in the corner. She also placed another tree in the front, on the left side. Finally, she placed a small cat in front of the sturdy house, and the cat was turning its head and looking forward. She then spent time making little uplifts in the sand with her small hands—sometimes patting the sand

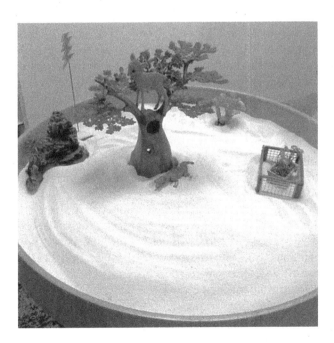

FIGURE 10.1. The quiet mother deer keeps guard.

down, at other times lifting it ever so slightly. She seemed very engaged in the process of creating the sandtray scenario, and she did not speak throughout. I sat facing her, but far enough away that I was not intruding. She looked up frequently to see what I was doing, and she saw me looking patiently at her tray.

Christine did not speak throughout this process, but we had long since broken silence in general and become comfortable with each other. Up to this point, though, Christine had not volunteered very much information except about her present-day activities: where she had gone on the weekend, how her cat was purring and hissing at her foster home, how she and her next-door neighbor were learning to ride bikes, and so forth. Sometimes I would ask whether she'd seen her mom, Sarah, and she would nod her head but offer nothing more. In the second session, we had started doing some work on affect identification, and she was able to point to feelings she had at different times (we used a poster with faces showing different emotions). Gerttie had led the way, pointing to how she was feeling at the moment or how she had felt at different situations. We first engaged Christine in showing us how she thought the baby doll was feeling, and later how she herself was feeling about different things. Eventually Christine was able to correct Gerttie and specify how she was feeling; later on, she could also say what size each feeling was, using a worksheet that shows feelings in smaller or bigger circles (Gil, 2013).

After Christine finished her sandtray, she stood up, and so did I. I walked around the sandtray, encouraging her to see it from different angles, and she followed me around the tray. I said, "The sandtray looks different from different sides." She stood at each of the four sides of the wooden box and stared at what she had made. I waited for spontaneous communication, but none happened. I asked her whether I could take a picture, and she agreed; she also wanted me to take a picture of her "holding it," with her arms thrown around the box. I took both pictures and gave her copies at our next meeting (these days, I send the .jpg files via email when kids ask for copies).

Given this child's usual withdrawal, and her anxiety and ambivalence, I decided to keep the sandtray intact and rolled it into another room. I had another sandtray in the room that other children could use during the week. By the time Christine returned for her next session, I would have processed the metaphor and prepared myself to invite her to "work the metaphor" with me—but I knew much would depend on how Christine reacted when she came into the office and found that her sandtray was intact and waiting for her.

My basic approach to "working the metaphor" is to consider it an externalization of very important and relevant material that cannot yet be addressed directly. In other words, I consider that if a client could tell me his or her problem explicitly, the client would do so. The metaphor is a way to tell without talking, and it is equally important that the client is telling him- or herself in tandem with telling someone who serves as an unconditional witness. Thus my exploration of the client's metaphor is done gingerly, in complete recognition of the trust that has been placed in me.

In order to prepare for engaging children in metaphor work, I first allow myself to spend time with the work that has been produced in therapy. When the work is a sandtray scenario, this means spending time taking in "the life of the tray"—looking at a photo, transcribing dialogues, whatever it takes to properly chronicle the therapy work of the client. In this particular situation, I sat in front of the tray after Christine had left (luckily, my next appointment was canceled, so I had ample time for reflection). I allowed myself to make free associations as I looked at the objects in the tray; I identified *points of entry* (target spots that aroused my curiosity); and I wrote down about six to eight pithy questions for three entry points. I also wrote comments and observations about the child's process in making the tray, as well as the content presented, and I crafted my language carefully to avoid eliciting defensive or distracting responses. My primary goal was to encourage Christine to reflect on what she had created, and to help her explore and amplify her own metaphor, which so clearly centered on attachment between the mother and baby deer (i.e., her mother and herself).

Amplifying the Metaphor

When metaphors appear in stories, art images, verbal language, or movements, some may be obvious, visible, and distinctive; others may be vague and convey a hint of something else. When we give children an opportunity to create sandtrays, we give them a chance to create metaphors by using miniatures to create tangible stories. These scenarios include important information about children's internal worlds.

I have stated elsewhere (Gil, 2011) that something important seems to happen when children externalize internal images, pictures, feeling states, and perceptions into a container (in this case, the sandtray). Children can be reassured by having the experience of placing miniatures in a contained space with firm boundaries (such as those provided in traditional wooden sandtrays). In addition, this externalization creates the "safe enough distance" that play therapists value immensely. In other words, children find a way to talk about themselves without taking risks that they may not yet perceive as possible (although this perception may not be a conscious, cognitive process, but a sensory and affective one in which they hesitate or feel uncomfortable). They begin to look at what is going on in their worlds in a way that allows them to maintain safety while approaching what they fear. In this fashion, children often use play to initiate gradual exposure—a way to expose themselves to feared or complex material in such a way that affect can be gradually tolerated and results in the feared material's losing its power.

It is of great importance to treat an externalized metaphor as just that—something that is standing for something else. As I have stated previously, if children felt comfortable discussing difficult experiences spontaneously, they would do so. I have had experiences in which children seem to be anxious to communicate verbally about what their parents did to them, or state openly how they feel, or make it clear that they want to go home. But when children seem reluctant or unable to commit to verbal language, an externalized metaphor provides them with an alternative method of approaching their traumatic experiences in a way that makes sense to them, and as such it often carries greater possibilities for integration of something that has changed.

Our first steps in this process are to encourage children's curiosity about what they have created, to redirect their attention back to what they've made, and to stimulate some introspection. We model therapeutic curiosity, and by doing so, we engage them in amplifying the metaphor in order to expand their awareness of their creation. The trick is to avoid interpretations and suggestions of things that our child clients have not already named or told us. As therapists, we may feel tempted to solve problems that appear in metaphors, to provide a reassuring ending, or to bring in a resource prematurely. Amplifying metaphors does not mean moving or manipulating them in any way. It means accepting what has come forward and simply attending to what is present, not necessarily to what it means narrowly or to what it could become. It means focusing on problems or worries or concepts that are presented, not those that we surmise or interpret as something else. When a child is describing a vulnerable deer, for example, it is less useful to wonder about who might be feeling vulnerable or afraid, and more useful to understand the deer's experience of vulnerability or safety (or whatever) as it is created by the child.

Identifying Points of Entry

Points of entry are areas of a story, sandtray, artwork, or the like with one or more identifiable objects that can serve as ways of entering the metaphor. For example, in Christine's sandtray, the house on the right, the tree in the front, and the cat looking forward were all entry points, as were the other animal objects. Clinicians can decide which entry point to work with in different ways:

1. They can consider the sequence in which the tray was made. Christine placed the large tree in the center of the tray first, so some clinicians might choose that; others might choose the last object placed to explore.
2. Clinicians may try to identify what are the most and least threatening aspects of the tray, and to start with the point of least resistance.

3. Clinicians can select a point of entry based on emergent issues, phase of treatment, or relationship to the client—in other words, intangible variables unique to each therapy case.

However the point of entry is selected, clinicians then develop some questions, comments, and observations in order to refocus the child's attention on a specific aspect of the tray (like using a wide lens on a camera and then focusing on the forefront or background). In spite of the fact that talking will occur and the left hemisphere of the brain is now activated, it is important to note that staying within the metaphor itself actually pulls for a *whole-brain* response, in which the left and right hemispheres are equally engaged and active (Siegel, Payne, & Bryson, 2012). If the child was being asked to answer questions related to real life, or to indicate how the metaphor stands for something other than what we see, the child might have to revert to left-hemisphere activity that could cause defensive mechanisms to come into play. The goal here is to have the child remain open and receptive, rather than need to use defenses because the material is crossing the "safe enough" threshold and begins to feel threatening.

Pithy Questions to Amplify Metaphors

In my clinical experience, careful and purposeful therapeutic language is the most challenging part of amplifying metaphors. Although there are only a few rules that guide this process of asking or commenting, clinicians are encouraged to "practice, practice, practice" creating these questions, because they do not come easily.

The rules are as follows:

1. Do not ask questions that require a "yes–no" answer (e.g., "Do you want to tell me about this?").
2. Do not ask "why" questions (e.g., "Why did you pick this particular miniature?").
3. Do not make interpretive comments (e.g., "So it seems that you might be feeling scared of your mom").
4. Do not rush ahead or go beyond what is presented to you by the child (e.g., "So how will this bear decide what to do next?").

Some ideas that may be helpful in creating amplifying questions are as follows:

1. Express your therapeutic curiosity about the object/metaphor.
2. Be patient and spend some time with the identified point of entry.
3. Questions are fine, but once you can see that the child is not responsive, try making comments or observing things instead, and take the emphasis off expecting the child to respond verbally.

When Christine returned to the next session after making her tray, she let out a huge sigh and covered her mouth with her hands as she walked over to the sandtray. "It's still here," she said with apparent excitement and pleasure. "I knew it would be here!" I responded by saying, "I thought we might take a longer look at it together." She seemed completely receptive as she started dusting sand off the house, making more fingerprints in the sand, and slightly rearranging how things were in the sandtray. Her first movement was to anchor the tree deeper in the sand and move more sand to surround its roots.

Here are the questions I prepared prior to this session for Christine's sandtray, after spending some time allowing myself to explore the tray. I identified three possible entry points and then created questions designed to amplify the metaphors in the tray:

Entry Point 1: The Cat in Front of the House

"I notice there is a cat in front of the house. What is the cat doing?"
"I wonder if the cat has been in the front of this house before?"
"If the cat were to turn his head the other way, what would he see?"
"What's the cat's favorite part of this house?"
"If the cat could use words, what would he say to the house?"
"When the cat is not in front of the house, where is the cat?"
"What does the cat see as he looks out?"

Entry Point 2: The Tree in the Center of the Tray

"What kind of a tree is this?"
"How long has the tree been in this place?"
"What's it like for the tree to be exactly in the place it is?"
"I notice this tree has a little open space. How does the tree like having that space there?"
"It seems there is something inside the tree. I wonder what that is?"
"If the tree could speak to that creature, what would it say to it?"
"I wonder how long that creature has been in that space?"

Entry Point 3: The Mother Deer

(Christine had placed two deer, a mother and a baby, in the branches of the tree. She had also placed another creature inside the tree, a porcupine "with needles.")
"What is the mother doing on the branch of the tree?"
"I notice there is a baby next to the mother deer. What's it like for the mother to be near the baby?"
"What's it like for the baby to be atop the tree?"
"What is the mother/baby thinking?"
"What is the mother/baby doing?"

"I wonder if they could speak to each other, what they would say?"

"I wonder if they know there is a porcupine nearby?"

"What do they think about the porcupine being nearby?"

"How do the branches feel about having company up high?"

"If the mother could be heard by the cat, what would she want the cat to know?"

Here is the dialogue that I had with Christine, based on some of the questions that I had prepared.

THERAPIST: What is the mother doing on the branch of the tree?

CHRISTINE: She's trying to be very quiet.

THERAPIST: So she's trying to be very quiet.

CHRISTINE: Yeah, she doesn't want to make too much noise.

THERAPIST: What will happen if she makes too much noise?

CHRISTINE: She'll get caught hiding, and then she'll be in trouble.

THERAPIST: So the mother deer is hiding right now.

CHRISTINE: Yep, right in the branches . . . but she's also watching, you know, keeping guard.

THERAPIST: Oh, so Mom is keeping guard.

CHRISTINE: Yeah, she's a good guard, too!

THERAPIST: It's great when moms can be good guards, and sometimes they hide so they don't get in trouble.

CHRISTINE: Yeah, you have to be really quiet.

THERAPIST: How does the baby feel when the mom is guarding and hiding?

CHRISTINE: She holds her breath. She is really quiet. She doesn't say anything and keeps real still.

THERAPIST: Oh, so the baby knows what to do. She's real quiet, holds her breath, keeps still.

CHRISTINE: Yep, she doesn't want to get caught because bad trouble comes . . .

THERAPIST: What kind of trouble comes?

CHRISTINE: You know, the porcupine. He has very sharp needles, and he shoots them out and hurts the mommy deer.

THERAPIST: Oh, so the porcupine has sharp needles and hurts Mom.

CHRISTINE: Yeah, we don't like him. He's mean all the time.

THERAPIST: What does the porcupine do when he's not being mean and shooting needles?

CHRISTINE: I don't know.

THERAPIST: How is the porcupine mean to the baby deer?

CHRISTINE: He hurts her mommy and screams at her too.

THERAPIST: I'm so sorry to hear that. I'm so sorry that the porcupine hurts and scares the mommy and baby. . . . What's it like for the baby to be atop the tree?

CHRISTINE: She likes it there. Her mommy likes it there too, because she's tricking the porcupine.

THERAPIST: So being away from the porcupine feels safe to the baby and mommy?

CHRISTINE: Yeah.

THERAPIST: I wonder if the baby and mommy deer can feel safe anywhere else?

CHRISTINE: Only if the porcupine isn't there. Sometimes the police take him far away, but he always comes back and finds them.

THERAPIST: Sounds like he's a very persistent porcupine. . . . I wonder if the mommy and baby could speak to each other, what they would say?

CHRISTINE: Just "I love you."

THERAPIST: The mommy and baby love each other.

CHRISTINE: Yep.

THERAPIST: How do the branches feel about having company up high?

CHRISTINE: They like the deer being there. That's funny . . . deers don't climb trees, but sometimes they do. And squirrels do, and caterpillars do.

THERAPIST: If the mother could be heard by the cat, what would she want the cat to know?

CHRISTINE: The mommy would thank the cat for being a good pet and tell her that we'll be back home soon, as soon as we can find a new place to live. Mommy says we're going to have a new home with a cat.

THERAPIST: I see you and your mom are going to live together in a new home with a cat.

I had chosen and prepared my questions in order from least to most difficult (at least, I surmised that it might be most difficult for Christine to talk about the experiences with domestic violence that I believed were being represented in the center of the tray). We spent about four sessions exploring her metaphor, and she developed more and more comfort as we spoke.

By the time we got to the third question, Christine was willing, even eager, to stay with the metaphor and answer questions or comments from that vantage point; however, she was almost always reluctant to say anything about her father and his violent behavior. It was almost as if she thought talking about it would be discovered by him and put her in danger. Christine's subsequent trays were typically developmentally appropriate, with princesses and fairylands. Apparently, the tray that first slipped out (the mother and baby deer up a tree) was closer to reality than she could tolerate for very long.

Dyadic Work with Sarah and Christine

One of the central aspects of our work was attachment-based. It was clear that the violence in the home had caused profound disruptions in the parent–child relationship. Specifically, Christine had experienced an environment of tension and violence, which increased her stress level and affected her ability to soothe or self-regulate. Her mother's attention was constantly diverted, and although Sarah was making her best efforts to protect Christine from harm, Christine was often neglected, pushed away, or simply left alone to fend for herself. Even when Sarah held or fed Christine, she did so in an anxious, frightened state that was visible in her eyes, her facial tension, her skirted glances, and the constricted muscles in her arms. In addition, Christine had learned that her mother was unable to protect herself from harm, and by extension, unable to protect her. The child's basic safety and security had been severely compromised, and this damage needed to be addressed in therapy.

This work had two stages: having mother and child share and reflect on the story that Christine had told in the sand, and having them use Christine's metaphor to rework the issue of safety.

When I first told Christine that I'd like her mother to see the sandtray she had made about the mother and baby deer and the porcupine, she looked a little uncertain. She wondered whether her mother might get mad at her for telling me the story. I told Christine that her mother and I had talked about the sandtray story, that her mother was looking forward to hearing about it from Christine, and that Sarah might even want to add to the story and might have some ideas about it. Christine was hesitant to show the tray to her mother, but quickly became excited about telling her the story that she had told me, adding some of the things she had discovered when she and I had talked together. Here is a paraphrase of what Christine told her mother and how Sarah responded to her child:

CHRISTINE: (*pointing to the recreated scenario in the sand tray*)
Mommy, look, the mommy deer and the baby are high, high on the tree. And the porcupine is there, but he can't climb up the tree; he can't come scare them. Mommy, look, the baby and mommy

love each other, and they live together in a tall tree where the porcupine can't get them!

SARAH: (*asking Christine to sit on her lap and holding her*) I see the mommy and the baby, and I am so sorry that they feel afraid of the porcupine.

CHRISTINE: (*stepping off and facing mother*) But he can't climb up the tree, Mommy, so the mommy and baby are safe now.

SARAH: (*putting her back on her lap and hugging her*) The mommy went up the tree because it was the only thing she could think to do, because she was afraid of the porcupine. But now the mommy deer has learned a lot—a lot about taking care of herself and getting away from the porcupine. I think this mommy and baby deer deserve to live on the ground, where they can find food for themselves, and they can build a house with a roof, so they don't get wet when it rains. And you know what else? The mommy deer has to stretch her legs and stand up straight, and help her little deer learn how to stretch too! What I'd like to do now, sweetie, is put that porcupine somewhere else, so that the mommy and baby deer can come down and see how much fun it is to be on the ground!

And with that, Sarah set the context for more attachment work as she began to present herself as capable (no longer a victim) to her child. She took the porcupine, held it in her hands, and in a firm voice stated, "I'm not afraid of you any more, and you are never allowed to come around us again!" She placed it in a box in the office and said, "You are out of our lives forever. I have a little deer who has a lot of safe living to do, and she and I are going to explore our nice forest together!" Christine looked at her mother with big eyes, and kissed her on the cheek. "Come on, Mom," she said, "come over and let's make a new world for them." They played together and moved things around, and the mother and baby deer made tracks in the sand as Sarah said, "They're on firm ground now. They are flexing their muscles now, kind of like you and me. I'm getting a place ready for us that will be safe and cozy. You'll see."

Reintroducing the Metaphor

Another option for amplifying the metaphor is to reintroduce it to the child in some other medium or in some other way. In this particular case, after the wonderful work Sarah and Christine did in the sandtray, I reintroduced the story of the mother and baby deer hiding from the porcupine by doing an art therapy project called the Safe Environment Project (Sobol & Schneider, 1998). Sarah and Christine did this work together, and I provided a paper plate, some paints and markers, and the mother and baby deer miniatures. I then asked them to create a safe environment for the two deer.

Mother and daughter produced an environment with foliage, color, a protective fence, a small covered area, food, water, and a friend for the deer.

This reintroduction of the mother and baby deer, in a completely different activity, allowed Christine to interact once again with the metaphor she had created earlier and to find ways to engage with the metaphor further on another level of resource building, now introduced by the clinician (myself), at this advanced phase of therapy. My integrated approach is documented elsewhere (Gil, 2006), but suffice it to say that therapy can include the purposeful integration of directive and nondirective strategies. In addition, consensus exists on the importance of integrating dyadic work with young children and their parents into play therapy with the children, and "attachment therapies" have been developed and well articulated in the last decade (Berlin, Ziv, Amaya-Jackson, & Greenberg, 2005; Booth & Jernberg, 2010; Greenspan & Lieberman, 1988; Hughes, 2000, 2007; Schore, 1994).

Conclusion

The use of clinical metaphor has been encouraged throughout the clinical literature on hypnotherapy as well as family therapy. Expressive therapists have long considered metaphor work pivotal to what they do; they recognize that children in particular find play and art natural ways of communicating and expressing themselves.

Art and play therapists understand the myriad benefits of valuing children's metaphors, and often engage children by creating clinical metaphors and introducing these into their own work with the children. Whether the metaphors are initiated by clients or their clinicians, they serve as projections or representations of something that cannot always be acknowledged or verbalized. Thus it behooves clinicians to learn to decipher the camouflaged communications imbedded in metaphors, and to help clients reflect, explore, and amplify these in order to become more interested in and curious about their creations and themselves.

Metaphors are, by definition, opportunities for transition, and clinicians using metaphor work believe in the potential of processed or managed metaphors to be reintegrated on a deeper level—taken back in, as it were, with new acquired meaning. Metaphors also offer opportunities for healing through processing of difficult experiences.

This chapter summarizes the importance of giving children (and their parents) the opportunity to do metaphor work, and it gives suggestions for amplifying metaphors in ways that facilitate self-reflection and exploration. An integrative approach allows for processing the metaphors both symbolically and verbally; therapists help children to externalize their thoughts and feelings by staying within their metaphors, rather than drawing too-quick correlations between the metaphors and real life. In fact, if children were feeling able or willing to speak about their distress, they would do so. Instead, they seem to find it much easier to "speak" through metaphor and amplification of their work. In the case described in this chapter, attachment-based work was central to improved health in the mother–child relationship, and both Christine and Sarah were able to stay with Christine's metaphors and receptive to guidance about deepening their understanding of their symbolic communication. In addition, it is important to note that no attachment work is complete without direct interventions with the parent–child dyad, and these can be delivered in a playful, energetic, and creative manner within an integrated (directive and nondirective) model. This case example illustrates a fluid methodology of individual and conjoint work, as well as a natural continuum from nondirective to directive work.

REFERENCES

Berlin, L. J., Ziv, Y., Amaya-Jackson, L., & Greenberg, M. T. (2005). *Enhancing early attachments: Theory, research, intervention, and policy.* New York: Guilford Press.

Booth, P. B., & Jernberg, A. M. (2010). *Theraplay: Helping parents and children build better relationships through attachment-based play* (3rd ed.). San Francisco: Jossey-Bass.

Davis, N. (1990). *Therapeutic stories that teach and heal.* Burke, VA: Author.

Erickson, M. H., & Rossi, E. L. (1979). *Hypnotherapy: An exploratory casebook.* New York: Irvington.

Esparza, D. P. (2012). Therapeutic metaphors and clinical hypnosis. *Purpose-driven hypnotherapy: A method for positive change.* Retrieved from *www. pdhypnosis.com/index.php/weblog/articles/181*

Gil, E. (2006). *Helping abused and traumatized children: Integrating directive and nondirective approaches.* New York: Guilford Press.

Gil, E. (2011). *Working with children to heal interpersonal trauma: The power of play.* New York: Guilford Press.

Gil, E., & Shaw, J. (2013). *Working with children with sexual behavior problems.* New York: Guilford Press.

Greenspan, S. I., & Lieberman, A. F. (1988). A clinical approach to attachment. In E. J. Blesky & T. Nezworski (Eds.), *Clinical implications of attachment* (pp. 387–424). Hillsdale, NJ: Erlbaum.

Guiffrida, D. A., Jordan, R., Saiz, S., & Barnes, K. L. (2007). The use of metaphor in clinical supervision. *Journal of Counseling and Development, 85,* 393–400.

Hughes, D. A. (2000). *Facilitating developmental attachment: The road to emotional recovery and behavioral change in foster and adopted children.* Northvale, NJ: Aronson.

Hughes, D. A. (2007). *Attachment-focused family therapy.* New York: Norton.

Lankton, S. (2004). *Assembling Ericksonian therapy: The collected papers of Stephen Lankton.* Phoenix, AZ: Zeig, Tucker, & Theisen.

Onnis, L., Bernardini, M., Giambartolomei, A., Leonelli, A., Menenti, B., & Vietri, A. (2007). *The use of metaphors in systemic therapy: A bridge between mind and body languages.* Paper presented at the Congress of the European Family Therapy Association, Glasgow, Scotland. Retrieved from *www.eftacim.org/doc_pdf/metaphors.pdf*

Ricoeur, P. (1967). *The symbolism of evil.* New York: Beacon Press.

Schore, A. N. (1994). *Affect regulation and the origin of the self.* Hillsdale, NJ: Erlbaum.

Siegel, D. A., & Payne Bryson, T. (2012). *The whole-brain child: 12 revolutionary strategies to nurture your child's developing mind.* New York: Bantam Books.

Sobol, B., & Schneider, K. (1998). Art as an adjunctive therapy in the treatment of children who dissociate. In J. L. Silberg (Ed.), *The dissociative child: Diagnosis, treatment, and management* (2nd ed., pp. 191–218). Lutherville, MD: Sidran Press.

CHAPTER 11

The Neurobiological Power of Play

Using the Neurosequential Model of Therapeutics to Guide Play in the Healing Process

Richard L. Gaskill
Bruce D. Perry

Children, like all human beings, are best understood in a social con-text. We humans are healthiest and most productive when we are born, grow, live, work, and raise our families in social groups (Ludy-Dobson & Perry, 2010). We have existed and thrived for thousands of years because of our neurobiological drive to form safe, nurturing, mutually rewarding, and lasting attachments (Szalavitz & Perry, 2010). In normative attach-ment relationships, children can safely explore new experiences and master developmental competencies, including the ability to regulate themselves cognitively, affectively, behaviorally, physiologically, and relationally (Blaustein & Kinniburgh, 2005). Secure attachments ultimately become the basis of resiliency in children exposed to distressing experiences (Sha-piro & Levendosky, 1999). When these important attachment systems are compromised through multiple and chronic lapses within caregiving systems, crucial neural systems can be altered. This alteration negatively affects key competencies, such as the ability to regulate emotions and expe-riences. These effects in turn can contribute to neuropsychiatric problems and result in enduring social and emotional difficulties across the lifespan (Blaustein & Kinniburgh, 2005). Zeanah et al. (2004) have reported the prevalence of attachment-disordered children to be as high as 35% of chil-dren entering foster care, and as high as 38–40% of high-risk infant and toddler populations. Such demographics suggest the need for play therapy intervention techniques that can appropriately target the neural networks involved in self-regulation and relational functioning.

Any discussion of the role of play in neurodevelopment must first address one core question: What is *play*? What are the key elements that distinguish play from other activities? For the purposes of this chapter, we use the three elements used by Burghardt (2005) to define play in animals. First, play mimics or approximates a common or important purposeful behavior; second, play is voluntary, is pleasurable, and has no immediate survival role or obvious "purpose"; and, finally, play takes place in a non-threatening, low-duress context. These key elements are often at odds with many well-intended (and typically ineffective) therapeutic experiences. It is no surprise that the core elements of play echo some of the essential ingredients of successful therapeutic interactions with maltreated and traumatized children—perceived control, reward, and manageable stress (see Perry & Szalavitz, 2006). Bringing play into therapeutic work, therefore, not only makes sense; it is often an essential element for therapeutic progress. Yet it is important to appreciate that "play" for the toddler looks different from "play" for the adolescent. Play is an effective therapeutic agent when it provides a developmentally appropriate means to regulate, communicate, practice, and master. As with other therapeutic approaches, however, we often select the manner of "play" that we bring into therapy according to a child's chronological age and to our specific training as therapists; there are thus times when the expectations we bring into the therapeutic relationship are unrealistic. The resulting mismatch between a therapist's expectation and a child's capability undermines the potential for true play (i.e., the interaction is not spontaneous or pleasurable for the child), and thereby therapeutic progress. When the therapist (or parent, caregiver, or teacher) understands the real developmental capabilities of the child and the child's current state (e.g., calm, alert, fearful), realistic expectations and developmentally appropriate activities (including the manner of play) can be used to help the child heal. This crucial awareness of the "stage" and the current "state" is informed by an understanding of neurobiology. This chapter provides an introduction to some neurodevelopmental principles that inform play therapy practice.

Play Therapy: Overview, Context, and Efficacy

Historical Overview and Scope of Play Therapy

The developmental importance of children's play has been recognized for hundreds if not thousands of years, beginning with the thoughts of Plato (427 B.C.–347 B.C.) and continuing later with Rousseau's (1762/1930) notions. In the 20th century, Freud (1924), Gesell and Ilg (1947), Erikson (1964), Piaget (1962), Kohlberg (1963), Vygotsky (1967), and other developmental theorists defined, articulated, and advocated for the role of play during childhood. Developmental theorists generally have viewed play as an essential experiential element of social, emotional, physical, intellectual, and psychological development. The somatosensory experiences in some play activities have been viewed as the neurological foundations for later advanced mental skills, such as creativity, abstract thought, prosocial behavior, and expressive language. Furthermore, Zigler, Singer, and Bishop-Josef (2004) have cited a growing body of research finding that "Vygotskian-type" play promotes development of self-regulation, a cornerstone of early childhood development across all domains of behavior (social, emotional, cognitive, and physical). Play has been considered so critical to healthy development that the United Nations recognizes it as a specific right for all children (Office of the United Nations High Commissioner for Human Rights, 1989). Since the period from birth to age 6 establishes the foundation for learning, behavior, and health throughout the lifespan, the United Nations has accorded play equal importance with nutrition, housing, health care, and education.

Landreth (2002) has suggested that talk and cognitively oriented therapies are inappropriate for children through much of their development, due to the relative underdevelopment of complex cognitive capacities in childhood. The powerful role of play in children's growth, and the slow attainment of adult mental and verbal abilities, both suggest play as a developmentally appropriate strategy for treating children's emotional and behavioral difficulties. Accordingly, play has been incorporated into therapies with children for years. Freud's treatment of "Little Hans" incorporated play into therapy at the turn of the last century (Bratton & Ray, 2000; Bratton, Ray, Rhine, & Jones, 2005; Landreth, 2002). From this time on, there has been significant growth of play therapy theory and practice— from psychoanalytic play therapy in the 1920s, to release play therapy in the 1930s, to relationship play therapy also in the 1930s, and finally to nondirective play therapy beginning in the 1940s and 1950s (Landreth, 2002). Play therapy variations continued to expand through the end of the 20th century with the development of Adlerian play therapy (Kottman, 1995), Jungian play therapy (Allen, 1988), gestalt play therapy (Oaklander, 1994), ecosystem play therapy (O'Connor, 2000), object relations play therapy (Benedict, 2006), experiential play therapy (Norton & Norton, 1997), cognitive-behavioral play therapy (Knell, 1995), developmental play therapy (Brody, 1997), Filial Therapy (Guerney, 1964), and others.

Studies have described play therapy strategies for social maladjustment, maladaptive school behavior, self-concept, anxiety, conduct disorder, aggression, oppositional behavior, emotional maladjustment, fear, developmental disabilities, physical and learning disabilities, autism, schizophrenia, psychoticism, posttraumatic stress disorder, sexual abuse, domestic violence, depression, withdrawal, alcohol and drug abuse, divorce, reading disorders, speech and language problems, and multicultural issues

(Bratton & Ray, 2000; Bratton et al., 2005; LeBlanc & Ritchie, 2001). Recent research has begun to address the efficacy of play therapy versus other treatments, using randomized controlled studies with large sample sizes (Bratton & Ray, 2000; Bratton et al., 2005; Pearl et al., 2012; Tsai & Ray, 2011).

Efficacy of Play Therapy

Over the past 30 years, a number of meta-analytic studies examining multiple play therapy studies have found play therapy to be effective with a wide variety of problematic issues. These studies demonstrated that children had improved prosocial behavior and decreased symptomatic behavior (Bratton et al., 2005; Casey & Berman 1985; LeBlanc & Ritchie, 1999, 2001; Ray, Bratton, Rhine, & Jones, 2001; Weisz, Weiss, Alicke, & Klotz, 1987). The treatment effect sizes ranged from a high of 0.80 (Bratton et al., 2005) to a low of 0.66 (LeBlanc & Ritchie, 2001), with most falling between 0.71 and 0.79. These results indicate that children receiving play therapy interventions performed much better than children who did not receive play therapy, and that play therapy demonstrated a large effect on children's behavior, social adjustment, and personality (Bratton et al., 2005; Ray et al., 2001).

Play therapy interventions appear to be equally effective, regardless of the presenting problem. Play therapy is effective across modalities, ages, genders, and theoretical schools of thought (Bratton et al., 2005; LeBlanc & Ritchie, 1999; Ray et al., 2001). Several studies suggest that the maximum effect size is achieved after 30–40 sessions, whereas shorter or longer treatment durations are less effective (Bratton et al., 2005; LeBlanc & Ritchie, 1999, 2001). LeBlanc and Ritchie (1999, 2001) suggest that short-term play therapy treatment models may obtain negative outcomes because children are acting out previously unexpressed feelings in the early stages of such treatment and have insufficient time to resolve these issues. These authors have observed that children participating in play therapy appear to take considerably more time to process information and make effective changes in thinking or behaving, compared to adults in conventional therapies.

Multiple studies (Bratton et al., 2005; LeBlanc & Ritchie, 1999, 2001; Ray et al., 2001) point to the importance of parental involvement as an essential predictor of positive outcome. When parents received structured play therapy supervision or guided interactions between themselves and their children, effectiveness rose dramatically. Bratton and colleagues noted that the Filial Therapy model (Guerney, 1964) and the child–parent relationship theory model (Landreth, 2002) yielded larger effect sizes than other studies. This is not surprising, given that play therapy with humanistic interventions produced a larger effect size than nonhumanistic treatments. Children learn through play, and this often requires a patient, supportive, and caring adult to scaffold that process (Vygotsky, 1967).

The Developing Brain and the Vulnerability of Childhood

The human brain is organized in a hierarchical manner. The higher regions in the brain mediate the more complex and executive functions, while the lower areas mediate the simpler, more regulatory functions. There are four developmentally distinct regions (brainstem, diencephalon, limbic, and cortical) that are woven together by multiple neural networks, some of the most important being the well-studied monoamine (i.e., norepinephrine and dopamine) and other related (e.g., serotonin, acetylcholine) systems. These networks originate in lower areas of the brain; have widespread distribution (collectively to all brain areas and the body); and have a direct impact on all motor, social, emotional, and cognitive functioning, as well as the stress response. When these networks develop normally, there is smooth functional integration. When these networks are impacted by intrauterine insults (e.g., prenatal alcohol or drug exposure), early life attachment disruptions, or traumatic stress, these networks will be dysregulated, resulting in compromise in all in the functions impacted by their wide distribution. These crucial networks play a role in integrating, processing, and acting on incoming patterns of information from the primary sensory networks (such as touch, vision, and sound), which monitor the external environment; somatic networks (such as motor–vestibular, cardiovascular, and respiratory), which monitor the internal environment; and cerebral networks (such as cortical modulating networks), which monitor the brain's internal environment.

The continuous input from the brain, body, and world, coupled with their widespread distribution, provides these networks with a unique role in the stress response—and in stress- or trauma-related dysfunction. Furthermore, as neurodevelopment progresses from lower (i.e., brainstem and diencephalon) to higher (i.e., limbic and cortical) areas, these regulatory neural networks play a key role in the development of the brain from the intrauterine period through adolescence. The timing and pattern of activation of these regulatory neural networks play a crucial role in shaping the functional capacity of all brain and body areas (see Perry, 2001).

Neurons and neural networks change in response to activity. In the case of the stress response networks, predictable, moderate activity leads to flexible and capable stress response capacity (with a potential for demonstrating resilience), whereas extreme, unpredictable, or uncontrollable activation leads to a sensitized, overly reactive set of stress response networks (see Perry, 2008, 2009; Ungar & Perry, 2012). Any developmental insult—such as prenatal alcohol or drug exposure, or extreme, prolonged activation of the stress response (such as that seen in maltreatment or other traumatic experience)—will alter the development of these crucial neural networks, and thereby disrupt functioning in all of the areas these regulatory networks innervate.

The resulting alterations in the regulation and functioning of both central and peripheral autonomic neural networks (as well as the neuroendocrine and the neuroimmune systems) will result in increased risk of significant and lasting emotional, behavioral, social, cognitive, sensory–motor, and physical health problems (Anda et al., 2006; Felitti et al., 1998; Perry, 2006, 2008, 2009; Perry & Dobson, 2013; Perry & Pollard, 1998; Perry, Pollard, Blakley, Baker, & Vigilante, 1995). Manifestations of the resulting sensitized stress response systems have been well documented. They include intrusive recollections; persistent avoidance of associated stimuli or numbing of general responsiveness; and arousal symptoms of hyperarousal, hypervigilance, increased startle response, sleep difficulties, irritability, anxiety, and physiological hyperactivity. Maltreated and traumatized children may exhibit behavioral impulsivity, increased muscle tone, anxiety, a fixation on threat-related cues, affect regulation, language disorders, fine and gross motor delays, disorganized attachment, dysphoria, attention difficulties, memory problems, and hyperactivity (Perry et al., 1995). Furthermore, these physical, emotional, psychological, and intellectual effects may persist across the lifespan (Anda et al., 2006; Spinazzola, Blaustein, & van der Kolk, 2005). Nearly two-thirds of traumatized children exhibit physical signs and symptoms indicating dysregulation in brainstem or diencephalic functions, such as inhibition of gastrointestinal processes, cardiac activity, blood pressure, respiration, anxiety, and hypervigilance (Hopper, Spinazzola, Simpson, & van der Kolk, 2006; Perry, 2001, 2008). The specific physical signs and symptoms will depend upon a multitude of contributing factors, including genetics, epigenetics, intrauterine environment, early bonding experiences, history of developmental adversity, and attenuating relational buffers (see Ungar & Perry, 2012). This creates a confusing clinical picture that does not fit neatly into our current inadequate model of categorization. The comorbidity of neuropsychiatric diagnoses associated with childhood maltreatment is so pervasive that it encompasses nearly all diagnoses in the new fifth edition of the *Diagnostic and Statistical Manual of Mental Disorders* (DSM-5; American Psychiatric Association, 2013), resulting in the inability of current diagnostic labels to capture the complex heterogeneous dysfunction adequately (Perry, 2008; Perry & Dobson, 2013).

Although traumatic experiences may have a negative impact on adult functioning, the same adverse experiences have a much more deleterious impact on children because of the pervasive impact on development. Traumatic stress in adulthood affects a developed and functioning brain; trauma in childhood affects the organization and functioning of the developing brain. Adults suffering a traumatic event have been found to attain asymptomatic posttreatment status 75% of the time, but children suffering a traumatic event have been found to achieve asymptomatic status only 33% of the time (van der Kolk et al., 2007).

The Stress Response and State-Dependent Functioning

The crucial regulatory neural networks involved in the stress response (and multiple other functions) are themselves modulated through patterned, repetitive, and rhythmic input from both bottom-up (i.e., somatosensory) and top-down (i.e., cerebromodulatory) systems. The brain processes (and acts) on incoming input at multiple levels; although the brain is essentially an open and interactive system, this multilevel process of sensing, processing, and acting on the environment basically begins at the site of initial input of sensory, somatic, or cerebral input to the lower areas of the brain. The primary regulatory systems that originate in the lower areas of the brain begin to sort, integrate, interpret, store, and respond to incoming stimuli long before conscious portions of the brain receive the information, if they receive it at all (Marteau, Hollands, & Fletcher, 2012; Perry, 2006). Primary somatosensory processing takes place below the level of consciousness, and only novel, significant, or potentially threatening stimuli are passed on to higher cortical centers for further processing (Perry, 2008; Sara & Bouret, 2012). When the input to these regulatory networks is unfamiliar (novel), disorganized (chaotic), or associated with potential threat (i.e., reexposure to a cue from a previous traumatic experience), there will be alterations in the activity of these systems. In the crucial norepinephrine-containing networks originating in the locus coeruleus, for example, a complex and graded response that is proportional (in typically functioning individuals) to the level of threat (Sara & Bouret, 2012) will begin. A key part of that response is a shift of "control" from higher, cortical systems to limbic, then diencephalic systems. Neuroimaging during highly emotional states demonstrates increased activation of subcortical regions and significant reduction of blood flow to the frontal lobe during intense arousal (van der Kolk, 2006). This shift in activation alters cognitive, social, emotional, and motor functioning. In other words, novelty, chaos and threat change the "state" of the individual. This shift in state involves shutting down the cortical modulatory networks that could typically be recruited and involved in conscious, intentional modulation of the feelings of anxiety, hunger, thirst, anger, and other "primitive" feelings and perceptions. The result is that less mature, more poorly regulated, more impulsive behaviors will result under perceived threat. And if child's developmental experiences have been such that they have fewer cortical-network-building experiences (e.g., neglect- or chaos-related poverty of touch, words, relationships), their cortical modulation networks will be relatively underdeveloped as well. The combination of a sensitized set of regulatory neural networks (i.e., the stress response systems are "locked into" a persisting state of fear) with a "shut-down" and underdeveloped cortex will result in a very impulsive, globally dysregulated child. This is worth remembering when one is interpreting trauma-related and attachment-related behavioral problems with maltreated children; exhausted and frustrated caregivers, teachers, and therapists are quick to personalize and infer deliberate intention to automatic, elicited behaviors. The capacity for self-reflection, planning, and intentional behavior requires a relatively organized, regulated, and accessible cortex.

Another crucial aspect of this shift is its impact on the capacity to feel pleasure. Release of dopamine in the two regions of the brain—the nucleus accumbens and the ventral tegmental area—can provide a sensation of pleasure. These "reward" areas can be stimulated in many ways, ranging from cortically mediated, intentional behaviors that are consistent with an individual's beliefs or values (e.g., sharing candy with someone) to primarily limbic mediated relational interactions (e.g., a laugh with a friend) to diencephalon-mediated appetitive experiences (e.g., eating sweet, salty, or fatty foods) to brainstem-mediated regulatory behaviors that decrease physiological distress (e.g., drinking cold water when dehydrated). As the individual moves down the arousal continuum, the reward "options" shrink. In a state of high arousal or fear, delayed gratification is impossible. Future consequences or rewards of behavior become almost inconceivable to the threatened child. Reflection on behavior is impossible for the child in an alarm state, and cognitive strategies to modify behavior (even if previously internalized and mastered) cannot be recruited in an efficient way because the cortex is relatively inaccessible under threat. Cut adrift from the internal regulating capabilities of the cortex, the individual acts impulsively to any perceived threat. The key to helping the child begin to move back to a more regulated state, making the child feel safe and thereby more available for cognitive engagement and therapeutic change, is to utilize the direct somatosensory routes and provide patterned, repetitive, rhythmic input. Therapeutic change starts from a sense of safety; in turn, the sense of safety emerges from these regulating somatosensory activities.

Finally, these complex children will be very resistant to traditional therapeutic (i.e., primarily cognitive-behavioral or cognitive-relational) interventions (see the case vignette below). Traditional psychodynamic or cognitive-behavioral play therapies that support the development of cognitive regulatory control are likely to fail when the lower brain networks are disorganized, underdeveloped, or impaired. A neurodevelopmentally informed assessment process and therapeutic strategy can help the clinical team better understand such a child's developmental stages and state reactivity; to be effective, the clinician must *know the stage and watch the state*.

Implications for Play Therapy

We (Gaskill & Perry, 2012) have previously outlined the primary challenges of integrating a neurodevelopmental perspective with traditional play therapies. Child mental health treatment models, including play therapy, evolved out of adult psychodynamic and cognitive-behavioral therapies that use primarily cognitive and verbally mediated (i.e., top-down) inter-actions focusing on executive processing, insight, understanding, plan-ning, and decision making. Ultimately, maltreated children will need to address cognitive issues such as guilt, shame, self-esteem, grief, and loss, and to gain understanding of, acceptance of, and a new perspective on their experiences—but these cortically mediated issues must be addressed in a developmentally sensitive sequence, and only after some modulation of the primary regulatory networks has been established (Perry, 2001, 2006, 2008, 2009; Cook et al., 2005).

Accordingly, the play therapists will often need to use bottom-up modu-latory networks (somatosensory) to establish some moderate self-regulation prior to the implementation of insightful reflection, trauma experience inte-gration, narrative development, social development, or affect enhancement. Doing so will require therapeutic methods to access and provide reorganiz-ing input to the regulatory networks of the lower brain areas (Kleim & Jones, 2008; Perry, 2008, 2009). The key to treatment is to be sure that the child is regulated and that relational and cognitive expectations are appropriate for the child's developmental age. Furthermore, this requires rethinking traditional "dosing" and context of therapy.

Complex, deeply troubled children need more than the traditional once-a-week play therapy model. They will require therapeutic environ-ments that immerse them in positive, repetitive rehearsals of healthy inter-actions and activities. These interactions and activities often need to be regressive in nature, requiring low adult-to-child ratios (often 1:1) and activities frequently associated with much younger children, as many foun-dational experiences (neural networks) have been missed or are incomplete (Perry, 2006, 2009, in press; Perry & Dobson, 2013). The numbers of inter-actions required to change ingrained low-brain patterns call for extensive commitment from parents, teachers, therapists, and extended family, as the time required exceeds the capabilities of a single individual (Perry, 2009).

Fortunately, many playful activities that provide the activation nec-essary to modulate and reorganize these regulatory neural networks can be integrated into play therapies and playful therapeutic experiences (most therapeutic change happens outside of therapy). Play therapists should never forget that if something is not fun, it is not play, and that it is impossible for a child to have pleasure in a relational interaction if the child's brain is in an alarm state. The key, therefore, to being true to the "play" in play therapy is helping the child become regulated and thereby safe. Once basic state regulation has been established, more traditional play therapies will be effective. Bottom-up interventions for children with state-regulatory dif-ficulties will consist of some variety of somatosensory activity (e.g., music, dance, walking, drawing). Although language will undoubtedly be neces-sary in the process of working with these children, play therapists must realize that in dysregulated children it will not be likely that words, rea-soning, or ideas will change the primary regulatory networks in the lower areas of the brain. Rather, regulatory organization and creation of normal homeostatic states depend more on the "primal language" of gentle tones of voice; comforting, repetitive sensory experience; and soothing repetitive and patterned movements by patient, safe adults. Providing this "primal language" may take the form of child-directed free play; repetitive, patterned sensory integration activities carried out at home, school, and clinic; or fine and large motor activities. All such activities will require an atmosphere of enjoyment, safety, and attunement between adults and children. As noted above, this work must often be done in very low adult-to-child ratios that match a child's functional age, often 1:1 (see Gaskill & Perry, 2012). For a child with severe dysregulation, the play therapist may need to restrict the environment as well, to control environmental stimuli to match the child's developmental age; otherwise, overstimulation of the child is likely to produce frustration, irritability, tantrums, aggression, and withdrawal (including dissociation).

Finally, the unique aspects of each child's history, genetic endowment, and epigenetic influences preclude a "one-size-fits-all" treatment model (Ungar & Perry, 2012). Such multifaceted symptomatology requires play therapists to incorporate neurobiological principles, comparing play therapy techniques, delivery methods, treatment frequencies, optimal numbers of treatment sessions, and outcome measures (Bratton et al., 2005; Perry & Dobson, 2013; Ray et al., 2001). A crucial element in any therapeutic approach with these children is patience. Neural plasticity is a primary neurophysiological process underlying therapeutic change; expressed plasticity (i.e., changing a neural network) requires adequate (sometimes thousands of) repetitions (Kleim & Jones, 2008). Play therapists, family members, teachers, and other caregivers who are not aware of this can often become frustrated/confused and give up (Perry, 2009).

The Neurosequential Model of Therapeutics

The Neurosequential Model of Therapeutics™ (NMT) is a developmentally sensitive, neurobiology-informed approach to clinical problem solving. NMT is not a specific therapeutic technique or intervention. As described by Brandt, Diel, Feder, and Lillas (2012),

> The Neurosequential Model of Therapeutics™ (NMT) (Perry, 2006) provides an integrated understanding of the sequencing of neurodevelopment embedded in the experiences of the child, and supports biologically informed practices, programs, and policies. As a global evidence-based practice (EBP) and coupled with the NMT's brain mapping matrix, the model supports providers in identifying specific areas for therapeutic work and in selecting appropriate therapies, including evidence-based therapies (EBTs), within a comprehensive therapeutic plan. Organized NMT-based intervention models, such as NMT therapeutic child care, can be EBTs. (p. 43)

A key component of the NMT is an assessment process that informs a clinician about a child's broad set of brain-mediated strengths and vulnerabilities. From this assessment process, the general direction for therapeutic, educational, and enrichment expectations and opportunities can be determined. In the case of play therapy, simply stated, the NMT can help the therapist appropriately design the most developmentally appropriate forms of play to bring into the therapy. The following case vignette illustrates the power of play in the therapeutic process. It also illustrates the specific value of selecting developmentally appropriate forms of play in a relationally safe context, and of using adequate "dosing" in a patterned, repetitive, rhythmic, and rewarding manner.

Case Vignette: Tom

History

Tom is a 7-year-old boy who has been living with a foster family for the last 13 months. He was the only biological child born to an 18-year-old mother who actively used multiple drugs (marijuana, nicotine, alcohol, and cocaine) during her pregnancy. He was born addicted to cocaine and spent 2 weeks in a pediatric intensive care unit following his birth at 36 weeks' gestation. Both of his biological parents had extensive family histories of mental health problems, substance abuse, and criminal behavior. The parents split up when Tom was 2 months old, due to domestic violence; he lived with his mother, who was described as "disengaged, withdrawn, and flat." Multiple reports of abandonment and neglect were made, and at 14 months child protective services placed Tom with his biological father. The father lived in a violent, drug-filled, chaotic world, with no stable housing. Visitations (both formal and informal) with the mother continued during this time. The father tended to drop Tom off when he was involved in a criminal activity or drug binge. During visits, Tom witnessed his mother having sex and being beaten up by various men; Tom was also physically (and possibly sexually) abused by several of these men. His mother locked him in a bedroom, only episodically feeding him and rarely interacting with him. At age 5, Tom was removed and placed in foster care after his father was arrested for armed robbery of a convenience store; the father had walked into the store with Tom and used him as a decoy during the robbery.

Original Presentation

At the time of removal, Tom demonstrated abnormalities in functions mediated by all areas of the brain, from brainstem to cortex. He had excessive salivation and blinking. He was extremely fearful, anxious, and hypervigilant; he had an increased startle response, as well as sleep difficulties and frequent nightmares. He was also aggressive and threatening: He lashed out at other children in placement and was cruel to the pets; he "plotted to trap and kill" the carers. Tom was violent to peers, strangers, and especially all of his foster parents (hitting, kicking). He demonstrated a wide range of primitive and unsocialized behaviors, including growling and snarling; smearing feces; urinating while standing and having meals; gorging food; and consuming soap, shampoo, and dishwater. He had extreme tantrums that could last for 3 hours. He picked skin to the point of bleeding when upset. Tom misread signals; he found smiles threatening. He tried to control others, would lie to do so, and would blow up when he did not get what he wanted. He had articulation problems, pressured speech, and echolalia. Finally, his cognition was very primitive: He could not demonstrate either literacy or numeracy (i.e., he could not recognize letters or numbers).

Clinical Course

Tom's difficult behaviors resulted in five disrupted placements over 14 months; all of the carers felt he was too dangerous (at age 6) to keep in their homes. During this time, he was in weekly therapy at a local mental health authority and had two therapists over this period. The notes indicated that "evidence-based" trauma-focused cognitive-behavioral therapy was used by one therapist (with no apparent improvement), and that play therapy was used by the second therapist. The play therapy was conducted in the office of this therapist, who primarily attempted to use sandtray work as part of the process. The therapist expressed frustration at Tom's limited "capacity for insight" and his "unwillingness" to share his fears or concerns. She documented that in the majority of the sessions he refused to sit and "do therapy," but insisted on standing, walking around, jumping, and making many attempts to leave the office. Tom did not seem to be having a lot of fun in the form of "play" that this therapist wanted to integrate into therapy.

NMT Assessment and Recommendations

Tom was ultimately placed with foster parents who were familiar with the NMT. Clinicians certified in the NMT consulted with the play therapist working with Tom. An NMT assessment was conducted (see Perry & Dobson, 2013 for more details). As part of the NMT assessment process, a brain map was constructed indicating functional status (fully developed and typically functioning relative to a mature adult brain, emerging or precursor capability or mild to moderate compromise, undeveloped or severely dysfunctional). Brain functions are localized to the brain region mediating the specific function (e.g., cardiovascular regulation is a brainstem function; sleep is a diencephalon function; attachment is a limbic function; and abstract cognition is a cortex function). This oversimplification attempts to localize function to the brain region that is the final common mediator of the function, with the knowledge that all brain functions are the product of complex, transregional neural networks. This approximation, however, allows a useful estimate of the developmental/functional status of the child's key functions, establishes the child's "strengths and vulnerabilities," and determines the starting point and nature of enrichment or therapeutic activities most likely to meet the child's specific needs. The map becomes a comparison with a typical, same-age child. The graphic representations allow a clinician, teacher, or parent to quickly visualize important aspects of a child's history and current status. The information is key in designing developmentally appropriate educational enrichment and therapeutic experiences to help the child. Not surprisingly, this assessment demonstrated that while Tom was chronologically 6 years of age, he was developmentally functioning below the level of a toddler in some domains, and in others at or below the level of an 18 month old. He was extremely dysregulated, and it was estimated that his baseline level of arousal was high alarm. This meant that he would have minimal access to any cortically mediated functions and would have minimal cerebromodulatory capability. In short, words were not going to change Tom's behavior. A shift in therapeutic strategy was recommended. The foster parents, Tom's teachers and the play therapist were willing to shift their expectations and interactions with Tom away from cognitive-predominant to an enriched somatosensory schedule. Therapy took place while Tom and his therapist walked, in parallel, in a park. The school allowed Tom to avoid small-group activities (for which he was not yet developmentally ready), and to pursue a schedule of primarily somatosensory activity with a 1:1 aide (walking, playing with clay, finger painting, rocking in a chair, swinging, kicking a soccer ball, etc.). In the home, time with caregivers was spent walking, running, helping groom the pets, giving and receiving hand massages, and sitting side by side in a rocking bench (while his foster mother read to another of the children). The number of "intentional" (i.e., scheduled) somatosensory regulatory and therapeutic hours in the week was increased from 3 (which had been somewhat random) to 18 in the first 3 months of placement, and then to 30 (set up in a more scheduled, predictable pattern).

This regulating set of activities had the effect of minimizing Tom's dysregulated, impulsive, and aggressive behaviors. The positive impact on his state resulted in improved relational functioning, with a corresponding decrease in the anxiety that the teachers and carers felt when Tom was around. The confidence and positive affect of the adults contributed to additional regulation and reward. The positive feedback cycle led to a remarkable cascade of improved functioning that reflected a shift in his baseline state (from high arousal at baseline to low arousal/high alert). This shift in state "unmasked" some previously unexpressed functional capability; moreover, there was improved internalization of new cognitive and relational experiences, which contributed to the building of new functional capabilities. Most remarkable was that Tom passively learned to read (and now loves to read) by sitting next to his foster mother as she read to another child. Certainly Tom has far to go. But prior to the 8 months (at this writing) of the developmentally targeted regulatory interventions, he had 14 months of traditional therapeutic work with minimal impact. Of primary interest to a play therapist is the joy Tom now feels while he is succeeding; play therapy is most effective when it can capture the core elements of true play. The neurobiological power of play can only be fully expressed, however, when the types of adult-imposed play activities match the developmental needs and strengths of the regulated child.

Conclusion

Children who have experienced trauma, chaos, and neglect exhibit complex functional compromise in multiple domains, including physiological, motor, emotional, social, and cognitive. The specific nature and presentation of this multidomain functional compromise will vary, depending upon such factors as genetics and epigenetics, as well as the timing, nature, and pattern of both stressors and relational "buffers" in a child's life. A central finding in these children is a sensitized set of regulatory neural networks that originate in lower areas of the brain and have a wide distribution in the brain and body. By integrating a neurobiology-informed clinical approach, play therapists can select and sequence developmentally appropriate play activities that will help regulate these children and facilitate therapeutic efforts to enhance their relational and cognitive capabilities. The NMT is an evidence-based practice that can provide a practical and useful clinical framework to help play therapists identify the strengths and vulnerabilities of maltreated children, and implement developmentally appropriate therapeutic, educational, and enrichment services.

REFERENCES

Allen, J. (1988). *Inscapes of the child's world: Jungian counseling in schools and clinics*. Dallas, TX: Spring.

American Psychiatric Association. (2013). *Diagnostic and statistical manual of mental disorders* (5th ed.). Arlington, VA: Author.

Anda, R. F., Felitti, V. J., Bremner, D. J., Walker, J., Whitfield, C., Perry, B. D., . . . Giles, W. G. (2006). The enduring effects of abuse and related adverse experiences in childhood. *European Archives of Psychiatric and Clinical Neuroscience, 256*(3), 174–186.

Benedict, H. E. (2006). Object relations play therapy: Applications to attachment problems and relational trauma. In C. E. Schaefer & H. G. Kaduson (Eds.), *Contemporary play therapy: Theory, research, and practice* (pp. 3–27). New York: Guilford Press.

Blaustein, M. E., & Kinniburgh, K. M. (2005). Providing the family as a secure

base for therapy with children and adolescents. In K. Blaustein, M. Spinazzola, & B. van der Kolk (Eds.), *Attachment theory into practice* (pp. 48–53).
Brookline, MA: Justice Resource Institute.

Brandt, K., Diel, J., Feder, J., & Lillas, C. (2012). A problem in our field. *Journal
of Zero to Three, 32*(4), 42–45.

Bratton, S., & Ray, D. (2000). What the research shows about play therapy. *International Journal of Play Therapy, 9*(1), 47–48.

Bratton, S., Ray, D., Rhine, T., & Jones, L. (2005). The efficacy of play therapy
with children: A meta-analytic review of treatment outcomes. *Professional
Psychology: Research and Practice, 36*(4), 376–390.

Brody, V. (1997). *The dialogue of touch: Developmental play therapy.* Northvale,
NJ: Aronson.

Burghardt, G. M. (2005). *The genesis of animal play: Testing the limits.* Cambridge, MA: MIT Press.

Casey, R., & Berman, J. (1985). The outcome of psychotherapy with children. *Psychological Bulletin, 98*(2), 388–400.

Cook, A., Spinazzola, J., Ford, J., Lanktree, C., Blaustein, M. B., Cloitre, M., . . .
van der Kolk, B. (2005). Complex trauma in children and adolescents. *Psychiatric Annals, 35*(5), 390–398.

Erikson, E. (1964). *Childhood and society* (2nd ed.). New York: Norton.

Felitti, V. J., Anda, R. F., Nordenberg, D., Williamson, D. F., Spitz, A. M., &
Edwards, V. (1998). Relationship of childhood abuse and household dysfunc-
tion to many of the leading causes of death in adults: Adverse Childhood
Event Study. *American Journal of Preventive Medicine, 14,* 245–258.

Freud, S. (1924). *A general introduction to psycho-analysis.* London: Boni & Liv-
eright.

Gaskill, R. L., & Perry, B. D. (2012). Child sexual abuse, traumatic experiences,
and their impact on the developing brain. In P. Goodyear-Brown (Ed.),
Handbook of child sexual abuse: Identification, assessment, and treatment
(pp. 30–47). Hoboken, NJ: Wiley.

Gesell, A., & Ilg, F. (1947). *Infant and child in the culture of today.* New York:
Harper.

Guerney, B. (1964). Filial Therapy: Description and rationale. *Journal of Consulting Psychology, 28,* 304–310.

Hopper, J. W., Spinazzola, J., Simpson, W. B., & van der Kolk, B. A. (2006). Pre-
liminary evidence of parasympathetic influence on basal heart rate in posttraumatic stress disorder. *Journal of Psychosomatic Research, 60,* 83–90.

Kleim, J. A., & Jones, T. A. (2008). Principles of experience-dependent neural plasticity: Implications for rehabilitation after brain damage. *Journal of Speech,
Language, and Hearing Research, 51,* S225–S239.

Knell, S. M. (1995). *Cognitive behavioral play therapy.* Northvale, NJ: Aronson.

Kohlberg, L. (1963). Moral development and identification. In H. W. Stevenson
(Ed.), *Child psychology* (pp. 277–332). Chicago: University of Chicago Press.

Kottman, T. (1995). *Partners in play: An Adlerian approach to play therapy.* Alexandria, VA: American Counseling Association.

Landreth, G. (2002). *Play therapy: Art of the relationship* (2nd ed.). Muncie, IN:
Accelerated Development.

LeBlanc, M., & Ritchie, M. (1999). Predictors of play therapy outcomes. *International Journal of Play Therapy, 8*(2), 19–34.

LeBlanc, M., & Ritchie, M. (2001). A meta-analysis of play therapy outcomes. *Counseling Psychology Quarterly, 14*(2), 149–163.

Ludy-Dobson, C. R., & Perry, B. D. (2010). The role of healthy interaction in buffering the impact of childhood trauma. In E. Gil (Ed.), *Working with children to heal interpersonal trauma: The power of play* (pp. 26–43). New York: Guilford Press.

Marteau, T. M., Hollands, G. J., & Fletcher, P. C. (2012). Changing human behavior to prevent disease: The importance of targeting automatic processes. *Science, 337*(6101), 1492–1495.

Norton, C. C., & Norton, B. E. (2002). *Reaching children through play therapy: An experiential approach.* Denver, CO: White Apple Press.

Oaklander, V. (1994). Gestalt play therapy. In K. O'Connor & C. E. Schaefer (Eds.), *Handbook of play therapy* (Vol. 2, pp. 144–146). New York: Wiley.

O'Connor, K. (2000). *The play therapy primer* (2nd ed.). New York: Wiley.

Office of the United Nations High Commissioner for Human Rights. (1989, November 20). *Convention on the rights of the child* (General Assembly Resolution No. 44/25). Retrieved from *www2.ohchr.org*

Pearl, E., Thieken, L., Olafson, E., Boat, B., Connelly, L., Barnes, J., et al. (2012). Effectiveness of community dissemination of parent–child interaction therapy. *Psychological Trauma: Theory, Research, Practice, and Policy, 4*(2), 204–213.

Perry, B. D. (2001). The neuroarcheology of childhood treatment: The neurodevelopmental costs of adverse childhood events. In K. Franey, R. Geffner, & R. Falconer (Eds.), *The cost of maltreatment: Who pays? We all do* (pp. 15–37). San Diego, CA: Family Violence and Sexual Assault Institute.

Perry, B. D. (2006). Applying principles of neurodevelopment to clinical work with maltreated and traumatized children. In N. B. Webb (Ed.), *Working with traumatized youth in child welfare* (pp. 27–52). New York: Guilford Press.

Perry, B. D. (2008). Child maltreatment: The role of abuse and neglect in developmental psychopathology. In T. P. Beauchaine & S. P. Henshaw (Eds.), *Textbook of child and adolescent psychopathology* (pp. 93–128). New York: Wiley.

Perry, B. D. (2009). Examining child maltreatment through a neurodevelopmental lens: Clinical application of the Neurosequential Model of Therapeutics. *Journal of Loss and Trauma, 14*, 240–255.

Perry, B. D. (in press). Applications of a developmentally sensitive and neurobiologically-informed approach to clinical problem solving: The Neurosequential Model of Therapeutics (NMT) in young maltreated children. In K. Brandt, B. D. Perry, S. Seligman, & E. Tronick (Eds.), *Infant and early childhood mental health.* Arlington, VA: American Psychiatric Publishing.

Perry, B. D., & Dobson, C. L. (2013). Application of the Neurosequential Model of Therapeutics (NMT) in maltreated children. In J. D. Ford & C. A. Courtois (Eds.), *Treating complex traumatic stress disorders in children and adolescents* (pp. 249–260). New York: Guilford Press.

Perry, B. D., & Pollard, R. (1998). Homeostasis, stress, trauma, and adaptation: A neurodevelopmental view of childhood trauma. *Child and Adolescent Psychiatric Clinics of North America, 7*(1), 33–51.

Perry, B. D., Pollard, R., Blakley, T., Baker, W., & Vigilante, D. (1995). Childhood trauma, the neurobiology of adaptation, and "use-dependent" development of the brain: How "states" become "traits." *Infant Mental Health Journal,* 16(4), 271–291.

Perry, B. D., & Szalavitz, M. (2006). *The boy who was raised as a dog: And other stories from a child psychiatrist's notebook.* New York: Basic Books.

Piaget, J. (1962). *Play, dreams, and imitation in childhood.* New York: McGraw-Hill.

Ray, D., Bratton, S., Rhine, T., & Jones, L. (2001). The effectiveness of play therapy: Responding to the critics. *International Journal of Play Therapy,* 10(1), 85–108.

Rousseau, J. (1930). *Emile.* New York: Dent. (Original work published 1762)

Sara, S. J., & Bouret, S. (2012). Orienting and reorienting: The locus coeruleus mediates cognition through arousal. *Neuron, 76,* 130–141.

Shapiro, D., & Levendosky, A. (1999). Adolescent survivors of childhood sexual abuse: The mediating role of attachment and coping in psychological and interpersonal functioning. *Child Abuse and Neglect, 11,* 1175–1191.

Spinazzola, J., Blaustein, M., & van der Kolk, B. A. (2005). Post-traumatic stress disorder treatment outcome research: The study of unrepresentative sample. *Journal of Traumatic Stress, 18*(5), 425–436.

Szalavitz, M., & Perry, B. D. (2010). *Born for love.* New York: HarperCollins.

Tsai, M., & Ray, D. C. (2011). Play therapy outcome prediction: An exploratory study at a university-based clinic. *International Journal of Play Therapy,* 20(2), 94–108.

Ungar, M., & Perry, B. D. (2012). Violence, trauma and resilience. In R. Alaggia & C. Vine (Eds.), *Cruel but not unusual: Violence in Canadian families* (2nd ed.). Waterloo, Ontario, Canada: Wilfrid Laurier University Press.

van der Kolk, B. A. (2006). Clinical implications of neuroscience research in PTSD. *Annals of the New York Academy of Science, 107*(IV), 277–293.

van der Kolk, B. A., Spinazzola, J., Blaustein, M. E., Hopper, J. W., Hopper, E. K., Korn, D. L., et al. (2007). A randomized clinical trial of eye movement desensitization and reprocessing (EMDR), fluoxetine, and pill placebo in the treatment of posttraumatic stress disorder: Treatment effects and long-term maintenance. *Journal of Clinical Psychiatry, 68*(1), 37–46.

Vygotsky, L. S. (1967). Play and its role in the mental development of the child. *Soviet Psychology, 5*(3), 6–18.

Weisz, J., Weiss, B., Alicke, M., & Klotz, M. (1987). Effectiveness of psychotherapy with children and adolescence: A meta-analysis for clinicians. *Journal of Consulting and Clinical Psychology, 55*(4), 542–549.

Zeanah, C. H., Scheeringa, N. W., Boris, N. W., Heller, S. S., Smyke, A. T., & Trapani, J. (2004). Reactive attachment disorder in maltreated toddlers. *Child Abuse and Neglect, 28*(8), 877–888.

Zigler, E. F., Singer, D. G., & Bishop-Josef, S. J. (2004). *Children's play: The roots of reading.* Washington, DC: Zero to Three Press.

PART III

Clinical Applications: Approaches to Working with At-Risk Populations

CHAPTER 12

Helping Foster Care Children Heal from Broken Attachments

Athena A. Drewes

This chapter addresses the impact of attachment difficulties that children and teens in the foster care system experience with their caregivers, and describes how therapists can utilize a prescriptive/integrative approach to treat them. Play therapists and other child therapists will be helped to understand the unique challenges these children/teens and their foster caregivers confront in forming attachments; ways to utilize play-based techniques that will directly address complex trauma suffered through loss of the biological parents, broken attachments, and other subsequent abuses; and ways to work with a caregiver and family in understanding a foster child's special emotional needs. I describe the need for both directive and nondirective treatment approaches in working with foster care children, as well as how and what expressive arts techniques can be successfully utilized to help heal the emotional hole in the heart of such a child.

Challenges to Attachment Formation in Foster Care

Children in foster care often have histories of complex trauma (primarily attachment-based trauma), which results in increased externalizing and internalizing problems. Those foster care children with externalizing behaviors are at particular risk for placement disruptions, resulting in multiple placements over time and creating a vicious cycle of breaks in attachment. Consequently, they are not likely to trust authority figures and other adults around them, and are guarded and disengaged (Earl, 2009). Engaging such children in treatment involves confronting a series of challenges.

Emotional walls are put up as inner fortifications, and these defenses make it extremely difficult to gain access to these angry young persons in therapy. However, we as play and child therapists play an important role as attachment figures and can be agents of change in reaching troubled attachment-disordered foster children and teens.

After an initial "honeymoon" period in treatment (and in the foster home), a foster child with a history of disrupted attachment generally begins testing limits, looking for vulnerabilities and weak spots within the foster parents to see how long they will tolerate the child's behaviors before sending him or her away again, as all the other foster parents have done. Difficulties with affect regulation; problems with feelings identification, expression, and integration; limited coping strategies; hoarding of food; poor hygiene; destruction of property; low self-esteem; and hypercontrol soon begin to manifest themselves. These behaviors in the foster home cause the foster parents, and even the therapist, to feel helpless, demoralized, emotionally exhausted, angry, frustrated, and hostile. In turn, these feelings lead to deeper feelings of inadequacy and guilt.

Moreover, treatment may need to involve not only the foster child and foster parents, but also the child's siblings, both biological and foster. These siblings can feel terrorized in their own home both physically and through verbal assaults by the foster child, along with feeling resentful that the foster child is getting more attention through negative behaviors than they do. Even family pets are not immune from negative actions by the foster child. Pets can be poked, kicked, teased, dropped, fed too much or too little, or even killed by a foster child.

Many foster parents have the mistaken view that "love will conquer all." Although in part this is true, since a caregiver's unconditional love is of course essential, other factors are needed as well: stability and security of the home, clear expectations, and concise directions, along with nurturance and encouragement of the caregiver by the therapist to remain in control. However, these factors do not create the most comfortable environment for the foster child, who will resist and engage in control battles that will spill into the therapy sessions. It is important for the therapist to work individually not only with the foster child on attachment issues, but with the foster caregiver, who may in time become the adoptive parent.

Treatment Approaches

Within the safety of the therapy room, much as in the safety of the new foster home, the foster child can feel secure enough to explore, identify, and make sense of thoughts, feelings, wishes, and intentions, along with discovering strengths and seeing him- or herself from a new perspective (Hughes, 2009). It is therefore critical for the therapist to sincerely accept and respect the inherent worth and dignity of the foster child, while offering a safe and genuinely supportive environment. This will be especially important when the foster child begins testing the therapist and the limits of therapy, and resists getting emotionally attached during treatment. We therapists need to give foster children control over their physical environment—allowing them to determine how close to or distant from us they want to be, whether they need a physical barrier (e.g., a hoodie pulled over the head, a pillow or stuffed animal to hug), and at what pace they wish to engage with us or try to navigate the intensity of the one-to-one relationship (Earl, 2009). Indeed, the child-centered play therapy philosophy of following a child's/teen's lead and pace allows the young client to feel that personal boundaries and protective defenses are being respected.

Offering invitational expressive arts and directive play-based activities within the sessions not only will allow the child or teen to experience fun, but will give him or her a sought-after sense of control. The use of expressive arts materials allows the therapy to move at the level of the foster child's emotional rather than chronological age. It also allows the therapist time to get to understand and respect the vulnerable foster child's avoidant, withdrawn, or aggressive defensive behaviors, which were created to protect the child from perceptions of an unsafe and betraying world (Earl, 2009). In addition, the play therapist offers through the shared activities an emotional nurturance, or what Miller (2005) terms "nourishing communication." Through the therapist's playfulness, acceptance, curiosity, and empathy, the foster client begins to experience *intersubjectivity*, feeling nourished and enhanced by another person—experience lacking while the client was an infant. Child-centered, play-based therapy sessions can offer the child/teen the necessary time, space, and choice to begin exploring the treatment relationship along with his or her personal issues, in an atmosphere of unconditional acceptance. Such therapy sessions with an attachment-disordered foster child can also reduce verbal demands on the child through the use of expressive arts materials (e.g., sandtray work, drawing, collage making, clay work, painting, music, movement, drama, mask making, etc.). Working with expressive arts allows for communication to stay within a metaphor while the child or teen explores intimate and often painful material nonverbally. The creation can contain what has been experienced without causing the young client to feel exposed.

It is particularly critical for us as therapists to convey to foster children that we are equally interested in all aspects of their lives, not just the problems. We are not merely interested in "fixing" them, but are genuinely interested in their interests, worries, strengths, challenges, and successes, as well as the past and future, with all on an equal level. Through attunement to and matching of a foster child's or teen's affective state, along with a shared focus of attention, a relationship and a dialogue can begin to develop.

Treatment Issues

Issues that surface in working with foster care clients include grief and bereavement over the loss of their biological parents (at birth or later in their lives), difficulties with affect regulation (particularly anger), and difficulties with forming and keeping relationships and friendships. Consequently, the treatment of choice can be dyadic therapy with the foster parent/caregiver (if possible) or family therapy, but often it is individual therapy with collateral contact with this caregiver. For younger foster care children (especially those under the age of 10 for whom therapists are trying to build a relationship with their foster caregivers), the use of developmental play, Theraplay, parent–child interaction therapy, the Circle of Security, dyadic developmental psychotherapy, child–parent relationship therapy, or Filial Therapy can be most helpful, along with individual therapy as needed.

Once a safe environment is established in therapy, and trust begins to develop between a foster care client and a therapist, use of a prescriptive/integrative approach should be considered for individual therapy. In such an approach, the therapist takes responsibility for guiding the therapy process and for challenging the foster care client to address specific concerns. An integrative approach uses both directive and nondirective approaches—respecting the traumatized foster child's competing drives for mastery and control, while they may at the same time want to suppress and avoid painful and conflicted material that needs to be dealt with. The therapist assesses prescriptively what treatment approach and techniques should be utilized, based on the client's symptoms and current concerns. As treatment progresses, the therapist may change treatment modalities (e.g., may bring in dyadic work more or may move more into individual work) as indicated by the needs of the client. Therefore, treatment is custom-made for each client and evolves over time.

The use of play-based techniques and expressive arts interventions is often the most successful method of engaging a foster care client and working through many issues. The way I handle an integrative session is to use the first 5 minutes as a "check-in" on issues or homework from the last session, reports from the school or foster parent, unfinished issues from the last session, and so on. Then we spend the next 15–20 minutes on directive expressive arts and play-based techniques that address various issues facing the foster child. The remaining time is left for nondirective play, in which the child can choose an activity or use the playroom in any way he or she would like (as long as safety and other basic requirements are respected). The foster parent can be brought in during any of these time slots to join in the activities, or alternate sessions may include dyadic work with the foster parent, or a once-monthly session can be held alone with the foster parent to work on parenting skills, as needed.

Addressing Allegiance Issues

Allegiance is a big topic that often arises with regard to foster children or teens and their current caregivers versus their biological parents. Often a foster child has ambivalence about connecting with or loving another "mother," which results in difficulty bonding with the current caregiver or future adoptive parent. Loyalty to the biological mother remains, regardless of how much or little a foster child or teen knows about the birth parent or of the treatment the child received from that parent. Some foster clients may not want to be adopted because of their strong feelings of allegiance to their birth parents. Therefore, it is always critical that the foster caregivers not force the teen or child into calling them "Mom" and "Dad" upon entering their home. It is also crucial that the foster caregivers not speak poorly of either birth parent, as the foster client has 50% of each birth parent within him or her! Any negative comments that are made about the birth parent(s) are interpreted as though they are made about the client and become integrated into the child's sense of self, further decreasing his or her already low self-esteem.

Expressive Arts and Play-Based Techniques

Letters to Birth Parents

In addressing foster children's loss of and grief for their birth parents, I explore with them whether they ever wonder about their birth parents. Do they ever wonder if they look like them? On their birthdays, do they wonder if their birth parents are thinking about them? Foster caregivers are encouraged to ask these questions too, and to make statements such as "Your birth parents would be proud of you, just as we are," or "I wonder if your birth mom has curly hair like you," or "I'm so glad they gave you to us!" (Eldridge, 1999).

I also wonder (and encourage foster parents to wonder) to the foster clients about the various confusions that could arise from having two sets of parents, the biological and the foster parents; or about their mixed-up feelings on birthdays when they remember their birth parents; or what questions they might have about why their birth mothers placed them for foster care or adoption. It is important to normalize the common feeling among foster children that they should not love another mom. Many children and teens feel anger at their birth mothers and want to punish them for abandonment, while at the same time they are crying from the depths of their broken hearts for a reunion. But I assure my foster clients that their hearts are big enough for two moms.

I often work with a foster client on writing a letter to a birth parent (whether or not the child knows anything about this parent) that the client can then keep. The letter can be short or can elaborate on such issues as these:

> "Why didn't you keep me? Is it because you didn't like me? What is your name, and what do you look like? I feel really mad because I didn't get to know you. Is there something wrong with you? Is that the reason I can't see you? Is there something wrong with me?"

Case Vignette: Candace's Letter to the Court and Grief Box

Sometimes children do not want to be adopted and want to stay in foster care. Advocating for their right to decide is an important job of the therapist. Here is an example of one foster teen's feelings about allegiance issues. Candace was 12 years old, and recounted that she had been in seven foster homes and two group homes prior to coming to our program to be in a therapeutic foster home. She had initially been placed in regular foster care at around 4 years of age; she numbered only three of her homes as favorites. Her birth mother was involved in drugs, and her parental rights were terminated. Candace was removed from her last foster home (with her sister) because she kept running away, mainly to be able to have contact with her mother. In therapy, she wrote the following for the judge:

> "I have been living with [the foster family] about one year and a couple of months. Many of my foster parents are the type of parents that I wouldn't mind being adopted by them. The only problem is that I only have one mother, and I don't want anyone else to be my real mother. She is my birth mother. Many people also tell me that just because you get adopted doesn't mean you can't go looking for your birth mother. But the way I feel is that you could only have one real mother. And only one. But that is my very own opinion. I don't mind living with a foster parent for a couple of years or so, but for me, I don't want to be adopted by anyone. I have a mother. But I am thankful for those who think of me as their child. And I think of them as my parents, but not my real parents."

Being able to tell the judge her feelings helped Candace to feel empowered.

Our sessions were spent on Candace's grief for and loss of her biological mom. Candace made up collages of things she remembered about her biological mother, as well as things she could enjoy about her foster mother. We also created a "grief box" (Eldridge, 1999). This is a box that can be decorated on the outside. We made a list of the various losses she had in her life: the loss of her birth parents, her personal medical history, her birth family's history, a sense of belonging, and a sense of having a continuous life narrative. Candace was encouraged to select from magazines pictures of a mother and child and of a father and child to represent the loss of her birth parents; to use a Band-Aid for loss of her full medical history (she often could not answer questions the doctor would ask about allergies and medical history of her family); to draw a picture of a tree or to find a blank family tree chart for the loss of her birth family's history; to use a drawing or magazine photo of someone who looked sad for her loss of belonging; and to use a broken cord or string for the loss of a continuous life story. Throughout treatment, we referred back to the grief box and the various objects, decorating it, and we sometimes added other things to it. This box became the storage place for all the emptiness Candace felt and the hole in her heart that was created by the loss of all these things.

I became the caretaker of these heavy burdens and losses, and we kept exploring them gently and slowly throughout treatment. Throughout our work together, through expressive art and play-based techniques, we explored ways to fill the hole in Candace's heart. At various points in treatment, I would repeatedly stress how her parents had done the best they could with the abilities they had at the time they were living together. Her birth mom's own problems got in the way of being the parent Candace wanted her to be, so she just could not be the parent she needed her to be. I stressed to Candace that she was lovable and was born lovable. Unfortunately, however, there was no magic to be able to make her parents into the people she needed them to be and wanted desperately for them to be.

Wall around the Heart

Daniel Hughes (1997) writes of a technique that Foster Cline (1991) has developed for therapy with foster children. Cline draws sequential pictures of babies from birth, at the age of their broken attachment and their placement in foster care, and then at their current age, to help emphasize how they create a "wall around the heart." I have adapted this technique and prefer to use drawings of hearts, but I use the same time sequence. In the first picture, I have the foster client draw a small heart and write under it his or her name, with "One day old" next to it. I ask the child, "Do you know what the heart is for?" Most kids say that it is necessary to keep them alive. I agree that it helps the blood to keep moving, but that it also is for loving and feeling love, an emotional heart. I suggest that when a child was born, his or her heart worked quite well, and the child was probably pretty good at being able to give and receive love. Then the next picture drawn is a somewhat larger heart, again with the child's name, and then with the child's age at about the time the child was neglected or the parent(s) abandoned him or her. I speak briefly about the pain of being treated that way and indicate that such pain hurts the heart. We then draw cracks on the heart. Drawing a third heart, larger still, I talk about how the pain in the heart is so great that the child has worked out a very smart way of saving the heart from any further pain. We then draw a wall around the heart. We create arrows of pain by crumpling up paper and then throwing it at the heart, but it all bounces off the wall and cannot cause any more cracks. I praise the child for saving his or her heart from breaking further by creating that strong wall. Then the child is asked to draw a fourth heart and date it at a time since he or she has been living in the current foster home. I ask the child to draw the cracks again, but to make many of them smaller; we also put Band-Aids over several of the bigger cracks (see Figure 12.1), representing how the cracks are healing or have healed. I then have the child draw the wall around the heart again in pencil. I tell him or her,

> "You no longer need the wall. And in fact, the wall stops love from reaching your heart. You may not be sure that your foster parents really do love you, but there is no way to experience the love, because the wall is there. The best solution is for us to find a way to take down the wall. Instead of the wall being a fort that helped to keep pain out, it has now changed into a prison wall. Now it keeps you from getting the love that you want."

I tell the child that the foster parents and I are willing to help him or her learn how to take down the wall. I ask for suggestions on how we can do this, and we then can start to erase the wall a little at a time.

Letter from the Biological Mother

As noted earlier, many foster children feel that they cannot love two mothers. In such cases, I reflect that their birth mothers would want them to

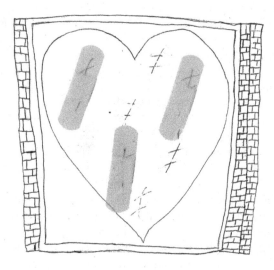

FIGURE 12.1. A re-created example of the fourth heart in the Wall around the Heart exercise, showing the partial healing of earlier cracks/wounds.

have mothers who loved them, since they could not raise them, and that the children's hearts are big enough to love two mothers. I ask them, "What would you imagine your birth mother saying to you, if she found out when you were 18 years old that you had continued to fight your foster or adoptive parents and refused to be close to anyone during your entire childhood?"

Then I make up a letter:

> "[Child's name], I am so sad that you were unhappy and angry during your whole childhood. I know that I was not able to provide you with a good childhood. I could not be the parent you needed me to be. But I also wished that you had let yourself get close to another mom who could have loved you, laughed with you, taught you and kept you safe. I know that [the foster mother's name] could have been that mom. I'm sad that you did not let yourself get close to her. You could have loved her and me too your whole life."

The child can then write his or her own letter from the birth mother, or even a letter back to the birth mother. It is important to help the child get in touch with the grief for and loss of the hoped-for parent—the idealized parent.

Techniques for Affect Identification and Regulation

Allan Schore (2003a, 2003b) writes that the most far-reaching effect of relational trauma is the loss of the ability to regulate the intensity of affect. Therefore, I usually work with foster children on building up a feelings vocabulary, being able to physically identify where they have their feelings, and learning how to integrate their feelings with better choices for problem-solving and coping skills when they are angry and upset. The Gingerbread Person Feelings Map (Drewes, 2001) is a variation of the Color Your Life technique (O'Connor, 1983), but uses drawing of a gingerbread person with arms outstretched, and with eyes, nose, and smile. It can be used with teens, as well as younger children, and in caregiver/parent–client dyads. The technique is used in order to assess (1) the overall range of feelings the client has and can verbally identify; (2) how aware the client is of where he or she physiologically feels these emotions; and (3) how well integrated the client's emotions are. The Gingerbread Person Feelings Map allows this information to be gathered in a nonthreatening and play-based way; it only takes a few minutes and can be used as an icebreaker in a first session, or at any time during treatment when appropriate.

Next to the shape of a gingerbread person, I add the words, *happy, sad, angry, worried, afraid*, and *love*, one under the other (see Figure 12.2). I then ask the foster child or teen to choose a few other feeling words to add. (I am often surprised at what children include, such as *petrified, stupid,*

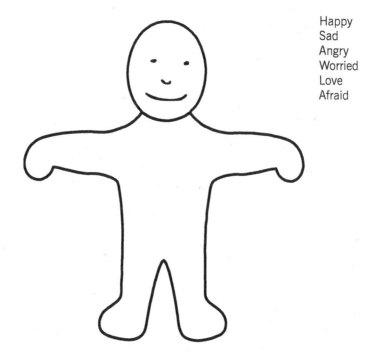

Happy
Sad
Angry
Worried
Love
Afraid

FIGURE 12.2. Gingerbread Person Feelings Map.

anxious, wishing I was somebody else, etc.) I write these words underneath the standard emotion words. This helps the child to expand his or her "emotional vocabulary." It also helps to give the child some control over the task and a feeling of being an active participant in the process. Next, I have the child choose a color for each feeling. It does not matter what colors are chosen (sometimes I get black for happy!). I also have the child or teen put a little line using the color chosen next to each of the feeling words, like creating a legend for a map.

Then I ask the client to use each color to indicate where inside the gingerbread person he or she may physically experience each feeling listed. The client can shade the colors in, scribble, draw hearts, or the like. Next, I go through each feeling and have the client imagine where he or she feels each one (so that none are left out). Once this task is completed (usually after less than 5 minutes), we process the drawing together. I pay particular attention to where in the body anger is expressed and how this might play out in the foster child's or teen's world in responding to situations, and I point this out to the client. I also look for how many feelings are integrated, and for how much color is used and where. In addition, I look for discrepancies: for instance, the child may have colored in happy feelings on the face, but anger in the hands, feet, or body; or may have placed a spot of color representing anger outside of the figure (possibly signifying difficulty toler-ating that emotion). In such a case, I process how the client may present to others as calm, but inwardly he or she is seething, or perhaps is manifesting anger through hitting others or restlessness in the legs. Also, where does the child or teen put love (often drawn as a heart), and is it "walled off" by lay-ers of scared, hurt, or angry feelings? If so, I explain how we each can have more than one feeling at a time within us; sometimes we feel ambivalent (e.g., angry and loving) at the same time toward someone. And sometimes one feeling is so strong that it can hide other feelings that we are feeling too, making us feel confused and unsure of what we are feeling.

This technique can be used with a foster parent and the teen/child together, with each working independently of the other. At the end, the par-ent and child/teen can share their finished products and compare similari-ties and differences in the ways anger and other emotions are felt. Another adaptation of this technique involves using two gingerbread figures (Gil, 2006). The child or teen colors in each figure according to the various feel-ings experienced when with each parent, either foster parent or biological parent.

Young clients who may be uncomfortable thinking about their bod-ies and using a person-like shape (especially if they were sexually abused) may prefer using a heart shape. Heartfelt Feelings Coloring Card Strate-gies (Crenshaw, 2008) are preprinted cards, each with a drawn heart and feelings words to add colors to, in order to help children identify, label, and express their feelings about "heartfelt" issues and relationships with the important people in their lives. As with the Gingerbread Person Feel-ings Map or Color Your Life, a teen or child picks colors to match various feelings listed and fills in the amount of each feeling he or she has, thereby quantifying how he or she is feeling at the moment or at some other point in time. The client can also write on the card a response to a time when he or she had this feeling. Color Your Heart (Goodyear-Brown, 2010) is another variation utilizing a heart shape, which is colored in proportion to the amounts of feelings in the child's heart.

Use of Clay as a Metaphor for Clients' Lives

I ask foster clients to take a small piece of Play-Doh or oogly clay (*www.theooglykit.com*), which is easily malleable and softens up quickly; to close their eyes (or, if they do not feel safe enough to do that, to stare off at something across the room); and, without looking or speaking, to create something within a 2-minute time period. Once the time is up, I have them look at what they created. Is it as they had imagined it would be? Did it turn out the way they expected?

I then process with the clients how their clay creations are much like their lives. Things happen in their lives, many of which are beyond control (being put into foster care, having parents who were unable to care for them, being unable to magically change their lives, having other abuses happen to them, etc.). But just as they are now able to change their creations, improve on them, make them more like how they want them to look, or start all over, so too they can do that with their lives. Some things may take until they are 18 years old or older, such as living on their own or looking for their biological parents. But they can make changes in other things now, such as how they react when they are angry, how they cope, whether they want to let others into their hearts and trust them, or whether they can keep from being sent away to another home. And just like their creations at this moment, they too can decide whether they want to continue with what has turned out or be an active force in making a difference in their lives and in the lives of those with whom they come in contact.

Magical Smiles

I teach my foster clients that they have magic within themselves. This is something that no one can take from them, that is within them and with them all the time, and that is so magical it can make others do things. Intrigued, the foster clients inevitably become interested. I tell them, "It is your smile. You have the most beautiful smile." (And, truly, I have not met anyone who does not have a beautiful smile that makes me respond in turn with a smile!) Of course, once I say this, a bright smile forms on every client's face! I then challenge the clients with homework of going out in the next week and smiling at three people that they choose (and we talk about people they know that they might try this with). The catch is that the clients need to look each person in the eye, so the other person knows they are looking at him or her. Then, when eye contact is made, they smile and see what happens. I always start the next session by checking on this homework and seeing the results of their smiles. Inevitably, even if they only tried it once, magic occurred in making another person smile back!

Case Vignette: Kayla's Jenga Session

Jenga is a game that taps physical and mental skills and can be played by children ages 5 and up, as well as by teens and adults. It is played with 54 small wooden blocks stacked in groups of three, which are criss-crossed to create 18 levels. Moving in Jenga consists of taking one and only one block from any level (except the one below the incomplete top level) of the tower, and placing it on the topmost level in order to complete it (see Figure 12.3). The game ends when the tower falls. The child/teen can go first, but it does not matter if the foster parent or therapist goes first, at the child/teen's request. Usually the client wants to go first, but if the client is unsure of the game and how to play it, it is sometimes helpful for the therapist to go first to model how it is played.

    Kayla, age 9, was placed in foster care at age 5. Kayla's biological mother had a history of psychiatric problems, along with alcoholism, and

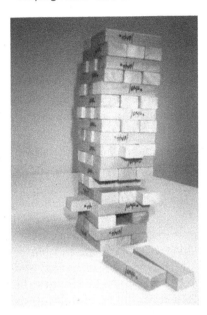

FIGURE 12.3. A Jenga session in progress.

there was no known history on the biological father. Kayla entered therapy because of attachment and bereavement issues related to the loss of significant people in her life, as well as systemic family issues in her foster home that were affecting her emotional and behavioral functioning.

After several sessions, Kayla spontaneously decided to use the Jenga game and wanted to go first after setting up the tower. Kayla carefully removed each of her blocks, putting them on the top and building the tower up. She was proud of her ability to build up the tower without making it fall. When it finally did fall, after many layers, it was due to my removal of a block. Kayla was delighted, clapping and laughing with glee when this happened. She quickly built up the tower to play another game. At this point, I decided to use Jenga metaphorically to help represent Kayla's losses and begin to address her attachment and loss issues. After about five or six blocks had been removed, leaving holes in the tower, and being placed on top with the tower higher, I began a discussion:

THERAPIST: You know, Kayla, when each block gets taken out, there is a hole that remains behind that makes the tower not very solid and strong. It reminds me of losses children experience and how it feels like there are emotional holes in their heart, which make their reactions to people and situations off balance. It makes me think of the experiences that you have had in your life.

KAYLA: Yeah?

THERAPIST: Yep. You have had many losses in your life. Let's see, each hole could represent your bio-mom, your bio-dad, and your foster dad, along with Tim, Fred, and now John.

KAYLA: My foster mom has a lot of boyfriends.

THERAPIST: And each time you make a friendship, then they leave. It must be hard to trust and try to get close to people, like the next boyfriend.

KAYLA: Yeah. Mom wants me to call them Dad, but I don't like that. And sometimes they act like they are the boss of me.

THERAPIST: So sometimes it makes you angry and maybe even confused. And then when they leave, sometimes you are left with a feeling hole in your heart, missing the people you cared for. And then there are some important people that you didn't even get to know well, like your bio-mom and bio-dad, who put you into foster care. (*Kayla appears interested and is actively watching and listening.*) So when you take out the block from Jenga and it makes a hole, it results in an unstable foundation. And the tower can fall down. Just like when people leave your life, they make a feeling hole in your heart, which results in not trusting others and acting out your feelings.

KAYLA: Yeah!

THERAPIST: But then you can rebuild the Jenga tower again the way you want it to be. You can take blocks from the top to make a secure base. Just like in therapy, we can help to start to fill in the holes in your heart by talking about all your feelings and missing your bio-parents and your foster dad. And we can find out who in your life could help give you what you need when you are feeling upset. So for this first block, if we were to put it back in to make the tower stronger, who would it represent? Who in your life now could be there for you and help you feel better when you are upset?

KAYLA: My foster mom. Even though she makes me angry sometimes, I can talk to her, and she gives lots of hugs.

THERAPIST: Great. Let's think of another person.

KAYLA: This one can be Miss Higgins, my teacher. She always knows the right thing to say when I am feeling sad. And this other one is for you, because you are a good listener and care about how I feel. And this last one is for my best friend, Maria. I can share my worries with her, and she shares hers.

THERAPIST: Great. Let's now take some of the blocks out and write different feelings on them. I'll write *angry* on this one. What feeling do you want to put on this one?

KAYLA: *Happy.*

THERAPIST: I'll put down *sad.*

KAYLA: *Frustrated. (This process continues until about 15 of the blocks have been given different feeling words, sometimes with help from the feelings poster on the wall.)*

THERAPIST: Now let's play Jenga again, but this time let's mix up the blocks with these feeling words on them with those that don't have anything written. Each time we pull out a block, we can talk about a time we had the feeling, and what we did to feel better or show our feeling.

Kayla and I continued to play Jenga, talking about the various people who had left an emotional hole and ways that it could be filled. We then went on to discuss feelings that came up in particular situations, along with ways the feelings were handled successfully or not so successfully. Toward the end of the session, I took a few of the fallen tower blocks and showed Kayla how thoughts, feelings, and behaviors are connected, and how one action can lead to another and perhaps to a not-so-beneficial outcome.

I selected seven blocks and placed them in a row near each other, standing up. Using a recent example of something that happened in school that got Kayla in trouble, I identified each block as representing each step of the situation.

THERAPIST: So first the girl bumps into you while you are near your desk, which is this first block. Then the second block represents you feeling angry and yelling back at her. The third block is when you push the girl back. The fourth block is when the teacher comes over. The fifth block is when you get upset at the teacher and yell at her for telling you to quiet down. The sixth block is when you kick over your chair. And the last block is when your teacher tells you to go down to the principal's office. So if we push over this first block (*the therapist does this*), see how it quickly knocks down each of the other blocks to the end.

But now we can set them up a bit differently. (*The therapist stands two blocks close together, and the remaining five blocks much further apart from each other, so they will not knock each other down if they fall.*) This first block is where the girl knocks into you and you feel angry. The second block is where you feel angry but decide instead to do something else, like take a deep breath and say, "Hey, don't push me," instead of pushing her back. If we knock over the first block, it hits the second block, but all the rest of the blocks still remain standing, and you don't get sent to the principal's office.

Our work together in therapy is going to help you in identifying your feelings and figuring out other ways to react early on, so that you don't get yourself in trouble. How does that sound to you?

KAYLA: Great. Thanks! I don't like getting in trouble in school. This is fun. See you next week!

By using the Jenga game in these ways, a therapist can help explain attachment deficits and their impact on a client's emotional life, explore the resources available to the client, and increase the client's feelings vocabulary. The therapist can also expand the game to include coping strategies that could go with angry and sad feelings, and the blocks can be used to match up feelings with strategies. Also, the therapist can write sentence stems on pieces of paper (these stems may reflect misperceptions about being in foster care, questions about why the birth parents gave the client up, self-esteem statements, etc.). Some examples of sentence stems are "Only bad children get adopted," "I am lovable," "Parents always love their children," "The color of my hair is ugly," and "I am beautiful and smart." Each time a block is taken out (leaving a hole behind), the child/ teen or therapist chooses one of the slips of paper and reads it. The therapist can then explore which thoughts are helpful and accurate and which are unhelpful and inaccurate by asking, "How does that sentence make you feel?" or "What if your best friend said that? What would you say back?" The child is then encouraged to come up with alternative statements that are more helpful or accurate: "What could you say that would help to make you feel better?"

In Kayla's particular case, Jenga was used to help understand the child's view of being in foster care; to access her deep feelings of loss, bereavement, and broken attachment; and to assess resources in her life, along with the depth of Kayla's feelings and her ability to make use of feelings vocabulary. However, Jenga can also be used for assessing and developing fine motor skills, increasing impulse control and task-oriented behavior, building self-esteem and competence, encouraging acceptance of rules, and modeling losing as well as winning. My hope in this session and subsequent ones was that Kayla would be able to better understand and visually grasp the concept of having "emotional holes in her heart" with regard to her losses and multiple placements, and the related feelings associated with the experiences. The foster parent could also be invited in to play the game and also help fill in the missing information to make the tower stronger.

Guided Relaxation

To aid children with deep breathing/relaxation and to help them avoid acting out when angry, the guided relaxation exercise known as Safe Place

(Drewes, 2011a, 2011b; James, 1989) is an effective tool they can use at any time. As clients sit with eyes closed, they imagine being a movie director. They are directed to breathe slowly in and out and to think of a time and place when they felt safe. It could be lying in the sun at the beach, hiding under their covers, snuggling with a favorite pet, or the like. They are told to zoom in their camera and film the location, taking in all that there is. Then they freeze the camera shot. As they continue to breathe slowly in and out, they look around and notice what they see, smell, hear, and feel, and whether or not there are any people or animals there. As they continue to breathe slowly in and out, they are instructed to feel how safe they are and how relaxed they feel in their bodies while in their safe space. Next they give their special safe place a name, preferably one word. It is the key that will get them back to their safe place any time they wish to go. All they have to do is remember the name. The clients continue to breathe in and out slowly, focusing on how relaxed and safe they feel. Then after a few minutes, they are directed to move the camera slowly back, and in another minute they will be back in the room with the therapist with their eyes open. The goal is to use operant conditioning to link the deep breathing with the experience of feeling safe and with the word chosen. Then, when the clients are upset or anxious, they can remember the word and their bodies will automatically begin to relax.

Conclusion

In general, the important key to entering the world of an attachment-disordered foster child or teen is integrative use of directive and nondirective expressive arts and play-based techniques that are both enjoyable and engaging, and that prescriptively meet the needs arising from the child/teen's symptoms and issues at the moment. It is also important to work on the issues of loss/bereavement resulting from separation from the biological parents, along with affect regulation and expression to help in dealing with underlying attachment and allegiance issues. Inclusion of the foster parent(s) is also critical in reinforcing gains and helping to generalize learned techniques for coping, as well as in building the bond of a new attachment.

REFERENCES

Cline, F. W. (1991). *Hope for high risk and rage filled children.* Evergreen, CO: Evergreen Consultants in Human Behavior.

Crenshaw, D. A. (2008). Heartfelt Feelings Coloring Cards Strategies. In L. Lowenstein (Ed.), *Assessment and treatment activities for children, adolescents, and families* (pp. 80–81). Toronto: Champion Press.

Drewes, A. A. (2001). Gingerbread Person Feelings Map. In H. G. Kaduson & C. E. Schaefer (Eds.), *101 more favorite play therapy techniques* (pp. 92–97). Northvale, NJ: Aronson.

Drewes, A. A. (2011a, April 29). *A skill-building workshop: Effectively blending play-based techniques with cognitive behavioral therapy for affect regulation in sexually abused and traumatized children.* Workshop presented at the Annual Conference of the Canadian Association for Child and Play Therapy, Guelph, Ontario, Canada.

Drewes, A. A. (2011b). Working with attachment disordered teens in foster care. *Play Therapy: Magazine of the British Association for Play Therapy,* No. 68, pp. 6–9.

Earl, B. (2009). Exterior fortresses and interior fortification. In A. Perry (Ed.), *Teenagers and attachment: Helping adolescents engage with life and learning* (pp. 97–121). Richmond, UK: Worth.

Eldridge, S. (1999). *Twenty things adopted kids wish their adoptive parents knew.* New York: Dell.

Gil, E. (2006). *Helping abused and traumatized children: Integrating directive and nondirective approaches.* New York: Guilford Press.

Goodyear-Brown, P. (2010). *Play therapy with traumatized children: A prescriptive approach.* Hoboken, NJ: Wiley.

Hughes, D. (1997). *Facilitating developmental attachment: The road to emotional recovery and behavioral change in foster and adopted children.* Northvale, NJ: Aronson.

Hughes, D. (2009). Principles of attachment and intersubjectivity. In A. Perry (Ed.), *Teenagers and attachment: Helping adolescents engage with life and learning* (pp. 123–140). Richmond, UK: Worth.

James, B. (1989). *Treating traumatized children.* Lexington, MA: Lexington Books.

Miller, P. W. (2005). *Body language: An illustrated introduction for teachers.* Munster, IN: Patrick W. Miller and Associates.

O'Connor, K. J. (1983). Color-Your-Life technique. In C. E. Schaefer & K. J. O'Connor (Eds.), *Handbook of play therapy* (pp. 251–258). New York: Wiley.

Schore, A. (2003a). *Affect regulation and the repair of the self.* New York: Norton.

Schore, A. (2003b). *Affect dysregulation and disorders of the self.* New York: Norton.

CHAPTER 13

Chronic Early Trauma as a Childhood Syndrome and Its Relationship to Play

Steven Tuber
Kira Boesch
Jessica Gorkin
Madeleine Terry

As Donald Winnicott described so beautifully (Winnicott, 1971; see also Tuber, 2008, 2012), the capacity for play is both an exalted hallmark of human development and yet something that is not an automatic outgrowth of the developmental process. A "good enough" degree of reliable, predictable, nontoxic caregiving must occur for an infant to develop the "luxury" of being able to take the caregiver for granted while beginning to show curiosity and playfulness in the world around him. When children experience chronic neglect or abuse, the effects are often devastating and far-reaching in restricting or even preventing this capacity for play. van der Kolk et al. (2009) propose the term *developmental trauma disorder* (DTD) to capture the comprehensive clinical picture of these children. DTD is an overarching concept intended to subsume the numerous consequences for a child who has suffered chronic deprivation, neglect, and/or abuse in the context of inadequate caregiving. In this chapter, we place DTD within a specific context: describing how these afflicted children's patterns of affect and defense, neurological functioning, and burgeoning self-concept are all drastically disrupted, and in turn disrupt the children's capacity to play.

Affect and Defense in DTD

The experience of trauma, by definition, implies intolerable distress and a resulting affective overload that can easily become overwhelming. In the case of children who endure chronic traumatic stress, the development of tools necessary for the seamless regulation of emotion is especially affected. When caregivers are absent or are unable to tolerate distress themselves, children are not helped to attend to their internal states and therefore do not learn to differentiate among them or label them. Research has shown that abused and neglected children evidence deficits in their ability to detect and accurately label emotional states in experimental vignettes (Pollack, Cicchetti, Hornung, & Reed, 2000). The children's inability to understand emotion in these external situations also reflects their difficulty in comprehending their own internal emotional landscape. When children do not learn to differentiate among internal states, they do not learn to associate their bodily sensations with affect and cognition (van der Kolk, 2005). As such, van der Kolk et al. (2009) propose that DTD is, at its core, a disorder of affective dysregulation. Traumatic stress overwhelms maltreated children's ability to regulate, effectively preventing the retrieval of relevant sensations, affects, and cognitions, and thereby prohibiting the children from understanding or acting upon what is happening to them (van der Kolk, 2005).

Pearlman (1997) describes feelings as "the underpinnings of needs" (p. 22). Without adequate affect regulation, children with DTD are likely to have difficulty identifying and accepting their needs. At the same time, children who cannot verbalize and make sense of their own emotional responses cannot rely on affect states to serve as accurate signals (Krystal, 1978). The result is that many children with DTD may suffer from an inability to distinguish threatening from nonthreatening situations, and may consequently present with emotional lability caused by an extreme, excessive response to minor stressors (Cook et al., 2005). Indeed, children exposed to violence have been shown to exhibit higher levels of mood and behavioral problems than children in control groups (Liberman & Knorr, 2007). However, as van der Kolk (2005) points out, many of the behavioral manifestations associated with DTD can be understood as efforts to minimize objective threat and to regulate emotional distress.

Defenses are cognitive strategies that alter veridical perception to protect an individual from overwhelming affect (Cramer, 2006). Given their difficulty in labeling affect and their tendency to overreact to even trivial stimuli, it follows that children with DTD mobilize defense configurations that are also impaired and subject to distortion and disruption. Like other cognitive abilities that emerge early in life, defenses develop from more primitive to more nuanced over the course of development (Tuber, 2012). Most children are able to use increasingly advanced defenses characterized by flexibility and discreteness of focus as they move toward adulthood.

However, the experience of chronic interpersonal trauma inherent to DTD disrupts the development of defenses, so these children may not learn to utilize more sophisticated and advanced defenses flexibly. Instead, during the first years of life (when boundaries between self and other are not yet fully differentiated), children may come to overrely on so-called "primitive" defenses, which appear anew at times when overwhelming experiences must be completely evaded (Tuber, 2012).

Although evasive defenses serve to protect children with DTD from overwhelming negative affect, the overuse of such defenses can result in affective numbing. Furthermore, primitive defenses are rarely able to protect the children completely from negative emotions. Rather, blocked affects such as terror, betrayal, and pain are likely to return in uncontrolled bursts or reenactments, which further contribute to the chronically traumatized children's affect regulation difficulties (Hegeman & Wohl, 2000). When children are not able to learn to use more sophisticated defenses to regulate affects, it is not uncommon for affects to be discharged through action such as aggression (Pearlman, 1997).

Children with DTD may learn to employ higher-level, more advanced defenses, but often in maladaptive ways. For example, identification is considered to be a higher-level defense and a developmental achievement. In their use of this defense, children with DTD may identify with their aggressors. Identification with the aggressors involves role reversal in fantasy, which may then be enacted in behavior, allowing the children (victims) to gain mastery by transforming themselves into the persons who create the threat. Thus even high-level defenses such as identification may come to be used in ways that are ultimately counterproductive for children with DTD.

DTD is also characterized by the use of dissociative defenses. Unlike denial or identification, dissociation is not considered part of a normal developmental process; it serves to automatize behavior, compartmentalize negative affects, and allow the individual to detach from awareness (Blum, 1987). Dissociation involves alterations in the capacity to integrate identity, memory, consciousness, and perceptions of the environment (Waller, Putnam, & Carlson, 1996). As we discuss further in the section on the development of selfhood, dissociative defenses are often essential in an environment of chronic trauma in order to protect the self from overwhelming and damaging affects. However, use of dissociation also robs children of an adaptive strategy with which to contain strong feelings. In such a situation, children tend to alternate between blocking affects entirely and becoming flooded by painful feelings (Hegeman & Wohl, 2000).

It is important to remember that defenses, which operate as protective mechanisms, may interfere with the development of emotional closeness, attachment, imagination, and readiness to learn (Lieberman & Knorr, 2007). This is of crucial importance in its impact on the capacity to play, stunting its arrival and linking it to fears of becoming overwhelmed if imaginary musings should become all too real.

Neuropsychological Implications of DTD

Particular adjustments at the neuropsychological level constitute a foundation for the aforementioned difficulties with disrupted affect regulation and maladaptive patterns of defense seen in children with DTD. These changes structurally diminish the capacity for play. Structural changes in the brain allow a growing child to interpret new sensory input, and to perceive, process, and integrate new experiences (van der Kolk, 2003). When complex developmental trauma invades and disrupts the maturational process, brain function is drastically affected (D'Andrea, Ford, Stolbach, Spinazzola, & van der Kolk, 2012).

The changes to the course of neurodevelopment that occur in complex developmental trauma are part of the immature brain's adaptation to a malevolent or neglectful environment, and constitute an alternative pathway that prioritizes survival behavior (Ford, 2005; Teicher et al., 2003). Experiencing chronic maltreatment or inevitable repeated traumatizations during sensitive stages leads to particular stress-induced changes in the mind and brain that render children vulnerable to reexperiencing early maltreatment in several ways (van der Kolk, 2005). A tendency toward dysregulation predominates. An examination of current neurobiological and neuropsychological research situates developmentally traumatized children within a context of struggle and disorientation. Difficulty with integrating sensory, emotional, and cognitive information can be traced to particular neurological structures and pathways that fail to facilitate the construction of meaning and grounding of experience so desperately needed by these children (van der Kolk, 2003, 2005).

Chronic trauma causes a breakdown in communication between the brain's two hemispheres. It is thought that this ongoing exchange of information can be disrupted by early trauma (Teicher et al., 2003). Teicher and colleagues assert that early exposure to high levels of stress hormones eventually results in deformities in the bundle of neural fibers called the corpus callosum, which connects the two hemispheres to facilitate their communication.

Children who have suffered abuse and neglect show impaired cognitive functioning by late infancy when compared with children who have not been maltreated, and the sensory and emotional deprivation associated with neglect seems to be particularly detrimental to cognitive development. Traumatized children are bombarded by excessive subcortical activation. This hyperactivity is compounded by decreased cortical inhibition, which leads them to disregard incoming information. High levels of the neurotransmitter norepinephrine, a catecholamine that acts as a stress hormone and neurotransmitter, add to the difficulties these children have in exerting executive control. Their perception of incoming information is distorted by deficient capacities to modulate and achieve the calm that is necessary to formulate a response (van der Kolk, 2003). As such, neglected infants and toddlers show delays in expressive and receptive language development, as well as deficits in overall IQ (Cook et al., 2005). According to O'Neill, Guenette, and Kitchenham (2010), children who have experienced chronic abuse and neglect in early childhood will struggle to learn across the lifespan, due in large part to the environment in which they were raised.

The noradrenergic alarm system is activated when children feel threatened. This is the system that organizes the release of norepinephrine; it has been associated with arousal and impaired prefrontal cortex activity. Activation of this system engages the "fast tracks" of the limbic system, which fire before the gradually responding prefrontal cortex has time to evaluate the stimulus and engage in planning action (van der Kolk, 2003). When a developmentally traumatized child becomes hyperaroused, activation of the orbitofrontal cortex (another structure of the limbic system that is necessary for discriminating stimuli) is disrupted, so that the child not only struggles to learn and assess, but also may lose control over behavior (van der Kolk, 2003). Chronic abuse and neglect may also be detrimental to the electrophysiology and development of the limbic system by leading children to experience excessive neural activation when faced with minor stimuli. This produces the extreme, emergency response patterns in reaction to minor stressors that we have discussed in the section on affect regulation (van der Kolk, 2003).

Different rates of maturation in the amygdala, hippocampus, and prefrontal regions also affect posttraumatic reactions in the developing child. The amygdala starts to function just after birth, so that infants rapidly become able to experience fear and assess danger. The hippocampus, which puts danger in a spatial context in a child's mind, matures comparatively slowly over the first 5 years of life (van der Kolk, 2003). As a result, children under normal conditions gradually acquire the capacity to identify and organize the nature of a threat, whereas victims of early abuse lack these cognitive skills at the time of severe trauma (van der Kolk, 2003).

As previously described, chronically traumatized children are also prone to dissociation and alterations in consciousness. Dissociative states are likely to arise from imbalances in cerebrospinal fluid levels of neurotransmitters and their metabolites; over time, chronic trauma exposure perpetuates neurochemical imbalances and may lead to a dependence on dissociation as a way to cope with emotional arousal.

When a chronically traumatized child experiences unrelenting threat, whether actual or perceived, physiological changes unfold to affect the body and brain, slowing brain growth and suppressing the immune system (Cook et al., 2005). Children with DTD are affected at multiple levels, but perhaps most strikingly in terms of their physical, somatic experience. Given that successful development can be thought of as the "transformation of external into internal regulation" (Schore, 2003, p. 180), these children must ultimately learn to notice and reflect on their bodies as a means of access to their internal selves. It is here that the impact on the capacity to play is most dramatically engendered. Play is perhaps children's greatest tool for learning to understand their bodies and themselves. Helping these children to identify, understand, and trust the connections among bodily sensations, inner feelings, and thoughts constitutes the foundation from which they can make sense of and master their own unique, human experience. Furthermore, their bodies act as containers of experience. Despite the terrifying and chaotic nature of their surroundings, these children may be helped to gain a sense of the divide between the body and the outside world, fostering a newfound capacity to differentiate within the play setting. It is this body–self unity that forms a critical foundation for ego integration. When a child presents with a deficient or nonexistent capacity for play, a premium is placed on the part of the play or art therapist to act as a catalyst in the reparation of the child's impaired ability to link mind, body, affect, and behavior. Through play and imagination, the therapist can foster the child's sense of and trust in the integrity of the self within the matrix of internal and external worlds.

The Development of a Self in DTD

As mentioned above, children with DTD lack a sense of coherence among their bodily perceptions, feelings, and thoughts. Another way of conceptualizing this is to consider the impairments in DTD at the level of the development of a viable sense of self. A coherent and consistent sense of self is a developmental achievement that depends upon early relationships with specific characteristics (Williams, 2004). The first of these characteristics is the caregiver's contingent response to an infant's expression of need (Fonagy, Gergely, Jurist, & Target, 2002). A second crucial aspect of caregiver behavior is consistency. A caregiver's consistent response patterns help the infant to experience the caregiver as an organized and cohesive other who is separate from him- or herself, even as the caregiver plays a major role in the infant's self-regulation. Finally, in infancy and beyond, development of the self is facilitated by caregivers who mirror and reflect children's inner states and behaviors, thus reinforcing the children's emerging self-states (Pearlman & Courtois, 2005).

Children who have suffered early relational trauma are deprived of many of the optimal circumstances for selfhood development described here. Caregivers who are themselves traumatized or experiencing extremely adverse life circumstances may not be able to reflect their children's emerging self-states back to them accurately and reliably. In the subsequent absence of having their bodily sensations acknowledged, symbolized through language, and regulated by their caregivers, the children miss opportunities for becoming aware of their agency and having their experience of themselves symbolized and represented to them by a close other.

In some situations of relational trauma, children are in the position of becoming attached to adults whom they perceive to be dangerous or negligent. It is a ubiquitous part of development that representations of the other are internalized before the self fully forms, laying the groundwork for identification. These alien parts within the self-structure are universal precisely because no caregiver is perfectly sensitive to a child's mind (Fonagy & Target, 2006). However, especially in response to caregivers who project their own unsymbolized feelings and thoughts onto their infants, traumatized children may more insidiously incorporate the invasive objects' characteristics, including malignant aspects, as part of their own selves and identities (Williams, 2004).

As a result, traumatized children can lose awareness of the boundary between internal and external reality, slipping into what is called *psychic equivalence mode*—the belief that their own thoughts are no different from external reality. In this state of mind, these children can easily come to feel that their memories of trauma are real, and come to fear their own minds. It is easy to imagine the consequences of such a state on the capacity for play. If one's mind is above all else to be feared, than how can one afford to let it "wander" playfully? Indeed, the avoidance of imagination becomes paramount in such a scenario, creating a vicious cycle of concrete thinking in the face of concrete, all-too-real adversity. This vulnerability often results in dissociation and shame, which in turn pose further threat to a cohesive sense of self and to adaptive relationships with others.

As we have discussed in both prior sections, the prevalence of dissociation in DTD is rampant. Here we highlight its impact on the growth of a sense of self. Dissociation is seen as the opposite of an integrated self and has been described as a void of subjectivity (Schore, 2002), such that in moments of dissociation both self and other cease to exist. This is exemplified by case studies of complex trauma survivors, in which patients are frequently represented as needing and wanting regulation from the outside (West, 2011) and seeking external references as a source of self-organization (Pinheiro & Viana, 2011).

Victims of relational trauma frequently cannot fully avoid a sense of responsibility for what has been inflicted upon them. Self-blame can even be a coping mechanism that allows these children to preserve a more positive image of their parents and preserve their attachments to them. However, the shame that results from this approach can become part of a growing child's very personality structure and sense of self (Herman, 1992).

The profound shame resulting from early traumatic experience not only becomes part of the self-structure, but also exerts a profound effect on relationships with others. This is because shame implies an imagined judgment of the self on the part of the other. The ubiquity of shame as a major threat to the self is striking in case studies focusing on adults with a history of relational trauma (Grossmark, 2009; Pinheiro & Viana, 2011). Pinheiro and Viana (2011) suggest that traumatized individuals may in fact organize their subjective experience around shame.

In sum, the formation of a secure sense of self is hindered in the phenomenon of developmental trauma, both because of deprived early relational experiences and because of challenges to the nascent sense of self that are above and beyond the trials of normative experience. In developmental trauma, an infant is faced with a sensory and emotional overload that cannot be processed within the caregiver–infant dyad. As a result, emotions cannot be symbolized, and behaviors, feelings, sensations, and cognitions are dissociated from one another, so that a unified personality cannot be fully formed. As we have discussed, children with DTD may lack the capacity to play for several reasons. Playing increases children's sense of agency in the world and helps them master how their own feelings and thoughts affect their external world. Children with DTD who have already been deprived of opportunities for self–other differentiation and agency thus continue to be deprived through their inability to engage in play. However, through play therapy, they can learn to differentiate self from other and experience validation of their feelings and nonverbal traumatic experiences (Young, 2008).

Case Vignette: Chang

Perhaps a clinical vignette from the treatment of a child whose history featured many components of DTD would be relevant to our discussion. I (Steven Tuber) met the patient (whom I will call Chang) very early in my training at an adolescent residential treatment center. Chang was 15 years old at the time, and as a consequence of his parents' substance dependence difficulties, he had spent the bulk of his early years in and out of multiple foster homes. Random separations from parental figures, and episodic, unpredictable violence both witnessed and felt by this child, were also marked features of his early life. I met him the day before treatment would formally begin, shook his hand as I introduced myself, and told him we would meet the next day. Chang had sufficient privileges on his unit to walk to treatment on his own the following day, and he came to my opened door with an excited, hopeful look on his face and a card in his hand. It was an 8½- by 11-inch piece of colored paper, folded in half, to which he had painstakingly glued scallops of aluminum foil around the edges. In elaborate italics was written "*To Steve*" on its cover, and when opened, in equally detailed italics was written: "*Would you be my friend?*" I was completely blindsided by this elaborate gesture of "love," and my bewildered, indeed frightened facial expression must have made this all too apparent to Chang. When I looked up and began to stammer some faint disclaimer, his face turned floridly enraged and he leapt at my throat, knocking me over and landing on top of me, forcing his hands around my neck in an effort to choke me. I reacted with panic, threw him off me, pinned his arms and legs with mine, and screamed at him, "Back off!" After a few tense moments, he calmed down, I calmed down (somewhat!), and I could let go of him. He quickly returned to his unit.

What had happened in that exchange? To use some of the prior wording of this chapter, Chang had taken my warm greeting of the previous day and turned it into an "all-or-none" expectation of deeply longed-for symbiosis, hoping for some way in which our possible "friendship" could replace his history of neglect, chaos, and abuse. He had apparently worked for hours on the unit making this card and telling his peers and counselors that "someone" was going to "really help" him this time. The precariousness of this longing, precisely because it had never been reliably fulfilled in any sustaining way, could not withstand even the slightest of disappointments. When he saw my frightened, overwhelmed reaction to the presentation of his "gift," his capacity to modulate or defend against his rage surrounding abandonment could not be accessed. Within a true "psychic equivalent" mode, I became the embodiment of all who had ever attacked and rejected him, leaving him with no alternative, in his mind, but to kill before being killed. As described above, Chang's thinking became concrete; his shameful rage became omnipresent; his limbic system became overwrought; his defenses became nearly nonexistent; his need to act rather than think or feel became mandatory; and the cycle of attack and counterattack became manifest within our first moments together.

It is crucial to emphasize, both for Chang and for other patients suffering from DTD, the intertwining nature of DTD's impact on affect–defense configurations, infant and child neurophysiology, and the development of the sense of self and other. Self–other experience occurs within a "bath" of affect; affects in turn inevitably evoke defenses to modulate them; all of these manifestations cause and are reciprocally caused by shifts in brain chemistry and physiology. For children with DTD, the resulting combination of difficulties stifles the use of imagination and play—usually the two great allies of children who are wrestling with psychological conflicts. The now feared capacity for play is atrophied in such children, furthering a cycle of maladaptation. This creates a toxic concoction that wreaks havoc on the child, the family, and society at large. For Chang, the result was a sudden, violent enactment of his need to destroy before being destroyed.

A Brief Nod to History

This chapter has sought to reorganize a great deal of research and theory on the impact of chronic early abuse and neglect into the burgeoning literature on DTD as a new, overarching syndrome in child psychopathology. As with all "new" diagnostic concepts, however, it is crucial to note its historical antecedents, since indeed there is nothing new under the sun. In the case of DTD, its roots lie squarely in the theoretical writings of Winnicott (1971; see also Tuber, 2008). In his seminal paper "On the Location of Cultural Experience," Winnicott wrote of the baby's experience:

> The feeling of the mother's existence lasts x minutes. If the mother is away more than x minutes, then the imago fades, and along with this, the baby's capacity to use the symbol of the union ceases. The baby is distressed, but this distress is soon *mended* because the mother returns in $x + y$ minutes. In $x + y$ minutes the baby has not become altered. But in $x + y + z$ minutes the baby has become *traumatized*. In $x + y + z$ minutes the mother's return does not mend the baby's altered state. Trauma implies that the baby has experienced a break in life's continuity, so that primitive defenses now become organized to defend against a repetition of 'unthinkable anxiety' or a return of the acute confusional state that belongs to disintegration of nascent ego structure. (1971, p. 97)

What we (and others) are calling DTD as a syndrome is thus a reconceptualization of Winnicott's depiction of $x + y + z$ time. Note how he discusses the impact in terms of self, other, affect, and defenses, which we mirror in the discussion above. Crucially, Winnicott also provides DTD with a temporal, phenomenological dimension. If the child's attempts at affect regulation (defenses) do not permit sufficient self-soothing while waiting for the caregiver's arrival in $x + y$ time; if brain chemistry and physiology "conspire" to reduce the child's capacity for cognitive and emotional flexibility during this time frame; if the child's experience of self has been linked to hopelessness regarding the reemergence of "good enough" caregiving by an attuned "other"; and if the "other" cannot be attuned enough to return to the child's needs within these all-too-real time constraints, then the child will indeed experience $x + y + z$ time—a time of trauma. In Winnicott's words, confusion and disintegration become the child's primary experience. In our present attempt to make sense of the child's experience, we are calling the manifestations of this $x + y + z$ state DTD. In Chang's experience, we can see how it played out all too violently and chaotically. We believe that this notion of DTD does diagnostic justice both to the remarkable distress of such a child's early experience and to the often life-long adverse sequelae of this experience. We thus are in favor of using DTD as an appropriate term to describe children who have experienced chronic early trauma, but we encourage practitioners to link this "new" syndrome to its earlier theoretical antecedents for the best understanding of its etiology and prognosis.

It should also be noted how adversely DTD can affect the capacity to use play therapy. If the very capacity for playfulness has been made toxic by the aftermath of DTD, then the experience of being encouraged to "play out" one's feelings can create a milieu of dread and panic instead of a forum for repair and replenishment. Chang's first session can be seen as a dramatic example of the consequences that occur when a child has no access to play and thus experiences dread with no buffer or respite. In the terminology used in this chapter, such a forum can overpower affect regulation, engender the rigid use of primitive defenses of avoidance and expulsion, and wreak havoc with the fragments of selfhood that may exist. For such children, the play therapy experience must be presented with great caution, often with a specific structure, and always with a strong sense by the therapist of how terrifying being alone with one's feelings may be for these children, across the domains of intrapsychic, neurophysiological, and interpersonal experience.

REFERENCES

Blum, H. P. (1987). The role of identification in the resolution of trauma: The Anna Freud Memorial Lecture. *Psychoanalytic Quarterly, 56*, 609–627.

Cook, A., Spinazzola, J., Ford, J., Lanktree, C., Blaustein, M., Cloitre, M., . . . van der Kolk, B. (2005). Complex trauma in children and adolescents. *Psychiatric Annals, 35*(5), 390–398.

Cramer, P. (2006). Coping and defense mechanisms: What's the difference? *Journal of Personality, 66*(6), 919–946.

D'Andrea, W., Ford, J., Stolbach, B., Spinazzola, J., & van der Kolk, B. A. (2012). Understanding interpersonal trauma in children: Why we need a developmentally appropriate trauma diagnosis. *American Journal of Orthopsychiatry, 82*(2), 187–200.

Fonagy, P., Gergely, G., Jurist, E. L., & Target, M. (2002). *Affect regulation, mentalization, and the development of the self.* New York: Other Press.

Fonagy, P., & Target, M. (2006). The mentalization-focused approach to self pathology. *Journal of Personality Disorders, 20*(6), 544–576.

Ford, J. D. (2005). Treatment implications of altered affect regulation and information processing following child maltreatment. *Psychiatric Annals, 35*(5), 410–419.

Grossmark, R. (2009). The case of Pamela. *Psychoanalytic Dialogues, 19*(1), 22–30.

Hegeman, E., & Wohl, A. (2000). Management of trauma-related affect, defenses, and dissociative states. In R. H. Klein & V. L. Schermer (Eds.), *Group psychotherapy for psychological trauma* (pp. 64–88). New York: Guilford Press.

Herman, J. (1992). *Trauma and recovery.* New York: Basic Books.

Krystal, H. (1978). Trauma and affects. *Psychoanalytic Study of the Child, 33*, 81–116.

Lieberman, A., & Knorr, K. (2007). The impact of trauma: A developmental framework for infancy and early childhood. *Psychiatric Annals, 37*(6), 416–422.

O'Neill, L., Guenette, F., & Kitchenham, A. (2010). 'Am I safe here and do you like me?': Understanding complex trauma and attachment disruption in the classroom. *British Journal of Special Education, 37*(4), 190–197.

Pearlman, L. (1997). Trauma and the self. *Journal of Emotional Abuse, 1*(1), 7–25.

Pearlman, L., & Courtois, C. A. (2005). Clinical applications of the attachment framework: Relational treatment of complex trauma. *Journal of Traumatic Stress, 18*(5), 449–459.

Pinheiro, T., & Viana, D. (2011). Losing the certainty of self. *American Journal of Psychoanalysis, 71*(4), 352–360.

Pollack, S., Cicchetti, D., Hornung, K., & Reed, A. (2000). Recognizing emotion in faces: Developmental effects of child abuse and neglect. *Developmental Psychology, 36*(5), 679–688.

Schore, A. N. (2002). Advances in neuropsychoanalysis, attachment theory, and trauma research: Implications for self psychology. *Psychoanalytic Inquiry, 22*(3), 433–484.

Schore, A. N. (2003). *Affect dysregulation and disorders of the self.* New York: Norton.

Teicher, M. H., Andersen, S. L., Polcari, A., Anderson, C. M., Navalta, C. P., & Kim, D. M. (2003). The neurobiological consequences of early stress and childhood maltreatment. *Neuroscience and Biobehavioral Reviews, 27,* 33–44.

Tuber, S. (2008) *Attachment, play and authenticity: A Winnicott primer.* Lanham, MD: Aronson.

Tuber, S. (2012). *Understanding personality through projective testing.* Lanham, MD: Aronson.

van der Kolk, B. (2003). The neurobiology of childhood trauma and abuse. *Child and Adolescent Psychiatric Clinics of North America, 12,* 293–317.

van der Kolk, B. A. (2005). Developmental trauma disorder: Towards a rational diagnosis for children with complex trauma histories. *Psychiatric Annals, 35*(5), 401–408.

van der Kolk, B., Pynoos, R., Cicchetti, D., Cloitre, M., D'Andrea, W., Ford, J. D., . . . Teicher, M. (2009). *Proposal to include a developmental trauma disorder diagnosis for children and adolescents in DSM-V.* Unpublished manuscript.

Waller, N., Putnam, F., & Carlson, E. (1996). Types of dissociation and dissociative types: A taxometric analysis of dissociative experiences. *Psychological Methods, 1*(3), 300–321.

West, M. (2011). Attachment, sensitivity and agency: The alchemy of analytic work. *Journal of Analytical Psychology, 56*(3), 354–361.

Williams, P. (2004). Symbols and self preservation in severe disturbance. *Journal of Analytical Psychology, 49*(1), 21–31.

Winnicott, D. (1971). *Playing and reality.* London: Tavistock.

Young, M. E. (2008). Play therapy and the traumatized self. *Psychology and Education: An Interdisciplinary Journal, 45*(1), 19–23.

CHAPTER 14

The Princess and *Dal Bhat Tarkari*

Play Therapy with Children of Cross-Cultural Adoption

Henry Kronengold

ABBY: OK, here's what we're doing. You're trying to find the princess. She was taken captive by the witch, who locked her in the castle. The witch is hiding her there. You try to save her. But be careful, the witch has guards all around.

ME: OK. Here I go. (*I adopt a brave posture and head toward the castle.*) I'm coming to save the princess, I'm coming to save the princess. (*Abby looks at me and puts her finger to her mouth, gesturing that I should be quieter. My voice lowers to a whisper.*) Right. Now to find the entrance. Ah-ha, I think it's over here. (*I point to a small room inside my toy castle, and I pretend to burst in.*) Princess, are you here? I've come to save you!

ABBY: Thank heavens you made it. Now let's get out of here quick. We have to get past the witch's guards. Come on! This way!

ME: OK, let's go. (*We run out of the castle, heading toward freedom. We keep running, pursued by guards and a very angry dragon. At last, we make it out of the castle, where I pause to catch my breath and plan our next move.*) Princess, we're out of there, but we need to find a safe place to rest before we continue the journey back home. (*I pause for a second, but there's no response.*) Princess, did you hear me? (*Still no response. Concerned, I start to look around.*) Princess, Princess, where are you? Did you go for a walk somewhere? Princess? (*I start to look around some more, but I don't know where she is. My face takes on a look of worry; my voice is now rising and more pressured.*) Princess? Princess?

ABBY: She's gone, you know. She's disappeared.

ME: What? What do you mean? How? She was just here!

ABBY: Not any more. She's disappeared, and you need to find her again. Did you hear that sound? The laughing?

ME: Yes. It's . . . (*My voice slows now.*) It's. The. Witch.

ABBY: (*Looks at me with a knowing glance.*) It wasn't going to be that easy you know.

As Abby would remind me repeatedly in our sessions, trying to find her and her constantly shifting identities in our sessions was definitely not going to be easy. In the dialogue above (and in many others), a princess was captured by a witch, whose motives were never clear. Despite repeated attempts to rescue the princess, she would mysteriously disappear, leaving the heroic prince both hapless and helpless in his efforts to rescue her. Play with Abby was rich, stimulating, and often confusing as she kept developing stories with missing and disappearing characters who would often transform themselves within a single scene (see Kronengold, 2010, for a detailed description of Abby's case). Interestingly, she wasn't the only child who presented with this sort of play. In a strikingly similar scene, Alma created and directed me in her own story involving a prince and a princess.

ME: Princess, Princess, I'm here to rescue you! (*I pretend to barge into the castle dungeon.*)

ALMA: Hi, Prince. Quick, we have to get out of here. The witch is nearby, and her guards are everywhere. I know a good spot we can hide. C'mon, let's go (*as she points toward the side of the castle*).

ME: OK, are you all right? I missed you.

ALMA: Yeah, I'm fine. But hurry, we've got to get away from here.

ME: Right, let's go. Umm, where are we going?

ALMA: To the inn. It's in the middle of the forest. We can hide there for the night and then head back home tomorrow.

ME: (*I pause to consider the idea. I also have a feeling that I know where this is heading as I nod my assent to Alma's plan.*). To the inn! Let's go. (*We hurry to the inn, have a seat, and make plans to get some food.*) I'll go to the innkeeper and bring back some food for us to eat. What would you like?

ALMA: Anything. I'm starving.

ME: OK, I'll be back in a minute. (*I walk over to talk to the pretend innkeepers; get some pretend bread, chicken, and water; and head back to the princess.*)

ALMA: (*Gestures to me to come over to the side of the room, as she wants to tell me something. She leans toward me and speaks in a whisper.*) Henry, you come back, but the princess is gone.

ME: (*whispering*) Gone? Where did she go?

ALMA: She's gone. Just gone. You have to figure that out. She disappears. The witch's guards must have found her, or the witch cast a spell and brought her back to the castle.

ME: Seriously?

ALMA: Seriously. She's gone again.

Although Alma's storyline was similar to Abby's, Alma's princess was more assertive, and her role in the play differed from Abby's. Whereas Abby took great pleasure in my confusion, Alma broke character to tell me about the scene, almost joining me in wondering what might have just happened. As I thought of this scene alongside the one from Abby, my mind wandered to yet another scene played out with Sarah, a child I had seen some years earlier.

SARAH: Henry, you're the brother. Now look, you see this house over here. There are five different rooms. Each one is used for something special in the house. The sister's bedroom is here, and you go looking around for her, but she's not there. You have to try to find her, but she's not around. OK?

ME: OK. What do I do once I can't find her?

SARAH: You get very worried and start calling the police.

ME: Do they find her?

SARAH: No. And anyway, you have to play the game. OK, now let's start. You start looking for me.

ME: OK, I'm looking. (*I look searching around the room.*) Hmm, I wonder where she could be? Hello! Where are you? Are you in the house? (*I search the area.*) She's not there. Where could she be? Where has she gone? I hope she's OK.

SARAH: Now you call the police.

ME: (*I pick up an imaginary telephone.*) Hello, police? I need some help. I can't find my sister. I've looked everywhere.

SARAH: (*Takes on the deep voice of an imagined police officer on the other end of the line.*) Hello. This is the police.

ME: Hi, can you help me? I can't find my sister. She's supposed to be home, but she's gone, and I can't find her. (*My voice becomes more plaintive.*) I've looked everywhere.

SARAH: You have to keep looking for her.

ME: (*surprised*) Yes, but I'm calling for help. I need some help finding my sister. You see, she's disappeared.

SARAH: I can't really help. Sorry. You need to find her. But don't worry. You will.

ME: I'm glad you think so. I just don't know where she is. Well, OK, then. I'll keep looking. (*I hang up the phone and resume searching. As I look, Sarah motions for me to look near the closet area of the office, next to a large brown desk chair where she's hiding.*) Hmm. I think I saw something moving over there. Maybe it's her? Sister, Sister, is that you? It's me.

SARAH: Yeah, hi. I was wondering when you were going to find me.

ME: Well, I didn't know where to look. What were you doing here, anyway?

SARAH: I had to get away. I'll explain it all later, but for now, let's just get back home.

ME: OK, let's head back. I can't wait to hear the whole story. (*As we walk back, Sarah whispers to me.*)

SARAH: She disappears again.

ME: Again? But she was just with me. How did she disappear?

SARAH: She just does. Then you have to go find her again.

ME: That's a lot of searching.

SARAH: Yeah, I know. You'll find her again.

The three dialogues above are rich and evocative, each reflecting a child's journey as she tries to make sense of where she comes from, where she is going, and how she got there. What is also remarkable about these dialogues is that, on appearance, they could have involved the same child. Instead, the stories and themes were voiced by three different children, whom I worked with at different times over a period of 13 years. The similarity of the children's play speaks volumes about common themes among children, as well as the role of play in helping children better understand and explore questions and feelings about their past.

My discussion about the three children in this chapter is not meant to be exhaustive regarding therapy with children who have been adopted across cultures, or the attachment difficulties that pose a challenge to their families and therapists alike. Rather, it is meant to consider an element of working with children that frequently arises within play. In this case, I discuss excerpts from my work with Sarah, Abby, and Alma, with an eye toward how play (along with other expressive media) can serve as a powerful vehicle to foster a child's development and healthy transition to his or her adopted family.

When Sarah first began treatment, she was nearly 4 years old; she was living with her adopted parents as well as another child her parents had adopted, a brother. Her brother, 9 years old, struggled with explosive behavior. Sarah was an unusually verbal child who regularly spoke to her mother about her brother's challenges and used to watch him like a hawk, lest he lose control without anyone noticing. Sarah's precociousness had served her well in life, and she was often praised for her maturity and intelligence. Of course, there was another side to staying so vigilant: Sarah was highly controlled, rarely expressed her feelings to other people, and (as can be seen in the dialogue above) was most comfortable directing others.

Alma walked into my office as an extremely poised, verbal, and precocious 4-year-old. She played, chatted, painted, danced, and smiled. In short, she did everything one could imagine to be a good play partner. She was incredibly charming, funny, and creative. At the end of our first meeting, I thought how much I enjoyed our session and how much fun it was to spend time with Alma. As I explored my own reaction, I recalled other children who had made such an impact in our first meeting. Prominent among this group were, of course, Sarah and Abby. Abby had made herself at home almost as soon as she walked into my office, immediately announcing her playful presence as we began our work together. How unusual it was for these children to occupy this particular place in therapy and in my own mind. Working with each of them was great fun; their sessions were both creative and rich. At the same time, I wondered: Was the very reason they were coming to see me connected to their ability to connect so easily in their initial sessions? Other children would begin sessions warily, careful not to stray too far from their parents. But Alma, Sarah, and Abby were so different.

The answer seemed connected to their attachment histories and to the changes in each child's early experience. In a healthy situation, children born to biological parents typically become attached to those parents, depending on them for nurturance and support, while enjoying their time with each parent in a way that is both loving and reciprocal. There are of course lapses in a child's attachment to his or her parents—but in a typically developing and healthy child, there is what we refer to as a *secure* attachment (Ainsworth, Blehar, Waters, & Wall, 1978; Bowlby, 1969/1982, 1973), where the child feels safe in the presence of the parents and gradually internalizes that feeling of safety to explore the world. In a child's younger years, he or she is most comfortable with caregivers and is careful when meeting new people. In Alma's case, however, she hadn't developed this sort of connection at a younger age. She had been raised first in an orphanage and then by a loving foster family in the Himalayan Mountains. Alma's unusual ability to solicit attention, to lodge herself into another person's world, and to make that person want to get to know her had probably contributed to her winding up with a new loving mother in New York City. Her ability to engage others with such impressive skill and fearlessness stood out, just as it did for Abby and for Sarah. Each of them had come from a different part of the world, and each had developed a capacity to stand out from other children. These skills proved most useful on first impression, making initial sessions and meetings memorable. Based on my own experience in my initial session with Alma, I can only imagine how her adopted mother felt during and after their first meeting. Alma's adaptive abilities were extraordinary. But at what cost? What happened after the shine of the first meeting wore off? This little girl worked so hard to impress and engage others, presenting more as a young adult than a small child. What happened when she needed to be a child again? Could she? Perhaps there was a reason why Alma also couldn't sleep at night, calling as a younger child might for her mother's comfort. Perhaps there was a reason why when Alma became upset and her mother didn't respond with perfect empathy, Alma would say that she shouldn't have been adopted and didn't deserve to have a mommy. Whereas some of Alma's statements may have had a manipulative element, others suggested her lingering insecurity, manifested by the inconsolable flow of tears at those difficult moments.

Then there was Abby, playful and fun but struggling with her behavior. Abby acted out at home and at school, with frequent tantrums and difficulty following classroom routines. In our early sessions, she wished to control my every move, from how I played to where I stood in my office. The ever-vigilant, mature, and articulate Sarah was less overtly controlling, but she kept watch over everyone and everything in her home. At school Sarah adopted the role of a teacher's assistant, with a particular eye on helping struggling classmates. Once she personally referred a preschool classmate of hers who was struggling with tantrums. At the same time, Sarah also complained of headaches, stomach pain, and various other bodily ailments. For a highly verbal child, she was very uncomfortable expressing her feelings; when upset, she would become overwhelmed and shut down. In one memorable episode, Sarah became upset at school and fell to the floor, seemingly unconscious. Her teachers, worried that Sarah had had a concussion or possible seizure, immediately sought medical attention as attendants tried to figure out what happened and why Sarah was unresponsive. It was only an hour later, when her mother came to the doctor's office and spoke to her daughter, that Sarah opened her eyes, picked up her head, grabbed her backpack, and calmly walked out the door to head home. She had been awake the entire time.

In the cases of these three girls, their play offered details as to what they were struggling with, in terms of both their attachment and their confusion over their early experiences. Alma's play began quickly, as did Sarah's and Abby's. In our early sessions, Alma directed a version of her story about a princess who had been captured by an evil witch, was saved by the prince, was recaptured by the witch, was saved again by the prince, and so on and on. Alma played this game repetitively at home, although she maintained her enthusiasm no matter how many times she played out the drama.

> ALMA: I'll be the princess and you'll be the prince. Oh, and I'll be the witch also, and you can play some of the guards, OK?
>
> ME: OK.
>
> ALMA: (*In a most industrious mode, she sets up the castle and characters in exact positions.*) OK, I'm the princess now, and you're the prince, and we're about to get married. Ready, OK?
>
> ME: OK. What I am supposed to do?
>
> ALMA: (*in a friendly but assertive voice*) You're supposed to ask the princess to marry her, and then you'll walk back to all the people to tell them you're getting married, and they'll start to get everything ready for the big wedding, but before they have the wedding, the witch, she's going to set up a trap for them, and she'll capture the princess, and she'll bring the princess back to her house and keep her there. OK?
>
> ME: Yup, I think I have that. (*I'm impressed but also surprised by Alma's strength and efficiency.*)
>
> ALMA: Good, let's go. OK, c'mon.
>
> ME: Right, oh, yes. Hello, Princess, it is so wonderful to see you today. My princess, my princess, would you like to marry me?
>
> ALMA: (*Maintains her friendly voice.*) No, no, you're supposed to do that in this part of the castle, and you don't say, "Would you like to marry me?" You say, "Come, Princess, let's get married."
>
> ME: OK. Come, Princess, let's get married.
>
> ALMA: Right, but you do that when we start the play, not yet.
>
> ME: I was just practicing.
>
> ALMA: OK, let's start.
>
> ME: Oh, hello, Princess. (*I look back at Alma to make sure I'm getting this right.*) Princess?
>
> ALMA: Yes (*expectantly, waving with her hand to cue me.*)
>
> ME: Come, let's get married.
>
> ALMA: OK. (*She now gives me directions about where we're supposed to go to prepare for the wedding.*) Now we move over to this part of the castle, but the witch is going to be waiting for us.
>
> ME: OK, let's walk over there to get married, my princess.
>
> ALMA: (*Continues directing.*) We walk over here (*she points to the back of the castle*), and then the witch pops out and gets the princess.

ME: Got it.

ALMA: OK, now we're walking.

ME: Yes, we're walking. Soon, Princess, we shall be married.

ALMA: (*She now takes on the scary voice of the witch, who has appeared near the castle walls.*) Not so fast. Ha, ha! Away, Prince, the princess is mine! (*She goes back to her regular voice as Alma.*) The witch takes the princess away and disappears. Now you're supposed to go look for her. Everyone is looking for her. But they can't find her.

ME: Where has the princess gone? This is the work of that evil witch! Ah, I must find her. I must find my princess. I shall look over there, in the mountains (*as I point to the sofa in my office*).

Alma's play was notable for its theme of a missing princess, a witch who wanted the princess for herself, and a beloved prince who was looking to rescue her. Her play was also notable for its great detail and for precise stage and dialogue directions. At the same time that Alma gave me instructions as to what I was supposed to say, there hadn't been too much actual dialogue in our scenes. In the process, Alma hadn't given much of a clue as to the emotions behind our scenes and characters. Perhaps Alma was trying very hard to control these emotions, reflecting various degrees of loss and longing, or maybe she wasn't yet aware of them. In any event, the lack of emotional content may have been why Alma kept repeating this story in our early sessions and in her play at home with her mother. Maybe she was trying to locate the feelings that were likely to be resonating in her own experience, but so far she wasn't able to. Instead, she had latched onto this familiar fairy tale as a sort of proxy for her own experiences. I saw our play as an opportunity for Alma to begin either to better understand her emotional world or allow it to register. Now that I was the prince doing the searching, I had a bit more space to operate in our session. I expected that while Alma would offer direction, I could begin to narrate my own experience of looking for the princess, and in the process start to introduce more emotional themes into our play.

ME: Princess, Princess! Oh, Princess! My beloved princess, where are you? Where could you be? Where did that wretched witch take you? What has she done? (*I search around unsuccessfully.*) Ahh! (*I let out a sound that tries to capture both sadness and anger.*) Princess? (*I look around the sofa/mountain area longer.*) She's not here. This used to be the witches' lair. She must have moved and is holding my princess somewhere else. I will check back near the castle. Maybe there is some sort of magic area she has come up with. Those witches. Terrible creatures!

ALMA: He's going to look for her over there. But she's not there either. But then he goes to the forest and he hears a sound, and he realizes the princess is close by, so he looks over here (*she points near a playhouse in my office*), and then he sees the witch's house and he rescues the princess. But then they run away, and they stop at a place where they get something to eat and drink, and the witch's guards are there looking for them, and the guards recognize the prince and the princess and they have to run, and some people at the place try to help the prince and princess, but other people try to stop them.

ME: Got it.

ALMA: OK. Csshh! (*She makes a noise to show me the princess is nearby.*)

ME: Wait a second. I'm still over here near the castle. I haven't even walked over to the forest yet. (*I do this as I'm trying to slow this scene down—to allow it to simmer and resonate, rather than just playing out the details so quickly.*)

ALMA: OK. Well, go over there, then.

ME: I'm going to head over to the forest. Maybe I can find the princess over there. Oh, Princess! Princess! Where are you?

ALMA: (*Looks at me.*) OK, now I'm going to make the sound, and you'll go and realize it's the princess.

ME: (*I nod my head.*) Yes, I remember. I've got it. Go ahead, do the "Csshh" sound thing.

ALMA: (*Smiles.*) Csshh! Csshh!

ME: Two sounds!

ALMA: Just go ahead.

ME: What was that? A squirrel? A rabbit? An owl flying in the forest? Or, maybe it was a sign, a message! Perhaps the princess is nearby. I'm looking for her. (*My voice starts to slow down and lowers to a whisper.*) Maybe I'll hear another clue.

ALMA: (*in a faint, tiny voice*) Help! Help!

ME: I hear her. She's out there. Shh. I'll walk quietly and listen. (*I put my hand to my ear and walk carefully through the office.*)

ALMA: In here. Over here. It's me. She stuck me in the dungeon.

ME: Here I come. (*I arrive at the dungeon.*) Princess, it's me! I'm here to rescue you!

ALMA: (*Starts directing me.*) Now they escape and run back to the castle.

ME: (*Here I decide to nudge Alma to stay in our play—to stay with the emotion of the story rather than its direction.)* Wait a minute. I was in character.

ALMA: They escape.

ME: Yeah, but I was ready to act the whole thing out.

ALMA: So they try to get married again.

ME: But the escape?

ALMA: *(Looks at me sympathetically.)* OK. Let's go ahead.

ME: *(in a pleased voice)* Great. OK, um, where were we?

ALMA: You were rescuing the princess.

ME: Right, OK, back to our places. I'm . . .

ALMA: You're outside the dungeon, and I'm in the dungeon, and you rescue me, and then we run away, but the witch chases after us with her guards. We get to this inn where there's a place to eat and drink and stay there, but the guards find us and then . . .

ME: *(I playfully put my hands up, urging Alma to slow down a bit.)* I was kind of "in the rescue moment," you know. Like, this whole thing is a little way ahead here. Can I just, well—I mean no disrespecting the story, which of course is quite fascinating—but can we get back to the rescue? I feel like I'm kind of focused on that part right now, and then we can get to the rest of the story.

ALMA: Well, OK. Go ahead. Just remember where they go next.

ME: Totally. I got it. Clear on this. After the rescue, they go to the inn, get chased, the whole thing.

ALMA: Good. OK, go ahead.

ME: OK. *(I pause for a minute, as I'm feeling we went a little far afield. I also want to make sure I haven't lost Alma in my wish to keep the keep the scene going.)*

ALMA: Well?

ME: Sorry, just taking a second to get back into the scene. I was looking for you. I just found you in the dungeon after you called out, and now I'm trying to rescue you. Just getting back into the feeling.

ALMA: Can we just go ahead?

ME: Yes, yes. Just a second more. I'm the prince, and I just found you. Kind of a mix of excitement and, and . . .

ALMA: You're happy to find me, but you were also scared.

ME: *(My eyes open wider.)* That's good. That works.

ALMA: *(Sighs.)* Let's go.

ME: Ready. *(My voice rises.)* Princess, I'm here, I'm here to rescue you.

Oh, I thought I'd never find you again. (*I look around.*) We need to figure out a way out of here.

ALMA: The lock on the door is on the side. Open the lock, and I can get free. But beware of the witch.

ME: (*I fumble with the lock, making a few sounds of annoyance as I work at it.*) Almost got it, Princess. Almost. Getting there.

ALMA: Try turning it (*she motions with her hand*) that way.

ME: Got it. C'mon, Princess, let's get out of this place before the witch finds out and tries to catch us.

ALMA: OK, so now they run to the inn and . . .

ME: (*I sigh.*) We're in character, here you know.

ALMA: Oh, all right. All right.

ME: Let's go, Princess, through the forest. There's an inn at the edge of the forest. We can stop there to rest and eat something before we return to the castle. Princess, I can't believe I found you. I was worried the witch had made you vanish or put some sort of spell on you.

ALMA: She tried to. (*Now Alma is using her hands to gesture as she talks.*) She tried to put this spell on me to make me fall asleep forever, but I wouldn't let her, because I had learned magic to keep her from being able to put me under a spell.

ME: Magic? Hmm, what form of powerful magic is this that you learned, Princess?

ALMA: Just magic. I learned it from the fairies in the forest when I was younger.

ME: Remarkable. Very powerful, this magic is. Fairies, huh?

ALMA: (*Points to one of the chairs in the office.*) There's the inn.

ME: Yes, there it is. It will be good to get a chance to rest. All this running around has left me tired.

ALMA: I know, me too. And I'm more tired and hungry, because I was stuck in the dungeon all that time, you know. Let's go inside. (*She gives me some more information as to our setting.*) OK, so there are a lot of people inside and it's noisy, and we sit down to have something to eat and drink, but then the witch's guards come in, and they're looking for us.

ME: OK. (*I go back into character. I take a bit of pretend food and a drink from a pretend glass.*) Oh, it's good to eat something. I'm sorry, Princess, you must be really hungry and tired. Are you OK?

ALMA: Yes, I'm OK now. (*Starts to look worried.*) But look over there, I know those two guys. They work for the witch! We've got to get out of here!

ME: Uh-oh! C'mon, let's go out this way. (*We run to the side of the castle, trying to elude our pursuers.*)

ALMA: They're getting closer. I can hear them.

ME: I know, me too. Let's hide in those trees. (*We run over to the floor lamp in my office. Alma looks up at me, and I put my finger to my mouth.*) Sshh. (*I whisper, as Alma nods and we stand perfectly still for a minute. Alma makes an exaggerated gesture to show that she's not moving at all as she stands silently, almost holding her breath. Then I wave with my hand for her to peek out of the trees with me.*) I think they missed us.

ALMA: They could be back or close by.

ME: True. Let's head this way, but stay close to the trees in case we need to hide again. And let's be very, very quiet.

ALMA: OK. Let's go. This way. I'll lead. (*Alma starts to walk as I follow. We continue silently until she suddenly stops.*) I heard something!

For Alma, play was an opportunity to grapple with her prior attachment history and her fears. Her controlling, grown-up behavior belied her reality as a young and vulnerable child who had already experienced the helplessness that comes from confronting loss and confusion. Born in a small village, raised first in an orphanage and then in a foster home, Alma ultimately met a woman who would adopt her and become her mom. Dazzling on first impression, Alma grew bossier and moodier as she got to know people. As her play illustrates, she was also in a regular state of anxiety about how secure she could feel in her new home. I found that as Alma became able to use the play not just to make up stories, but to embody characters representing a range of feelings (such as anxiety, sadness, loss, and longing), she became calmer both in our sessions and at home. This was also the case with Sarah and Abby, who also created stories with trapped or missing characters who would pop in and out of the stories and transform themselves at any moment. All three children had been stuck in a loop of repeating the same story in their play. In Alma's case, she reenacted the same scenes when playing with her mother at home. Not surprisingly, her mom tired of this play and perhaps experienced some discomfort with Alma's focus on being kidnapped and taken by an evil witch. Alma's mother was certainly not such a person and was trying to create a loving and stimulating life for Alma in New York. But for Alma, there was still the fear that perhaps something could happen and she could be cast aside once more. When Alma first played out her stories with me, she was relatively removed from her play: She was happy to tell me about what was going to happen in the princess story, and was even happier to direct me. But I wanted Alma to become an actor in the story. I wanted her to be able to embody the emotions that had come with her experiences. I wanted Alma to have the opportunity to tell her story, and the fears it embodied, in a safe place with a degree of emotional investment that would allow her to begin to move forward and develop her attachments and relationships.

As play with Alma continued, she began to branch out with her themes. The prince and princess gave way to other stories, characters, and expressive media, as Alma enjoyed my castle, action figures, paints and markers, and particularly my fake food and kitchen utensils.

Food has played a role in understanding attachment since Harlow's (1958) early attachment research with rhesus monkeys. Influenced by Bowlby's (1951/1977) early theories of attachment emphasizing nurturance over biological sustenance as the most important factor in the relationship between a child and his or her primary caregiver, Harlow decided to test some of these theories in research with primates. He set up two groups of baby rhesus monkeys and put them in two separate cages. In one cage was a "mommy monkey" that was made of wire, but that had a feeding tube connected to it to provide milk. In the other cage was a "mommy monkey" also made of wire, but covered with a soft cloth material suited for cuddling. Harlow was interested in testing out how the baby monkeys developed and how they related to their respective "mommies." He found that the baby monkeys in the cage with the cloth monkey became attached to the "mommy monkey," and demonstrated improved health effects (e.g., they were better able to digest the milk dispensed to them). So began much of modern attachment research, as developmentalists started to focus on the nature of the relationship between mother and child and how that relationship was based on emotional attachment and psychological attunement rather than on a purely biologically based need for sustenance, as had previously been believed (Bowlby, 1969/1982). Since then, countless studies have been devoted to exploring the relationship between children and parents, with an eye on the importance of secure attachment in a child's healthy development.

But, as anyone who has ever felt comforted with a warm bowl of soup or a refreshing bowl of ice cream can attest, food still holds a certain sway in the world of psychological meaning. It certainly did for Alma, who had quickly developed a sophisticated palate, along with a near-compulsive need to finish her food and try out the dishes of her fellow diners. Alma was always hungry. I wondered what this hunger was about, as Alma ate as if she was worried that each meal might be her last for some time. Certainly this was an understandable stance for a child who had been through so many twists and turns in life. Not surprisingly, food started to make an appearance in our play as well, as Alma and I began to work on pretend recipes and kitchen organization.

ALMA: Let's take out the food. Do you have any kitchen things?

ME: Some. Take a look in that bin. (*I point to a blue bin in my toy closet.*)

ALMA: Hmm. (*She rummages through the bin, finding some small plates, utensils, cups, a tea kettle, and an egg beater.*) Do you have any big plates? Any more pots? There isn't that much here.

ME: Well, look, here's a pot, some plates, forks, and stuff. (*I pick up another utensil.*) And a teapot.

ALMA: (*Sighs.*) We'll use that stuff. You should really get a kitchen. (*She looks around the room, her eyes settling on a space near my bookcase.*) You could put it right over there. Then we could play with it.

ME: It's an idea. What kind of kitchen?

ALMA: You know, a kitchen.

ME: Yes, yes, but what should I have? I'm detecting a feeling that I may not have quite what I need here in the kitchen department, so I'm just looking for some input here.

ALMA: You'd have more pots and pans, and an oven, and an area for cutting stuff. Also a sink. You could have lots of pretend food. Even more than you have.

ME: Sounds impressive.

ALMA: Oh, and it should be pink.

ME: Pink.

ALMA: Yeah, that would look really pretty. C'mon, let's play.

ME: You want me to put a pink kitchen right over there, next to the nice rug.

ALMA: Uh-huh. We have to make the food now. C'mon.

ME: What are we making?

ALMA: Lunch.

ME: What's for lunch?

ALMA: We're making it. (*She starts to set up the tops of the bins as if they're trays, and with my help starts to use a couple of empty bins as an oven and a sink. I help her put things in place, noting her creativity and resourcefulness in using these everyday items to arrange nearly the same kitchen she has just recommended.*) I'm going to start cooking things. Let's see, let's make some pasta, some chicken, some vegetables. Oh, there's some steak. (*Alma notes the items as she begins to proceed through each and every food item in the bin. There are about 25 items in total, and Alma goes through each one, occasionally pausing to express her satisfaction with a smile and lingering gaze when she gets to a favorite item, such as ice cream or a piece of pretend pink frosted chocolate cake. Finally, every piece of food is sitting somewhat precariously, yet neatly, atop a flat blue plastic tray.)*

ME: Wow, that's a lot of food.

ALMA: *(with a satisfied look on her face)* Everything is there!

I looked at the platter, and I suddenly remembered similar play with Sarah over 13 years ago. I was in a different office with different toys. I also had pretend food, which Sarah would arrange carefully, and a large number of pretend animals, which she used to spend time arranging so that each animal was set up properly near its neighbor and no animals were ever left behind. Sarah had been particularly careful to make sure that all the baby animals were placed right atop one of their parents; this kept the babies safe and prevented the babies and the parents from getting separated. Sarah had accounted for every animal and every food item, perhaps to avoid leaving anything behind. Once everyone was lined up properly, the animals could partake of the food or go on adventures, but always together. Over time, Sarah had allowed the animals to separate from one another for periods of time. As the animals grew more adventurous, Sarah's anxiety and hypervigilance had cooled as well. Interestingly, as she became less anxious, she was better able to rely on her parents to take care of any issues at home with her brother or at school, while Sarah allowed herself to act more like a child. As I remembered the array of the animals and the food, another voice was calling out to me.

ALMA: Hello, are you listening?

ME: Yes. Sorry. My mind wandered for a second there.

ALMA: That was funny. I daydream sometimes, too. OK, let's make some food. Let's see, for breakfast we can eat . . . (*Alma looks over the food and starts picking items. As she does this, I start to associate to what she may have been eating back in her birth country before the adoption. I wonder about this association—is it my own projection, or is it connected to our play?)* We'll have some eggs, and some peaches . . . (*Alma is listing food again. As she does so, I'm still wondering about this girl who has only been in New York City for about a year and who's completely focused on arranging a meal that looks like the breakfast buffet at the Courtyard Marriott.)*

ME: What did you used to eat in India?

The question of when to stay in and when to step out of play is one of the most perplexing ones for any therapist. Staying in play allows the richness and fullness of a metaphor to take hold, uninterrupted by a therapist's need to make the metaphor linear. Linearity is comforting for adults and can make a therapist feel that he or she is being "therapeutic," but such linearity may not honor how a child comes to understand or manage his or her world (Engel, 2005; Kronengold, 2010). On the other hand, there are times when stepping out of a metaphor can deepen a child's capacity to reflect on experience and can allow the metaphor to take on a fuller shape (Carnochan, 2010). It would be wonderful to have a clear decision-making tree for when to wonder about a child's metaphor and when to follow it. But such decisions generally fall into the province of clinical judgment, which may vary considerably for any given child.

Abby had used all sorts of metaphors, as we played prince and princess, teddy bears, or brother and sister, and went on journeys and adventures. In her case, I trusted staying in the metaphor—what some may refer to as "trusting the process"—rather than stepping out and connecting her play to her life in any explicit way. But with Alma, I felt I was dealing with a different child. Abby was always younger in her style, always playful, rambunctiously so. Stepping out of her play felt inauthentic to how she approached the world. Alma, on the other hand, was another story. She was tremendously verbal and very comfortable expressing herself; she just didn't use words to express her feelings. With Alma, I wanted to help her reconnect to a developmentally appropriate place by using her capacity for fantasy and play—but I also realized that staying completely in play could in fact negate an important part of Alma. So I decided to ask my question and with it, perhaps open another world for us to explore: "What did you used to eat in India?"

ALMA: What do you mean?

ME: Well, what did you used to eat? Back in India, it must have been different from this food.

ALMA: Oh, yeah. We didn't have all this. No hamburgers or hot dogs like in here. It's different there.

ME: I can imagine. (*As we talk, we keep working on our pretend meal—arranging some food, putting dishes in our imaginary oven, and setting the table.*)

ALMA: We ate *dal bhat tarkari*. (*She says this very fast, as if swallowing the name of the dish in one gulp.*)

ME: What is it?

ALMA: *Dal bhat tarkari.* (*She repeats herself very fast, at least to my untrained ears.*)

ME: Huh?

ALMA: (*slightly annoyed*) *Dal bhat tarkari.*

ME: (*I still haven't actually heard what Alma was saying very well. I give it my best, knowing that I'm about to fail.*) Dabat taka. Taka, taka?

ALMA: (*laughing*) No, no. *Dal bhat tarkari.*

ME: (*I still don't know what she's saying, so I protest good-naturedly.*) Could you slow this down a little? I'm having a hard time here. (*As we slow down our pronunciation, I notice that our work in the pretend kitchen is moving more slowly as well, and Alma seems to be working on a dish unlike the ones I've seen her arrange before. She has a pretend fish in a bowl and only a couple of other ingredients near it.*)

ALMA: OK.

ME: Let's go piece by piece. What's the first part?

ALMA: *Dal.*

ME: *Dal.*

ALMA: *Bhat.*

ME: *Bhat.*

ALMA: *Tarkari.* (*She says this so it sounds more like "tree."*)

ME: What? (*I scrunch my face and look at her hopefully.*)

ALMA: *Tar-ka-ri.*

ME: Ah! *Tar-ka-ri.* I've got it. Da, umm, wait. (*I'm trying to remember the first parts of the name now, but I'm having a hard time.*) I can do this. Um, *da, ba, tarkari?*

ALMA: (*Rolls her eyes and laughs again.*) No, silly. *Dal bhat tarkari.*

ME: You do realize I really can't keep up when you say that. *Dhal, tak, tak, tak,* umm, I don't know.

ALMA: I'm working on dinner now.

ME: Yeah, I'll help.

Alma and I kept on preparing dinner. I made some vegetables, and it became clear to me that Alma was working on a particular dish rather than just using every ingredient in the office. As we talked about her home country and the food she used to eat, her relationship to the pretend food shifted. Alma was now comfortably moving back and forth between play and talking—or, better yet, imagination and reality. In fact, she appeared to be integrating the two. Our conversation shifted what Alma was making, and as she prepared the salmon, a dish with an added emotional resonance, our conversation shifted in turn. The humor between us allowed a playful quality to our back-and-forth, and the added connection between Alma and me allowed us to talk about a snippet of her life in India.

ME: Do you ever miss the food from your old home?

ALMA: Not really. I think about it sometimes. We have a lot of food here.

ME: Oh, OK. I was just wondering. You know like that dish, the . . . (*I'm still having trouble with the pronunciation. I feel at first a bit silly, but then I realize that there's an opportunity here, as my difficulty means that Alma gets to be my guide to entering this part of her world.*) . . . *bhak* something or other.

ALMA: (*Laughs.*) *Dal bhat tarkari.* We thought of making it. But then we didn't. One day we will. OK, this dinner is almost ready, I'm making salmon in a pot. There's salmon, and I cook it in soy sauce.

ME: (*I'm intrigued by how different this dish is from other pretend food creations.*) Salmon and soy sauce.

ALMA: Yeah, we're making a salmon bowl. We need to make the soy sauce, and we need some rice. Hmm. Do you have any soy sauce?

ME: No, but we can make some of our own.

ALMA: How?

ME: We can draw it.

ALMA: Good idea. (*She and I turn our attention to a drawing pad and art supplies. I start sketching little grains of rice, while Alma draws the soy sauce. We spend a few minutes checking our designs and cutting out the pieces that we'll use for our dish.*) Can you make some more of those? We need a lot of rice. Just drop them in the pot; it's already cooking. (*Alma surveys the salmon pot.*)

ME: Sure. I'll make some more. (*I take a whiff.*) Smells good.

ALMA: Yup, it's going to be very delicious.

ME: I never made this sort of dish before.

ALMA: Really? Oh, I make it all the time. You should try it; it's really good.

ME: I'm sure.

We worked on our salmon dish, at an almost meditative pace. Our play was quieter. We talked with each other, but our exchanges, both verbally and nonverbally, were not as busy. There was a calm to Alma's play, as for the first time it felt as if she had plenty of time and didn't need to rush as much information and content as possible into a session. It was hard to miss the connection between Alma's talking about her life back in India, the shift in how her food play moved from arranging items to creating something of her own, and her increasing calm in the session.

For Alma, and for Sarah and Abby as well, our work was about finding a voice within the support of a therapeutic relationship. Alma could certainly hold her own, and was one of the most formidable 4-year-olds I've ever met. But some of what seemed like a strong voice to others could be a smoke screen; her regular chatter and poise served to obstruct a view of a child who had been through so many transitions and so much uncertainty. Alma needed to play out the dramas of the disappearing princess to connect with her earlier experiences. She needed to play out the making of the food, to reclaim a part of herself that would allow her to make a full transition to her new life in New York City with her adopted mother. In the same way, Abby needed to lead me on adventures to faraway places with characters who began to emerge from the shadows, and Sarah needed to bring me into her own family dramas and her desire to be found and never again lost.

Each of these children used play, in the context of a therapeutic relationship, to explore and understand elements of her past. All three of them created vignettes that were strikingly similar in their depiction of missing princesses, forlorn princes and mothers, and ambiguously evil witches. Each child was unusually controlling in her play, working very hard to maintain direction over scenes that in an earlier time, had been far out of their control. Of course there were clear differences among Abby, Sarah, and Alma in the content of their play, their relationships to me, and their own personalities. But their shared presentations and predilections spoke loudly of their shared experiences and attachment histories. And their play revealed a shared longing to understand, to connect, and to give voice to what had happened to them. It is precisely this longing that can be addressed and honored in giving such children an opportunity to engage and in treatment find their voices.

REFERENCES

Ainsworth, M., Blehar, M., Waters, E., & Wall, S. (1978). *Patterns of attachment: A psychological study of the Strange Situation.* Hillsdale, NJ: Erlbaum.

Bowlby, J. (1973). *Attachment and loss: Vol. 2. Separation: Anxiety and anger.* New York: Basic Books.

Bowlby, J. (1977). *Maternal care and maternal health.* New York: Aronson. (Original work published 1951)

Bowlby, J. (1982). *Attachment and loss: Vol. 1. Attachment.* New York: Basic Books. (Original work published 1969)

Carnochan, P. (2010). Earning reality. *Journal of Infant, Child, and Adolescent Psychotherapy, 9,* 26–33.

Engel, S. (2005). *Real kids: Creating meaning in everyday life.* Cambridge, MA: Harvard University Press.

Harlow, H. (1958). The nature of love. *American Psychologist, 13,* 573–685.

Kronengold, H. (2010). Hey Toy Man. *Journal of Infant, Child, and Adolescent Psychotherapy, 9,* 3–17.

CHAPTER 15

Turning Back the Clock

Life before Attachment Trauma

David A. Crenshaw
Jennifer Lee

Googling the phrase *turning back the clock* yielded some surprises to me (David A. Crenshaw), and I spent several hours perusing the search results. One surprise was the overwhelming number of results related to sports. Particular games were referenced where the outcome would have been totally different if someone had not fumbled a ball or not struck out, or had scored a goal or a basket. There were, of course, a number of references to *turning back the clock* at the times during the year when daylight savings time in the United States begins and ends. Another large number of results were related to loss of health, particularly in life-changing spinal cord injuries or accidents causing brain injury. There were also a number relating to regrets, sadness about the natural aging process, and loss of physical vitality. However, I was surprised that there were relatively few results related to posttraumatic stress disorder (PTSD) and traumatic events, which are the focus of this chapter. The few references to PTSD in the Google search hits were primarily related to combat injuries and the psychological fallout from such devastating experiences as loss of limbs or memory due to brain trauma. *Turning back the clock* in this chapter refers to the powerful wish of a child or family members to reclaim the life they once lived before a traumatic event occurred (or, in the case of attachment trauma, more often a series of traumatic events).

Usually the image of play therapy consists of a young child engaged with a therapist in imaginative play where the child's life dramas and sometimes traumas are played out in symbolized form that allows safe distance from the actual events. Over time, the child gains mastery over these experiences and becomes able to continue onward with his or her developmental path. Older school-age children and adolescents who find it hard to talk with a therapist may sometimes engage in various expressive arts therapies, such as artwork, sandtray work, storytelling, poetry writing, or work with symbols, but they don't typically engage in fantasy play. There are exceptions, however, when older children (even adolescents) get down on the floor, play in the family dollhouse, and enact events that need to be processed at the same cognitive and emotional levels that pertained at the time of attachment trauma. One such severely traumatized teen was 14 when he got down on the floor, began playing with the family dollhouse, and enacted scenes of traumatic events that took place when he was only 4 (Crenshaw & Hardy, 2007). The extremely limited cognitive and emotional processing that he was capable of at age 4 required him to revisit these events therapeutically via symbolic play—the natural language of the preschool child. This case is discussed in more detail in the next section.

Longing for the Pretrauma State

Play therapists and family therapists are familiar with a child or family enacting patterns of behavior and interaction more appropriate to an earlier developmental stage in the life of the child or family (Crenshaw & Hardy, 2007; Fussner & Crenshaw, 2008). Interpersonal trauma can result in developmental arrest for a child (Billings, Hauser, & Allen, 2008; Hennighausen, Hauser, Billings, Schultz, & Allen, 2004), as evidenced by stunted ego development. A review of the research literature revealed that terms like *developmental arrest* were far more prevalent in the literature of the 1970s and 1980s, but have rarely been discussed in more recent literature except by the above-cited researchers. The paucity of literature on ego or developmental arrest may coincide with the declining popularity of psychodynamic approaches in recent decades. This is surprising in light of Shedler's (2010) meta-analytic review of the research indicating not only that psychodynamic therapy compared favorably with other evidence-based treatments, but, importantly, that its benefits lasted longer. Shedler explained the greater duration of benefits as probably due to increased insight, which resulted in improved adjustment after therapy ended.

An alternative or additional explanation for the striking enactments of behavior reflective of earlier developmental norms is the compelling longing in a child or even in a whole family to turn back the clock to the time before the trauma occurred. Consider this example: Janice (fictitious names are used throughout the chapter), age 14, in a session with the Reese family, was acting more in keeping with the developmental norms of a 10-year-old child. The therapist noticed that the other family members were also treating her as if she were 10. What was happening in this family? The therapist was curious about the developmental history of the family. In this instance, Janice was 10 when her mother went into a substance abuse rehabilitation program. Since then, there had been frequent crises and relapses requiring further inpatient treatment for the mother, and the family had been struggling to regain a stable footing for the past 4 painful years. The adolescent girl and her entire family burned with desire to turn back the clock to before the family trauma occurred. In time, they were able to express this longing in words and grieve together for the loss of the earlier happy times as a family.

In the case of severe attachment trauma previously described (Crenshaw & Hardy, 2007) and referred to above, a 14-year-old boy, Roberto, left his chair, sat down on the floor, and pulled the toy family house off the shelf. For close to a year, neither Roberto nor the therapist returned to their chairs in the office they had occupied during the first 6 months of the therapy. Roberto enacted the horrific violent scenes that he and his family had experienced at the hands of his alcoholic father, who had since been imprisoned for killing Roberto's mother. It is highly unusual that Roberto at age 14 would spontaneously take to the floor and play out his earlier experiences, but Roberto had been "incubated in terror" (Perry, 1997). Roberto processed the traumatic events in the experiential mode characteristic of children age 6 and under, which coincided with the time in his life when these horrifying events occurred. At age 6, finding words to tell any painful story would have been difficult; it was particularly so when the events were so terrifying in nature. The therapist served as a respectful and mostly "silent witness" (Gil, 2010) during the enactment of trauma scenes, except when Roberto became stuck in *revivification* rather than progressive mastery of the trauma events (Gil, 2006). It is essential for the therapist to intervene in the case of revivification, where the anxiety is increased rather than reduced by the enactments of the traumatic play. Gil (2010) has distinguished between *dynamic* and *toxic* posttraumatic play. Dynamic posttraumatic play displays movement, even if gradual, toward a sense of mastery. Toxic posttraumatic play indicates a stalemate: The child is stuck in repetitious play that does not relieve anxiety. When the child is stuck in posttraumatic play (Terr, 1990), intervening actively in a manner outlined by Gil (2006) is recommended. In the case of repetitively violent scenes, for example, when the character that Roberto was most closely identified with was immobilized by terror, the therapist would take command and call in the police and rescue vehicles to halt the violence and attend to the injured.

Creating the Trauma Narrative through Play

Roberto used the language of play that was available to him at the developmental age of 6 to create his trauma narrative, which allowed him to move forward with his development and become more invested in age-appropriate adolescent interests and concerns. After he achieved a sense of mastery through the play enactments, Roberto and the therapist returned to their chairs, and he focused largely on appropriate concerns for a 14-year-old (such as worries about girls liking him, body image, and academic pressures). Among the most striking features of symbolic therapeutic play are its compelling value when a child's issues remain to be resolved, and the complete loss of interest once the child can move on to other concerns.

In recent decades, the value of a narrative approach has been embraced in much of psychotherapy, including family therapy. Attachment research has revealed that narrative coherence is an important index of resolution of previous trauma and loss and leads to increased attachment security (van IJzendoorn, 1995). In the Reese family described above, multiple steps were required for the family to move forward. The mother's stopping her drinking was a crucial one, but also essential was the creation of a coherent family narrative that would allow them to grieve together for the loss of the pretrauma family life that they all in their own ways wanted to reclaim.

Work with trauma narratives in adult psychotherapy has received considerable attention in recent years (Schore, 2012; Siegel, 2012). Creation of trauma narratives in play therapy through developmentally appropriate language (the right-hemisphere language of play, symbol, and metaphor) has received less attention. It is helpful in the service of generalization for children to be able to verbalize their trauma narratives eventually, and play therapists can facilitate verbalization as they narrate and reflect on the children's play and its possible meaning. Although verbalization will be the ultimate goal many younger children—and older children who have suffered severe attachment trauma—will need to rely initially on creating meaning, perspective, and coherence of the narrative through the safe haven provided by the symbolism in play.

Developmental Kaleidoscopes

A serious drawback to the concept of developmental arrest (which has largely gone out of favor, as noted earlier) is that rarely is development blocked across the board at the point of the onset of attachment trauma. Typically children will present with a wide variety of developmental configurations, which are more reminiscent of a kaleidoscope than the linear developmental progression we expect to see. An adolescent boy may be an accomplished athlete and an adequate student academically, but when it comes to emotional regulation, he may be so variable in his control that his explosive behavior reminds his teachers of a preschool child. An adolescent girl may be abusing alcohol/drugs and may be sexually promiscuous, but she may only be able to sleep with a night light and a host of stuffed animals arranged in a specific order, which would be more common for a 3- or 4-year-old girl. In both cases, the symptomatic behavior results from poor emotional regulation that may stem from attachment trauma, but passes more easily for adolescent rebellious behavior than the more dependent longings expressed by the teenagers' actions. The actions point to the approximate age of the developmental trauma.

In the case of the 14-year-old girl, Jaime, her father left the family when she was 5 and gradually disappeared from her life. Her mother had a series of relationships with alcoholic and abusive men, which led to the mother's psychiatric hospitalization when Jaime was 13; this pushed Jaime into a kind of exaggerated pseudoindependence, because she no longer felt she could depend on anyone.

Jaime was immediately drawn to the family playhouse in the therapist's office with no detectable self-consciousness. The therapist, aware of the presenting problems, was initially taken aback that this would happen in the first session. Jaime engaged in ordering and organizing play in the first session, setting up the house, the furnishings, and the people in just the way she wanted them. She was quite decisive and didn't deliberate or agonize over her placements of people or furniture. The therapist asked whether he could join her on the floor, and she nodded approvingly. He sat at a distance that seemed comfortable and not intrusive to Jaime. He simply joined her as a silent, interested witness in the emotional space she inhabited upon entering the therapeutic context.

Over time, Jaime enacted numerous scenes that reflected the harrowing losses she had experienced when the parents separated and divorced, followed by the chaos stemming from her mother's choice of abusive partners, and finally her mother's depressive collapse and subsequent psychiatric hospitalization. She played out early memories of family picnics and vacations when she was quite, young before the divorce. Some of these scenes were actual memories; others may have been longings for and idealized images of the family she had hoped for but never really experienced. Unresolved grief and anger accompanied these unmet longings, along with the wish to turn back the clock to before things started to unravel in the family.

Necessary Grieving

Since the clock can't be turned back except in fantasy, in order for developmental progress to resume in the emotional life of a traumatized child, the long-avoided but necessary grieving needs to be undertaken. Since the pain of recognizing that one will never have what one longs for is so intense, it is no wonder that children and adults alike avoid the necessary grieving for as long as possible. The difference is that adults usually have more cognitive and psychological resources available to them for undertaking grief work. In order for the grief process to be fully therapeutic, it needs to be holistic. All child therapists encounter children who are able to talk about the sudden death of a sibling in a detached, nonemotional way. In these instances, there is cognitive awareness of the death, and the children are able to talk about the death in an intellectual way, but the affect is detached. The opposite can also occur: A child may experience waves of intense sadness, without a clue as to what the sadness is about. This is an example of internal emotional attunement without the cognitive awareness. If either the cognitive or emotional awareness is detached, the therapeutic benefit of talking about the grief will be limited.

The death of a parent for a young child can result in attachment trauma, but the rejection, neglect, abuse, or abandonment of a child by a parent can also constitute attachment trauma and in some ways may be more challenging to resolve. Although the death of a parent is exceedingly painful, it is also final and clear. In the case of rejection, neglect, abuse, or abandonment, the loss is sometimes ambiguous. Parents may come in and out of the lives of their children, for example, in cases of substance addiction. An abusive parent may at times be engaged with a child in positive ways. Perhaps the hardest to grieve for is a parent who rejects or neglects a child. As long as the parent is still alive, the child may hold out hope that the parent will someday be the parent the child needs. Disconnection can be harder to grieve for than death; it is a more confusing loss.

Children in the foster care system are particularly likely to experience disenfranchised grief (Crenshaw, 2002; Doka, 2002). Foster children carry within them a huge burden of unattended grief. The trail of disrupted attachments and broken-off relationships may be so long that no one loss can be adequately addressed in terms of its meaning and impact on a child. Unattended, often never grieved-for losses can be the emotional underpinnings of rage externalized, and profound sorrow internalized. A typical case history of children suffering from severe attachment trauma is replete with loss and repeated interpersonal injuries (often rejections, neglect, and abandonment).

In some instances, the effort to turn back the clock is driven by self-reparative attempts to recapture needed stimulation of the brain during an earlier critical period. A poignant example of such a child has been provided by Bruce Perry (Perry & Szalavitz, 2006) in his description of Connor, a 14-year-old boy who rocked and hummed to himself; was socially isolated, lonely, and depressed; failed to make eye contact; and had violent temper tantrums typical of a 3- or 4-year-old boy. Perry discovered that this child had suffered a history of early neglect by a caregiver hired by the family, who left him alone in the dark repeatedly for hours each work day. Perry saw the rocking, humming, and tantrums as desperate attempts by Connor to seek the stimulation that his brain had needed during the early months of life. As in many other cases of children who seek to turn back the clock because of neurobiological reparative needs, it was not one event that caused the damage but a cumulative deprivation suffered over time.

Case Vignette: Kai

When Kai, a 15-year-old girl, came to the office for her initial therapy sessions, she was immediately drawn to fantasy play activities expected of a much younger child. She eagerly played with dolls, created jungle scenes with plastic animal figurines, and held tea parties with her loyal cadre of teddy bears. She excitedly arrived to subsequent sessions bringing pictures of animals, many of which adorned her bedroom walls, or stuffed animals from her personal collection to incorporate into her play.

Kai and I (Jennifer Lee) consciously chose a pseudonym for her that reflected her background and history. The name Kai is somewhat ambiguous to reflect her cultural and mixed racial identity. It is symbolic of her complex history and those layers of identity and personal experiences that are not immediately apparent to others. Upon first appearance, Kai's heritage is not immediately apparent until one inquires about the meaning and significance of her name. This was symbolic of the deeper levels of Kai's personal history and the underlying vulnerability beneath her behavioral difficulties. Among these layers were the immeasurable losses and traumas she suffered, which led to her placement in residential care. Yet even after I worked with Kai for close to a year, there were many unknown layers, leaving an incomplete narrative that brought up more questions than answers.

Kai's early childhood was significant for multiple losses and disrupted attachments. When Kai was 4, her mother left the family (for reasons unknown) and had limited, sporadic contact with her children thereafter. Several years later, at the age of 8, Kai was orphaned when she lost both parents in the same year: Her father drowned in a boating accident, and her mother died of chronic illnesses. The death of her mother followed the death of her father by 3 months. Throughout her early childhood, moreover, Kai had had periodic psychiatric hospitalizations because of her dangerous behaviors in the home—specifically, temper tantrums, acts of self-harm, and extreme mood lability. It appears that Kai demonstrated an early vulnerability toward emotional instability, which was further compounded by the mother's abandonment, the death of both parents, and subsequent placements in foster care. Her foster placements were numerous and short-lived prior to her referral to residential care.

Kai rarely spoke about her parents and tended to avoid any discussions about her family. It was a rare clinical moment when she shared a lucid childhood memory; these moments, cobbled together, provided a hazy portrait of her early family life. Kai recalled endearing times at home with her mother, who was a weaver and made beautiful rugs and shawls. She also fondly recollected times listening to her father as he played a piano. Perhaps as a way to honor her father's memory and preserve an elusive yet heartfelt connection, Kai studied the piano as a teenager, taking lessons and practicing with patience and determination.

Necessary Grieving

Kai's clinical team was aware of upcoming dates that held personal significance, such as her parents' birthdays and the anniversaries of their deaths. Kai was able to articulate that these were important dates, but she could rarely find the words to express the depths of her sadness and longing. As we have discussed earlier, necessary grieving is critical for developmental progression in the emotional life of a child. Kai, however, had understandably limited cognitive, emotional, and psychological resources to process the multitude of her complex losses. As a child in foster care with severe attachment trauma, she was particularly vulnerable to disenfranchised grief (Crenshaw, 2002; Doka, 2002). With this seemingly endless list of disrupted attachments and splintered relationships, the meaning and impact of each of these losses were impossible to address. Working through unresolved grief in one relationship was likely to trigger a traumatic grief reaction from another disrupted relationship. The cascading effect of grief upon more grief felt insurmountable. Yet the impact of the avoidance of necessary grieving was manifested in Kai's repeated hurt and rejection in interpersonal relationships. She desperately wanted to have friends, but found that her desire for connection with same-age peers was not often reciprocated. While she struggled to fit in with other teenagers, she found camaraderie with younger children whose play interests were more compatible with hers. The absence of necessary grieving was further evident in the ambivalent way Kai related to adult figures in her life. Kai typically grew attached to staff members, sometimes requesting extra time for sessions and seeking as much contact as she could get. At other times, she would be inconsolable and unreachable, yelling at staffers to go away and insisting that she be left alone.

Developmental Kaleidoscope

With her intense interest in fantasy play with dolls and stuffed animals, Kai might be mistaken for a child of latency age or younger. At other moments, however, she was eager to talk about the fashion trends, her new hairstyle, and the boys at school like a typical teenager. Although it might appear as if Kai was stuck in the vacillation between her developmental and chronological ages, we are reminded that development for children like Kai does not necessarily progress in a linear fashion. As discussed earlier, their developmental configurations are more dynamic and complex, like the view through a kaleidoscope. There were strong variations in Kai's capacity for emotional self-regulation and interpersonal relatedness. She sometimes demonstrated adequate ego strengths when handling conflict and stressful interactions with her peers, yet she could immediately unravel into tantrum-like behavior at the slightest stressor without warning. At times, she would not know how to reciprocate in social interactions, being consumed by her own needs at the expense of ignoring important social cues. At other times, she would show genuine concern for the well-being of others and do whatever she could (e.g., bring food or offer personalized artwork) to ease their apparent suffering. Her ongoing tension between independence and dependence could readily be contextualized as typical adolescent behavior. Yet through the developmental kaleidoscope, we need to recognize the underlying longings for protection and security that were most likely unavailable when Kai was a young child. Similarly, her tension between fulfilling self-needs and the needs of others probably reflected a deeper desire for nurturance stemming from emotional deprivation from early caregivers. Although it would be convenient to embrace a global view of arrested ego development, a kaleidoscopic perspective allows for a deeper and expanded understanding of adolescent development for traumatized youth.

Creating the Trauma Narrative

The dollhouse was a central apparatus in Kai's play therapy sessions. She constructed a household of an extended family consisting of a single mother, her three young children, and elderly grandparents. Kai typically took on the role of the youngest boy, whom she named "Ted." In fact, Kai was so identified with Ted that she became visibly upset when she wasn't able to find the boy figurine at the beginning of one session. Once she located the figurine, she expressed great relief and was able to move forward in her play. Kai sometimes referred to this character as Teddy, a 5-year-old boy, Ted, a 15-year-old teenager; once she described him as "a 5-year-old boy who thinks that he is 15." This age confusion aptly reflected Kai's developmental arrest, perhaps indicating actual or recollected trauma occurring at or about the age of 5.

Whether Kai was Teddy or Ted, there was consistency in her character's behavioral issues. In one of her early sessions, Ted was charged with assaulting his grandmother and was sent to a group home because his behaviors were "too difficult" for the family to manage. In the course of Kai's play, Ted was often described as being aggressive with his siblings, running away from home, being sent to the psychiatric emergency room, or being removed from the home to live with another family. In the beginning, when her therapist alluded to exploration of the character's feelings, Kai's play became increasingly aggressive. It became clear that she did not possess the language or the verbal capacity to express her emotions safely. Her therapist adapted to the situation and learned to communicate with Kai through symbolic play and representation—the intuitive language of a much younger child.

Although Kai played out repetitive themes of removal, there was often a resolution through reunification with the family. This engagement in dynamic posttraumatic play compared to toxic posttraumatic play (Gil, 2010) suggested a gradual movement toward mastery of past trauma. These positive outcomes of being reunited with family members appeared to represent Kai's wish and longing to be with those she had loved and lost. Furthermore, it was a hopeful sign that Ted could always be contained by either caring grandparents or compassionate mental health professionals, who were often played by the therapist. Perhaps this was Kai's intuition that no matter how frequently she tested the limits and acted aggressively, her primary caregivers in her residential placement were not going to abandon her.

Kai generally demonstrated an ambivalent relationship with caregivers and authority figures through her play. She characterized "Cary," the mother, as a neglectful and incompetent parent with virtually no authority over her own children. Cary would often leave the house unannounced to spend time with her boyfriend, leaving the elderly grandparents to care for her young children. This enactment probably represented Kai's actual mother's physical and emotional abandonment of the family when Kai was 4 years old. Kai also personified ancillary authority figures as distrustful, dishonorable characters with ulterior motives. For example, a burglar masqueraded as a uniformed police officer in order to gain access into the family's home. A lawyer presiding over Ted's trial was later found to have an extensive criminal history. A worker from the ASPCA was an imposter who kidnapped and abused animals for his own amusement. However, her therapist, playing the role of the benevolent, empathic grandparents, was able to soothe Ted during an emotional crisis; the grandparents were strong and resourceful enough to contain the family unit and protect the children from outside threats and dangers.

A central theme in therapy was Kai's search for a safe place. In one dramatic scene, wild animals surrounded the house, leaving the family trapped inside and unable to escape. Impingements on the family's security were often dramatized with aggressive, violent overtones. The resolution of these scenes usually involved rescue to a secure location with outward expressions of love, gratitude, and belonging among family members. Again, Kai's engagement in dynamic posttraumatic play not only helped relieve tension and decrease anxiety, but was a hopeful indicator of her continued movement toward mastery of her past trauma.

About 6 months into treatment, there was a notable shift in Kai's play. She requested that she and her therapist switch characters and stances from the ones they normally played. When Kai took on the role of the mother, she embodied a different posture as a caregiver who loved and nurtured her children. This was in contrast to Cary's typically hostile, angry demeanor and her frequent abandonment of her young children. With greater frequency, Kai created family-oriented scenes (e.g., the adults baked holiday cookies and the children helped decorate the Christmas tree). Rather than the usual scenes of being chased by wild animals or running away from home, Kai became interested and invested in cultivating domestic scenes where the family was participating in everyday activities such as playing games and going out for ice cream. These scenes, either real or idealized perceptions of family life, reflected a deeper longing for quiet moments of connection and belonging.

Kai engaged in less posttraumatic play for several sessions, but this shift was temporary. At this time, Kai began to experience greater difficulties in school and in her residential placement. The next few months were marked by periodic hospitalizations and school suspensions, which also disrupted her course in therapeutic treatment. The causes or precipitants of this shift were unclear. Kai vehemently expressed her desire to leave her residential placement and merely explained that she did "not want to be here." Although Kai's request to be transferred to another facility was granted, there were lingering concerns about her eventual disappointment when faced with similar circumstances. When the therapist tried to process this transition with Kai, there was no sense of attachment or grief over the attachments already made. It was as if Kai was sealing herself off from any more loss, because loss in itself, as familiar as it was, felt unbearable. In the days before her discharge, Kai could be heard intermittently screaming and running away from staff members. It was as if she were trying to run away from her own shadow. If she ran fast enough, her shadow would go away. If she screamed loud enough, her shadow would leave her alone. She often reported not feeling safe, and yet it appeared little to do with her external environment. Her experiences and perceptions seemed to reflect an internalized fear and profound lack of safety she felt deeply within herself.

During her final session, Kai created a scene where the children were involved in a car accident and kidnapped by an unsavory character and his accomplices. The perpetrator, initially thought to be the mother's boyfriend, turned out to be the boyfriend's "evil twin brother." The real boyfriend was a kind and loving man who wanted nothing more than to care for the family. The split between "good" and "evil" appeared to reflect Kai's internalized dilemma between needing closeness and distance—wanting to stay in care and wanting to leave, and her desire to be compliant but having no real choice but to act out in defiance. Her characterization of the "good, real" brother might represent her desire to repair and salvage personal relationships, yet in the end, she left abruptly without saying goodbye.

During Kai's course in treatment, she was able to utilize the language of play to construct the beginnings of a trauma narrative. It appeared to be a safe avenue for her exploration to delve into the symbolism of play, where she could direct the actions of her characters and work toward some resolution of prior losses. Although it was an incomplete narrative, her treatment team can only hope that it was an initial step in the important process of her healing and recovery.

Conclusion

In our work with children who suffer from severe attachment trauma, we may also long to turn back the clock and help them reclaim their lives before the series of traumatic events began. As therapists, we may feel overwhelmed by the magnitude of the losses that our clients have suffered; these losses often seem like a seemingly impossible mountain to traverse before any real therapeutic outcome can be achieved. We may feel as helpless as the children we treat, and may fear that no amount of therapeutic work can resolve the tremendous, inconsolable grief they experience deep within themselves. And yet we can never magically turn back the clock, reverse the sequence of traumatic life events, or have the power to change any preexisting vulnerabilities. Nevertheless, we may be able to help our clients access a safe, symbolic language through play to help reach the inner recesses of their emotional life.

The developmental kaleidoscope is a dynamic, multifaceted process. As mentioned earlier, one configuration may show us a competitive athlete. Another configuration may reveal a dedicated student who takes pride in academic achievements. Yet another formation may unveil a gifted artist, musician, or writer. With each turn of the kaleidoscope, another image appears, and another perspective is realized. We may recognize developmental arrest in areas of emotional regulation, the capacity to tolerate distress, and interpersonal relatedness; yet these delays are part of a broader landscape. In the words of Robert Brooks (1993), we can faithfully search for "islands of competence" in the children we serve. As clinicians, we can adopt a strengths-based approach and honor the resilience our clients have demonstrated to make it through to this moment in time. We certainly don't have the power to turn back the clock, but we can remain sure-footed in our efforts to work through complicated grief and trauma by building on our clients' strengths and holding onto hope for their necessary healing and growth.

REFERENCES

Billings, R. L., Hauser, S. T., & Allen, J. P. (2008). Continuity and change from adolescence to emerging adulthood: Adolescence-limited vs. life-course-persistent profound ego development arrests. *Journal of Youth and Adolescence, 37,* 1178–1192.

Brooks, R. (1993). *The search for islands of competence.* Paper presented at the Fifth Annual Conference of CHADD, San Diego, CA.

Crenshaw, D. A. (2002). The disenfranchised grief of children. In K. J. Doka (Ed.), *Disenfranchised grief: New directions, challenges, and strategies for practice* (pp. 293–306). Champaign, IL: Research Press.

Crenshaw, D. A., & Hardy, K. V. (2007). The crucial role of empathy in breaking the silence of traumatized children in play therapy. *International Journal of Play Therapy, 16,* 160–175.

Doka, K. J. (Ed.). (2002). *Disenfranchised grief: New directions, challenges, and strategies for practice.* Champaign, IL: Research Press.

Fussner, A., & Crenshaw, D. A. (2008). Healing the wounds in a family context. In D. A. Crenshaw (Ed.), *Child and adolescent psychotherapy: Wounded spirits and healing paths* (pp. 31–48). Lanham, MD: Aronson.

Gil, E. (2006). *Helping abused and traumatized children: Integrating directive and nondirective approaches.* New York: Guilford Press.

Gil, E. (2010). Children's self-initiated gradual exposure: The wonders of post-traumatic play and behavioral reenactments. In E. Gil (Ed.), *Working with children to heal interpersonal trauma: The power of play* (pp. 44–63). New York: Guilford Press.

Hennighausen, K. H., Hauser, S. T., Billings, R. L., Schultz, L. H., & Allen, J. P. (2004). Adolescent ego-development trajectories and young adult relationship outcomes. *Journal of Early Adolescence, 24,* 29–44.

Perry, B. D. (1997). Incubated in terror: Neurodevelopmental factors in the "cycle of violence." In J. D. Osofsky (Ed.), *Children in a violent society* (pp. 124–149). New York: Guilford Press.

Perry, B. D., & Szalavitz, M. (2006). *The boy who was raised as a dog: And other stories from a child psychiatrist's notebook.* New York: Basic Books.

Schore, A. (2012). *The science of the art of psychotherapy.* New York: Norton.

Shedler, J. K. (2010). The efficacy of psychodynamic psychotherapy. *American Psychologist, 65,* 98–109.

Siegel, D. J. (2012). *The developing mind: How relationships and the brain interact to shape who we are* (2nd ed.). New York: Guilford Press.

Terr, L. (1990). *Too scared to cry: Psychic trauma in childhood.* New York: Harper & Row.

van IJzendoorn, M. H. (1995). Adult attachment representations, parental responsiveness, and infant attachment: A meta-analysis on the predictive validity of the Adult Attachment Interview. *Psychological Bulletin, 117,* 387–403.

CHAPTER 16

Integrated Play Therapy
with Childhood Traumatic Grief

John W. Seymour

Many children at some point in their lives will experience some sort of potentially traumatic event (Copeland, Keeler, Angold, & Costello, 2007). Much less commonly, one of those traumatic events involves a child's loss of a loved one, increasing the child's risk of complicated bereavement and persistent trauma symptoms. Cohen and Mannarino (2010; Mannarino & Cohen, 2011), have summarized the recent history of efforts by researchers and clinicians to define this combined experience, and have suggested the term *childhood traumatic grief* (CTG), defined as "a condition in which children whose loved ones die under traumatic circumstances develop trauma symptoms that impinge on the children's ability to progress through typical grief processes" (Mannarino & Cohen, 2011, p. 24). The combined experience of grief and trauma can become very challenging for children, families, support systems, and child mental health professionals.

With CTG, as a traumatized child moves through the grief process, thoughts and feelings of the loved one trigger trauma memories and symptoms, making it difficult for the child to sustain the experience of grieving sufficiently to achieve resolution. The grieving child becomes stuck in grief, blocked by what can become an increasing list of trauma symptoms, such as hypersensitivity, avoidance of trauma and grief cues, and withdrawal from supportive relationships. Trauma symptoms disrupt the grieving process, leading to further distress for the child, family, and support system, and hampering their ability to address either the trauma or the grief (Gil, 2006, 2010; Mannarino & Cohen, 2011).

There are strong interactions between a child's attachment pattern and the experiencing of CTG, as both the child and probably the parent(s) and/or other close caregivers will also be experiencing the trauma and loss (Blaustein & Kinniburgh, 2010; Crenshaw, 2007; Dozier, Bick, & Bernard, 2011; Mannarino & Cohen, 2011). Children and families with histories of loss, grief, or attachment injury will be particularly vulnerable to the effects of CTG. When the lost loved one is a parent or caregiver, the child has lost a proven resource for coping from the past as well as for the future. The surviving parent(s) or other key caregiving adults face the challenge of managing their own responses to trauma and loss, as well as trying to respond to the child's needs (Crenshaw, 2007). Typically, the younger the child, the more the child will be affected by the well-being of these grieving adults. Assessment and treatment approaches for CTG will need to include a thorough understanding of the attachment histories of the child, parent(s), and close caregivers, which will be a part of the recovery period (Crenshaw, 2007; Dozier et al., 2011).

Child therapists working with these families can find it very difficult to make basic and ongoing decisions within the assessment and therapeutic process: what exactly is happening (trauma, grief, or both); who is being most affected (child, parent, other caregiver); and how to make wise choices among therapeutic relational responses and techniques (trauma-based, grief-based, directive, nondirective, child-focused, parent-focused, child- and parent-focused, etc.). Cohen, Mannarino, and Deblinger (2006) suggest a layered approach to the therapy process—one that alternates between grief and trauma work. Gil (2006, 2010) has pointed out that this layered approach will require a child therapist at any given moment to be both highly attuned to the child's needs and flexible in responding to those changing needs.

The child therapist will need to have a working knowledge of the current literature on childhood grief and trauma, and of the assessment and treatment methods most effective for the combination of both (Gil, 2006, 2010; Mannarino & Cohen, 2011; Webb, 2010). In this chapter, current research on child development and on best child therapy practices in grief work, trauma recovery, and attachment repair are first reviewed for applicability to CTG. To illustrate the challenges and opportunities in providing child mental health services to this special population, the reader is then introduced to Gail and her family, who experienced the traumatic loss of a family member. Gail's story is a distillation of therapeutic work with several children and their families who had similar experiences of grief combined with trauma. Her story will not be every child's story, so the reader is referred to more detailed resources for a broader understanding of the range of how children experience grief, trauma, and recovery, with examples from Gail's treatment narrative of specific therapeutic assessment points and therapeutic techniques. Finally, suggestions regarding further professional study and professional self-care are included, to support the child therapist in maintaining continued effectiveness in this type of therapeutic work.

Trends in Child Research Influencing the Treatment of CTG

In the past 20 years, there has been a surge of research and clinical interest in childhood bereavement, trauma, development, and psychotherapy. These recent findings have some common themes particularly applicable to the assessment and treatment of traumatic grief. The complexity of CTG suggests that child therapists will need a range of approaches adaptable to the changing features of the recovery process. Kazdin (2009) has pointed out that while there is a wealth of research literature on child psychotherapies, our empirical understanding of their processes and outcomes is still limited. There continue to be debates regarding the best methods of research and practice to support convincing research, but efforts have intensified to determine precisely which therapeutic processes are the most effective for particular problems of childhood (Reddy, Files-Hall, & Schaefer, 2005; Steele, Elkin, & Roberts, 2008). Until there is more clarity in the outcome research, child therapists looking for guidance on the best practices for addressing CTG can be informed by these recent trends in clinical research.

Childhood Bereavement

In *Helping Bereaved Children: A Handbook for Practitioners*, Webb (2010) has reviewed the historic and current trends in childhood grief research, which can serve as an excellent resource to a child mental health professional wanting to update skills in assessment, treatment, and serving special populations of grieving children. Contemporary models of childhood grief and recovery have moved beyond earlier understandings of childhood grief, which were frequently couched in the modernist assumptions of psychoanalysis and other early theories of psychotherapy. These models understood grief work as a fairly linear process of stages, with the assumptions that children lack some capacity for grief work, and that the goal of grief work should be autonomy of the bereaved from the loved one lost.

More recent studies, such as the ones summarized by Klass, Silverman, and Nickman (1996), have built on qualitative research in childhood grief and development. In these studies, grief work is understood as being a more circular process, with the goal of being more interdependent with memories of the deceased as well as the living support system. In this model, "maintaining an inner representation of the deceased is normal rather than abnormal" (p. 349). Therapeutic interventions focus on facilitating ways that children can maintain bonds with their living community while creating bonds with the deceased. These connections "are not based on physical proximity but with memories, dreams, internal conversations, and cherished objects" (p. 350). This approach assumes that children do have the capacity for grief work, encourages a more open and inquiring approach toward grieving children, and values each child's perspective and coping style. It also promotes a strengths-based approach that builds on the capacities of the child, family, and support system.

Webb (2010) has adapted several crisis assessment protocols for children into a tripartite assessment for a bereaved child, focusing on three areas (individual factors, factors related to the death, and family/social/religious/cultural factors), with particular attention to details that will best inform clinical work with the child. Suggestions are made for specific assessment tools, and sample interview questionnaires are provided. Individual factors include age-related factors; past coping and adjustment; medical history; and prior experience with death and/or loss. Death-related factors include the type of death; details of the child's prior contacts with the deceased and the time of death; prior relationship to the deceased; and grief reactions experienced. Family/social/religious/cultural factors include the grief responses of the immediate and extended family; school and peer responses; religious affiliation, traditions of grieving in the family, faith, or culture; sociocultural meanings of the loss; and cultural expectations for children's involvement in the grieving process.

Whereas earlier studies of grief identified a more linear stage model for the grief process (Webb, 2010), current research emphasizes tasks that will be completed in more of an ebb-and-flow model, particularly for children. Although there will be a great deal of variation from child to child, a general understanding of the grief process can help normalize the experience for the child and family members. Worden's (1996) four common tasks of the grief process—(1) accepting the reality of the loss; (2) working through the pain of grief; (3) adjusting to life without the loved one; and (4) finding a way to hold on to memories of the loved one while moving ahead with life—have been frequently used to help give people a better understanding of what they are experiencing. Wolfelt (1996), describing a process of reconciling the loss, has identified these tasks: acknowledging the reality of the death; embracing the pain of loss; remembering the person who died; developing a new self-identity; searching for meaning; and reaching out to receive support from others.

A thorough assessment not only will prepare the child mental health professional to deal with the expected grief process resulting from the loss of a loved one, but will provide an important baseline of information for understanding a child's trauma responses when the grieving process becomes disrupted. The assessment phase is also a time of establishing the therapeutic relationship, and creating a safe and trusting environment for the challenging work that will be ahead.

Childhood Trauma

The trauma-focused cognitive-behavioral therapy (TF-CBT) model has been widely used and studied in the treatment of child abuse and trauma (Cohen & Mannarino, 2010; Mannarino & Cohen, 2011). TF-CBT is a manualized treatment that uses trauma-sensitive cognitive-behavioral interventions to assist children, parents, and families. Building on TF-CBT, Mannarino and Cohen (2011) have proposed and begun researching a traumatic grief cognitive-behavioral therapy (TG-CBT) model, created by adding a specific grief recovery component for the treatment of CTG to the earlier model. Initial trials of TG-CBT have shown the integrated grief and trauma model to be effective in reducing the symptoms of children and adolescents with CTG.

Cognitive-behavioral approaches incorporated into play therapy can be used to structure more specific alternatives for emotional expression, changes in perspective, or the rehearsal of new risk-limiting skills (Drewes, 2009; Knell, 2011). Despite the demonstrated success of cognitive-behavioral models for trauma treatment, however, a growing body of trauma literature is now suggesting that the affective, sensory, and relational dimensions need to be included along with the cognitive dimension in understanding the dynamics of trauma and the methods of treatment (Gil, 2006, 2010; Malchiodi, 2008; Shelby, 2010; Shelby, Avina, & Warnick, 2010; Shelby & Felix, 2005; Steele & Malchiodi, 2012; Stien & Kendall, 2004). Steele and Malchiodi (2012) have summarized this concern in their recent book, *Trauma-Informed Practices with Children and Adolescents*; they explain that "trauma is a predominately sensory process for many children and adolescents that cannot be altered by cognitive interventions alone" (p. xix), and they argue for a more balanced approach to trauma treatment. Along with comprehensive assessment, they identify the importance of developing self-regulation, providing trauma integration, and building child resiliency as other important aspects of trauma treatment. Sutton-Smith (2008) describes the origins of natural play as the child's first efforts to regulate personal responses to real conflicts, and notes that play continues to be the major means of handling conflict throughout childhood. Gil (2006), noting that sensory experiences of trauma are processed primarily through the right hemisphere of the brain, has suggested that more emphasis be placed on treatment strategies with sensory and experiential components.

Child Development

Recent research in child development has focused on the growing understanding and appreciation of neurodevelopment and neurobiology. Schore (2012) and Siegel (2012) have chronicled this surge of research, which has been made possible in part by advances in biotechnology and imaging technologies that have provided new tools for understanding the interactions of brain and body as humans interact in and with their environments. These findings have deepened our understanding of the attachment process in the developing child, providing us with new insights on how trauma and loss disrupt normal development and how strong attachment relationships moderate the effects of trauma. Some of these findings have particular applicability to child therapy. Perry and colleagues (Barfield, Dobson, Gaskill, & Perry, 2012; Perry, 2006; Perry & Hanbrick, 2008) have developed the Neurosequential Model of Therapeutics, which describes a progressive process of providing therapeutic interventions in the order of brain development, moving from the brainstem to the frontal cortex. Initial therapeutic interventions, then, should be based more on sensory integration and self-regulation, and these interventions should lead into higher-order affective, cognitive, and relational work. When grief work is complicated by trauma symptoms related to the loss of a child's loved one, the child therapist will need to be prepared to address the more sensory-based trauma symptoms with interventions designed to help with calming and self-regulation.

The human brain has come to be understood as dependent on social experience for development (Perry, Pollard, Blakley, Baker, & Vigilante, 1995). Accordingly, greater emphasis is now being placed on emotional and relational aspects of development—a shift from a more strictly cognitive-behavioral approach. Siegel (2012) suggests that therapeutic models should be experientially and relationally based, aimed toward promoting integration of body and brain through relationships. Since this integration first begins as children form attachments with caregivers, Schore (2012) suggests that the work of psychotherapy "is not defined by what the therapist does for the patient, or says to the patient (left brain focus). Rather, the key mechanism is how to be with the patient, especially during affectively stressful moments (right brain focus)" (p. 44). The combination of attachment threat with the death of a loved one and the sense of danger from the trauma surrounding the loss can create a great deal of disruption in the brain, as it tries to make sense of the overwhelming fight–flight–freeze response of CTG. In Siegel's (2012) model of interpersonal neurobiology (IPNB), the child therapist "seeks to create an understanding of the interconnections among the brain, the mind, and our interpersonal relationships" (p. 3). These findings in IPNB add detail to our understanding of the effects of the therapeutic relationship in reducing trauma symptoms, as well as the therapeutic effects of relational-based psychotherapies that enhance the child's relationships with parent(s) and other close caregiving adults. Internal human development is mirrored in the interactions of children through their experiences and relationships, which are commonly mediated through natural play.

Child Psychotherapy

Recent developments in child psychotherapy have closely paralleled developments in the broader field of psychotherapy, which has been gradually shifting away from model-specific treatments to more integrated and prescriptive models (Drewes, 2011a, 2011b; Osofsky, 2004, 2011). These models focus more on the qualities that establish and maintain the therapeutic relationship; on multimodal methods of assessing children's needs; and on matching these needs with interventions based on an understanding of the therapeutic mechanisms common in most models of child therapy. These integrative approaches are well matched for addressing the complexities of CTG.

Crenshaw (2007) has reviewed the recent research in neurobiology and child therapy and has proposed a seven-stage IPNB-informed treatment model for CTG. This model moves from an initial stage of establishing safety, through steps of grieving, to finding meaning and a coherent narrative to understand the traumatic loss. Dozier et al. (2011) have developed and pilot-tested an attachment and biobehavioral catch-up (ABC) model for teaching parents of a young child how to (1) recognize the child's problematic coping strategies; (2) encourage the child to practice better coping strategies; (3) overcome any attachment and trauma issues of their own that may get in the way of their current relationship with their child; and (4) help promote the best setting for their child to achieve better self-regulation.

Stien and Kendall (2004) have proposed an integrative three-stage model for addressing childhood trauma, building on Herman's (1997) trauma model for adults, and incorporating recent research in neurodevelopment. In Stage One, safety and stabilization, the therapist works to create a safe and predictable environment for the therapy, and to address issues of safety and predictability beyond the therapy room. The children and parents are provided with basic psychoeducation on the effects of trauma and steps toward recovery. In Stage Two, the therapist focuses on the symptom list with interventions to reduce arousal, transform the affective state of the child and family members, reduce avoidance behaviors, and improve current functioning. In addition, memory work is done to help the child and family members reinterpret the experience of trauma in such a way as to build self-efficacy. Cognitive techniques may be used, along with teaching healing imagery. In Stage Three, the therapist addresses developmental skills of appropriate connectedness and relatedness with family and support system members, helping to develop better problem-solving skills, to develop or reestablish social skills, and to highlight common values. Therapeutic work in this model includes experiential and expressive therapies to help with self-awareness and self-regulation.

Applying the Research to a Child Experiencing CTG

Complexities of CTG and the Benefits of Play

A common thread through the recent research has been the role of play-based techniques in addressing the complex components of CTG. Play-based techniques constitute a key element in TG-CBT (Cohen & Mannarino, 2010; Mannarino & Cohen, 2011) for children experiencing CTG. Play is a crucial part in the natural development of a child's abilities to relate to others and respond to challenges in life; it promotes self-regulation and self-mastery in the face of these challenges (Brown, 2009; Sutton-Smith, 2008). Play includes a certain randomness and uncertainty, and when it is used in child therapy, it provides opportunities to reinforce successful ways of relating and problem solving, as well as opportunities to expand a child's personal repertoire of coping skills. Play therapy, along with other experiential and expressive child therapies, can provide an approach that incorporates cognitive, affective, and relational components for trauma recovery (Steele & Malchiodi, 2012). In play therapy, the play becomes transformative in providing a new perspective on self and environment. Physical activity, personal expression, interpersonal relating, and meaning making with symbols and metaphors in play can all be utilized in the therapeutic setting for dealing with CTG.

The integrative play therapy (IPT) model (Drewes, 2011a, 2011b) is a strengths-based model, focusing on qualities inherent in play that can enhance the therapeutic relationship, match therapeutic interventions to clients served, and be informed by research on the therapeutic mechanisms shared by various play therapy models. Schaefer (1993) originally identified 14 change mechanisms common in all play therapy models, and recently expanded the listing to 20 in a coedited book, *The Therapeutic Powers of Play: 20 Core Agents of Change* (Schaefer & Drewes, 2014). IPT allows the child therapist to be nimble in responding to the changing directions in psychotherapy when grief and trauma are co-occurring (Gil, 2010), since interventions are chosen according to a child's immediate needs, rather than the outline of a particular theory's model. It allows the therapist to choose between more and less directed approaches, to better match the ebb and flow of the child's ability to sustain the intense feelings needed to address CTG (Gil, 2006, 2010; Shelby, 2010; Shelby & Felix, 2005; Webb, 2007, 2010). In IPT, the child therapist can implement therapeutic interventions that fulfill all four of the broad functions of natural play identified by Russ (2004): providing a means of expression for the child; enhancing communication and relationship building; facilitating insight and working through; and allowing the child to practice new forms of expression, relating, and problem solving.

Gail's Journey through CTG Begins

One summer afternoon, Gail (age 11) and her brother Matt (age 6) were swimming and playing in the family's backyard pool, a favorite gathering place for family and friends. Mom watched from a nearby pool chair, chatting on the phone with Dad, who soon would be home from soccer practice with brother Sam and Sam's best friend, Russell (both age 9). Mom suddenly noticed that the pool had gotten very quiet. To her right, she saw Gail in the center of the pool, swimming a slow backstroke, enjoying the cool water on a hot afternoon. To her left, she spotted Matt, motionless, near the bottom of the deep end. She dove in, pulled Matt out of the pool, and began efforts to revive him. Gail grabbed Mom's cell phone and made a 911 call for help, next called Dad, and then went to help Mom with Matt.

The family home was in a rural area, some distance from the main road. As Gail and Mom attended to Matt, they heard a siren in the distance, seeming to come closer and then go farther away. Minutes passed, and they continued to hear the siren moving back and forth through the countryside as the driver desperately searched the back roads for the right address. Finally, they saw the ambulance coming down their dirt road, with a cloud of dust billowing behind. The emergency personnel went right to work attending to Matt, loaded him in the ambulance, and sped off to the hospital, just as Dad arrived home with Sam and Russell.

Gail and Mom jumped into the car with them and headed for the hospital. When they rushed into the emergency room, hospital staffers brought them to the family consultation room. Russell's parents joined them at the hospital to wait for news. Soon a somber-faced physician and nurse came to the consultation room to give them the news that they had done everything they could do to help Matt, but even their best efforts had not been able to revive him. Matt had died. Russell's parents took him home, and Gail and Sam remained with their parents at the hospital to view Matt's body and begin the paperwork and phone calls related to funeral preparation.

Each of these persons shared this moment of loss together, yet they came to this moment with very different life histories and their own unique experiences of the events surrounding Matt's death. Although they would continue to have much in common in their grief, their individual grief experiences would vary widely as time went on. Each would have experiences that significantly affected their future well-being, and the ups and downs of their grief experiences would significantly affect each of them. This part of the chapter primarily describes the experience of Gail, Matt's 11-year-old sister, who over the coming weeks began demonstrating several signs of distress as a result of Matt's death.

At home, Gail's sleep was disrupted with nightmares that often related to the drowning. She avoided being outside near the pool, and developed a routine in the house that would keep her from being anywhere that she might see the pool. She avoided Matt's room and was bothered by the many reminders of his life that were around the house. Always a good student, she was now struggling in school. Teachers reported that she did not have her usual enthusiasm for learning and being with friends. She often seemed distracted from class interactions, and began making occasional trips to the school nurse for stomachaches and headaches. Her energy level was low and her appetite poor. Now and then, she would have brief outbursts of tears or temper, and on several occasions she made tearful statements that she felt responsible for not watching out for Matt in the pool that day.

Gail was fortunate to have an existing caring support system of family, friends, and school personnel, as well as other helpful adults in her life, such as her pastor and Scout leader. Even with everyone's best efforts, however, Gail's distress worsened, and her parents made an appointment with a child mental health professional to seek further help.

IPT with Gail

The IPT sessions with Gail were held in a therapy room designed for family therapy and play therapy, consistent with the primary training of the child therapist providing the care. One corner of the room anchored a small sitting area arranged in a living room style; the opposite corner of the room anchored a play therapy area with a small set of chairs and table, and rows of shelves with a variety of play materials. Additional sensory-based and developmentally based play materials, along with a portable sandtray table with figures, were stored close by for use when needed. The play materials available reflected Webb's (2007) listing of materials for grief work, including art techniques, doll play, puppet play, storytelling, sandtray play, and board games.

Gail's mom had already begun seeing a psychotherapist a few weeks after Matt's death, concerned that she would not be able to care properly for her other two children while experiencing this terrible loss. Gail's mom had confided to her therapist that she was concerned with Gail's behaviors at home and school, and even though Sam seemed to be doing fairly well, she did not feel confident about knowing that for sure. The therapist encouraged Gail's mom to make an appointment for Gail to be seen. Gail's mom scheduled a first visit so that both parents could meet with the child therapist and give an overview of their concerns.

Gail's mom and dad had met with their pastor several times since Matt's death, so it was not a new experience for them to be together discussing that terrible day. However, it was a first visit with a new professional, and initially the conversation was fairly matter-of-fact—relating the basic story of Matt's death, providing details of the family's and children's histories, and explaining their observations and concerns (primarily about Gail, but secondarily about Sam). They saw themselves as still reeling from the experience, and experiencing some significant highs and lows, though they had both been able to return fairly quickly to their jobs and daily routines (not that anything seemed routine at that point). Later in the interview, the therapist provided some basic pointers on childhood grief, trauma, and the recovery process, to normalize the experiences they were having and to give them some predictability concerning what to expect next from both the grief/trauma and the therapeutic approaches to working with children to address these concerns. As Gail's parents turned their attention to the play area of the room and a sampling of some of the play materials, they grew quiet and tearful. The quietness of the play area and the array of unused toys reminded them of Matt's now very quiet bedroom at home. Some time was taken to allow them to grieve and reflect before completing the session. The agreed-upon plan was to begin work with Gail, accompanied by one of her parents, and later to consider including Sam if it was decided that this would be helpful for Gail or him.

Gail arrived for her first session with her mom, and for the next several sessions alternated between coming with her mom and her dad. She seemed reassured that her parents had already met me, and had a little curiosity about the play materials. She was not eager to talk directly about Matt's death, but she was able to acknowledge that she knew that was why her parents wanted her to come, so the therapist focused on getting to know about her interests, abilities, friends, and activities. Spotting a Connect Four game, she asked to play. Soon after play began, she reported that she was worried because "since Matt [no verb]," she had been feeling "hyper" and "creeped out." She also gave details of what were intrusive memories of the day Matt died. The therapist and Gail talked about what she called the "pictures in my mind," her observations of when they had been worse or better, and anything she had found that would make them stop and leave her feeling better. She had used some simple techniques of distraction, such as reading and watching TV; to build on those successes, a number of simple techniques were demonstrated for Gail and her mother to try and then implement at home. Near the end of the first visit, Gail spotted a large bin of Legos in the play area. She said that Legos were Matt's favorite toy, and that she knew what she would play with next time.

During the next several visits, each time Gail came in the room, she would scan the room for any new play materials. At a few points, the therapist provided some additional psychoeducation on the grief process and trauma recovery, and reviewed and expanded on the anxiety reduction skills that Gail was using (sometimes on her own, and sometimes when prompted by her mom or dad). She enjoyed starting sessions with a brief game, but then her attention would turn to the Legos and she would begin to build. For three sessions during her play, she carefully and thoughtfully built a deep, four-sided structure of Legos, never saying a word. The third time she built it, she made a slow, barely audible "woo" sound that went up and down in pitch. The therapist and her dad thought that this was a siren sound, but neither interrupted her play to ask, and she seemed not to notice that she was even making the sound. At the end, she asked the therapist to keep the Legos object until her next visit, and it was stored safely away.

She returned the next week and immediately asked for the four-sided Legos object. She took it over to the play area, and after pulling out and arranging the dollhouse, she placed the box in the back yard of the doll-house. After choosing a number of small doll figures and vehicles, she solemnly said, "I'm going to show you what happened," and went through the entire sequence of events of Matt's death. As suggested by Gil (2010), she had in her own way used the play materials to expose herself gradually to her traumatic experience, in such a way that she was able to manage her traumatic symptoms. Over the course of her sessions, she would periodically pair more challenging play enactments (repeating parts of the story of Matt's death and events surrounding the funeral) with self-nurturing and calming elements (e.g., playing quiet games, caring for a baby doll, or gathering up the stuffed animals to be cared for at her farm) or more energized play (e.g., rhythm games, ball toss games) that would release some tension through active play. At other times, the therapist, discerning her need, might suggest one or the other of these activities for her to try, or engage Gail and her parents in a conversation of choices on how she could achieve better self-regulation through her choice of play at home.

Gail had predictable ups and downs in her progress. As could be predicted, family events would sometimes trigger both grief and trauma responses. Holidays were particularly challenging, and the therapist worked with Gail and her parents to develop special play remembrances (usually referred to as *rituals* when used with adults and families) that gave them the opportunity to acknowledge both Matt's loss and his continuing presence with them. The arrival of winter, and the placement of the winter pool cover, seemed to help Gail feel that this part of their home had fewer unpleasant reminders of Matt's death. By the spring, Gail's parents had incorporated enough information about grief and trauma that they initiated a conversation prior to removing the pool cover for the season, to brainstorm ways that they might prepare themselves and the children for a new season of swimming. Their preparations made the day less stressful than expected, and gradually, they returned to their warm-weather routines around the pool. By then Gail was coming only for occasional check-in visits, and then she and her parents ended play therapy, with the option to reconnect if there were concern in the future.

Over the course of play therapy with Gail and her family, all the elements of the IPT model of directive and nondirective play therapy (Shelby & Felix, 2005) were implemented. This approach included the parents' involvement in both parent education and Gail's play therapy sessions. It was developmentally informed, matching Gail's age and abilities. Thorough evaluation of Gail and her family setting guided the work throughout. The therapist had specific training in play and family therapy, as well as in applications to grief and trauma. Finally, the course of treatment, while well defined by shared goals and by Gail's progress, was matched to her timetable of managing her recovery rather than arbitrarily defined by a therapeutic protocol.

Many other techniques were used over the course of Gail's care, with every effort made to match her interests and the timing of her recovery process. Play therapists seeking additional resources for techniques for the grief process are referred to books by Fiorini and Mullen (2006) and Webb (2010). For techniques for the trauma recovery process, play therapists are referred to books by Stien and Kendall (2004) and Steele and Malchiodi (2012). For incorporating the therapeutic powers of play into therapeutic work for CTG, see Schaefer and Drewes (2014) as well as Seymour (2009, 2014).

Self-Care of the Child Therapist and CTG

Whatever the therapeutic model used with children experiencing CTG, child therapists wanting to remain effective with this population will need to continue professional development to stay abreast of new trends in treatment approaches. Child therapists trained in one particular approach, such as play therapy or art therapy, will benefit from learning other expressive and experiential approaches, to provide themselves with the widest repertoire of therapeutic options. There are also many personal challenges for child therapists who do ongoing work with CTG, and so these therapists need to maintain good personal and professional care to reduce the likelihood of vicarious traumatization (Gil, 2010). Ryan and Cunningham (2007) have described 10 strategies that enable child therapists to help themselves. These include continued professional training; supervision and professional peer support; balancing the types of clients seen; using team treatment models; and practicing good self-care of physical, emotional, and relational needs.

Child therapists will find working with clients experiencing CTG both challenging and rewarding. The complexity of the symptoms, the wide range of feelings, and the sense of unpredictability will affect both children and therapists. Child therapists who are able to maintain personal and professional care will have for their use with clients like Gail a number of beneficial approaches to CTG, supported by a growing body of research efforts in child development and psychotherapy.

REFERENCES

Barfield, S., Dobson, C., Gaskill, R., & Perry, B. D. (2012). Neurosequential Model of Therapeutics in a therapeutic preschool: Implications for work with children with complex neuropsychiatric problems. *International Journal of Play Therapy, 21*, 30–44.

Blaustein, M., & Kinniburgh, K. (2010). *Treating traumatic stress in children and adolescents: How to foster resilience through attachment, self-regulation, and competency.* New York: Guilford Press.

Brown, S. (2009). *Play: How it shapes the brain, opens the imagination, and invigorates the soul.* New York: Avery.

Cohen, J. A., & Mannarino, A. P. (2010). Bereavement and traumatic grief. In M.

K. Dulcan (Ed.), *Textbook of child and adolescent psychiatry* (pp. 509–516). Washington, DC: American Psychiatric Association.

Cohen, J. A., Mannarino, A. P., & Deblinger, E. (2006). *Treating trauma and traumatic grief in children and adolescents.* New York: Guilford Press.

Copeland, W. E., Keeler, G., Angold, A., & Costello, E. J. (2007). Traumatic events and posttraumatic stress disorder in childhood. *Archives of General Psychiatry, 64,* 577–584.

Crenshaw, D. A. (2007). An interpersonal neurobiological-informed treatment model for childhood traumatic grief. *Omega, 54,* 319–335.

Dozier, M., Bick, J., & Bernard, K. (2011). Attachment-based treatment for young vulnerable children. In J. D. Osofsky (Ed.), *Clinical work with traumatized young children* (pp. 75–95). New York: Guilford Press.

Drewes, A. A. (Ed.). (2009). *Blending play therapy with cognitive behavioral therapy: Evidence-based and other effective treatments and techniques.* Hoboken, NJ: Wiley.

Drewes, A. A. (2011a). Integrative play therapy. In C. E. Schaefer (Ed.), *Foundations of play therapy* (2nd ed., pp. 349–364). Hoboken, NJ: Wiley.

Drewes, A. A. (2011b). Integrating play therapy theories into practice. In A. A. Drewes, S. C. Bratton, & C. E. Schaefer (Eds.), *Integrative play therapy* (pp. 21–35). Hoboken, NJ: Wiley.

Fiorini, J. J., & Mullen, J. A. (2006). *Counseling children and adolescents through grief and loss.* Champaign, IL: Research Press.

Gil, E. (2006). *Helping abused and traumatized children: Integrating directive and nondirective approaches.* New York: Guilford Press.

Gil, E. (Ed.). (2010). *Working with children to heal interpersonal trauma: The power of play.* New York: Guilford Press.

Herman, J. L. (1997). *Trauma and recovery: The aftermath of violence—from domestic abuse to political terror* (2nd ed.). New York: Basic Books.

Kazdin, A. E. (2009). Understanding how and why psychotherapy leads to change. *Psychotherapy Research, 19,* 418–428.

Klass, D., Silverman, P. R., & Nickman, S. L. (1996). *Continuing bonds: New understandings of grief.* Washington, DC: Taylor & Francis.

Knell, S. M. (2011). Cognitive-behavioral play therapy. In C. E. Schaefer (Ed.), *Foundations of play therapy* (2nd ed., pp. 313–328). Hoboken, NJ: Wiley.

Malchiodi, C. A. (Ed.). (2008). *Creative interventions with traumatized children.* New York: Guilford Press.

Mannarino, A. P., & Cohen, J. A. (2011). Traumatic loss in children and adolescents. *Journal of Child and Adolescent Trauma, 4,* 22–33.

Osofsky, J. D. (Ed.). (2004). *Young children and trauma: Intervention and treatment.* New York: Guilford Press.

Osofsky, J. D. (Ed.). (2011). *Clinical work with traumatized children.* New York: Guilford Press.

Perry, B. D. (2006). The Neurosequential Model of Therapeutics: Applying principles of neuroscience to clinical work with traumatized and maltreated children. In N. B. Webb (Ed.), *Working with traumatized youth in child welfare* (pp. 27–52). New York: Guilford Press.

Perry, B. D., & Hanbrick, E. P. (2008). The Neurosequential Model of Therapeutics. *Reclaiming Children and Youth, 17,* 38–43.

Perry, B. D., Pollard, R. A., Blakley, T L., Baker, W. L., & Vigilante, D. (1995).

Childhood trauma, the neurobiology of adaptation, and "use-dependent" development of the brain: How "states" become "traits." *Infant Mental Health Journal, 16,* 271–291.

Reddy, L. A., Files-Hall, T. M., & Schaefer, C. E. (Eds.). (2005). *Empirically based play interventions for children.* Washington, DC: American Psychological Association.

Russ, S. W. (2004). *Play in child development and psychotherapy: Toward empirically supported practice.* Mahwah, NJ: Erlbaum.

Ryan, K., & Cunningham, M. (2007). Helping the helpers: Guidelines to prevent vicarious traumatization of play therapists working with traumatized children. In N. B. Webb (Ed.), *Play therapy with children in crisis: A casebook for practitioners* (3rd ed., pp. 443–460). New York: Guilford Press.

Schaefer, C. E. (Ed.). (1993). *The therapeutic powers of play.* Northvale, NJ: Aronson.

Schaefer, C. E., & Drewes (Eds.). (2014). *The therapeutic powers of play: 20 core agents of change* (2nd ed.). Hoboken, NJ: Wiley.

Schore, A. N. (2012). *The science of the art of psychotherapy.* New York: Norton.

Seymour, J. W. (2009). Resiliency-based approaches and the healing process in play therapy. In D. A. Crenshaw (Ed.), *Reverence in the healing process: Honoring strengths without trivializing suffering* (pp. 71–84). Lanham, MD: Aronson.

Seymour, J. W. (2014). Resiliency as a therapeutic power of play. In C. E. Schaefer & A. A. Drewes (Eds.), *The therapeutic powers of play: 20 core agents of change* (2nd ed., pp. 241–263). Hoboken, NJ: Wiley.

Shelby, J. S. (2010). Cognitive-behavioral therapy and play therapy for childhood trauma and loss. In N. B. Webb (Ed.), *Helping bereaved children: A handbook for practitioners* (3rd ed., pp. 263–277). New York: Guilford Press.

Shelby, J. S., Avina, C., & Warnick, H. (2010). Posttraumatic parenting: A parent–child dyadic treatment for young children's posttraumatic adjustment. In C. E. Schaefer (Ed.), *Play therapy for preschool children* (pp. 39–87). Washington, DC: American Psychological Association.

Shelby, J. S., & Felix, E. D. (2005). Posttraumatic play therapy: The need for an integrated model of directive and nondirective approaches. In L. A. Reddy, T. M. Files-Hall, & C. E. Schaefer (Eds.), *Empirically based play interventions for children* (pp. 79–103). Washington, DC: American Psychological Association.

Siegel, D. J. (2012). *The developing mind: How relationships and the brain interact to shape who we are* (2nd ed.). New York: Guilford Press.

Steele, R. G., Elkin, T. D., & Roberts, M. C. (Eds.). (2008). *Handbook of evidence-based therapies for children and adolescents: Bridging science and practice.* New York: Springer.

Steele, W., & Malchiodi, C. A. (Eds.). (2012). *Trauma-informed practices with children and adolescents.* New York: Routledge.

Stien, P. T., & Kendall, J. (2004). *Psychological trauma and the developing brain: Neurologically based interventions for troubled children.* New York: Haworth Press.

Sutton-Smith, B. (2008). Play theory: A personal journey and new thoughts. *American Journal of Play, 1,* 82–125.

Webb, N. B. (Ed.). (2007). *Play therapy with children in crisis: A casebook for practitioners* (3rd ed.). New York: Guilford Press.

Webb, N. B. (Ed.). (2010). *Helping bereaved children: A handbook for practitioners* (3rd ed.). New York: Guilford Press.

Wolfelt, A. D. (1996). *Healing the bereaved child: Grief gardening, growth through grief, and other touchstones for caregivers.* Fort Collins, CO: Companion Press.

Worden, J. W. (1996). *Children and grief: When a parent dies.* New York: Guilford Press.

CHAPTER 17

Mending Broken Attachment in Displaced Children

Finding "Home" through Play Therapy

Jennifer N. Baggerly

Eric J. Green

> But to penetrate the darkness we must summon all the
> powers of enlightenment that consciousness can offer.
> —JUNG (1931/1969, p. 389)

"All my toys are in the garbage where we used to live." "I don't have any friends in this new place." "My dad had to go to another city to find work." These are common expressions of loss and grief for children who have experienced homelessness or displacement due to natural or human-made disasters. These responses could be temporary or could become complicated grief, contributing to attachment difficulties. What determines the outcome? In some cases, it may be a skilled and empathetic child therapist.

In this chapter, we show how mental health professionals using art therapy and play therapy can contribute to healing for children suffering from these types of displacement. First, we create a context by describing characteristics and challenges of children displaced by homelessness or by natural or man-made disasters. Second, we discuss how to use play therapy to help children who are homeless. Finally, we discuss how to use Jungian art therapy to help children who are displaced by disasters. Play and art therapy can help children create a new sense of "home" within their own hearts that will strengthen current and future attachments.

275

Characteristics and Challenges

Homelessness

Children who are *homeless* lack a fixed, regular, and adequate nighttime residence intended for ongoing shelter (National Coalition for the Homeless [NCH], 2009a). It is important to understand that homelessness is not due to moral inadequacy of a parent. Reasons why a family may be homeless are complex; they may include poverty, lack of affordable housing, low wages, cutoff of public assistance, lack of affordable health care, domestic violence, mental illness, or addictions. Overall, "homelessness results from a complex set of circumstances which require people to choose between food, shelter, and other basic needs" (NCH, 2009b, p. 7). Understanding these causes of homelessness will increase play therapists' empathy for families who are homeless and will help the therapists recognize children's play reenactment of events leading to homelessness.

In the United States, young children in families are the fastest growing segment of the homeless population (NCH, 2009a). As of 2007, children made up 39% of the homeless population. There are 1.35 million children who are homeless each year in the United States, which is approximately 1% of the general population (NCH, 2009a). The average age of a homeless child is 6 years old (Institute for Children and Poverty [ICP], 2007).

Disasters

Children who are displaced by a natural or man-made disaster have experienced an event that met the following criteria: It (1) caused destruction of property, injury, or loss of life; (2) had an identifiable beginning and end; (3) was sudden and time-limited; (4) adversely affected a large group of people; (5) was a public event that affected more than one family; (6) was beyond the realm of ordinary experience; and (7) was psychologically traumatic enough to induce stress in almost anyone (Rosenfeld, Caye, Ayalon, & Lahad, 2005). According to the World Health Organization Centre's for Research on the Epidemiology of Disasters, in 2010 "a total of 385 natural disasters killed more than 297,000 people worldwide, affected over 217 million others and caused $123.9 billion of economic damages" (Guha-Sapir, Vos, Below, & Ponserre, 2010, p. 1). In a representative sample survey of 2,030 U.S. children ages 2–17, Becker-Blease, Turner, and Finkelhor (2010) found that approximately 14% reported a lifetime exposure to a disaster, and 4.1% to a disaster in the past year.

Impact of Homelessness and Disasters on Children

Both children who are homeless and children who have been displaced by a natural or man-made disaster have experienced loss of physical and emotional safety, which can affect them in numerous ways. Neurodevelopment in children who are homeless can be hindered because of multiple losses and trauma (Kagan, 2004; Perry, 2001). Homelessness results in attachment disruption to children's important relationships, such as those with grandparents, teachers, and friends (NCH, 2009b). Attachment disruption may also occur between a child and a parent who is no longer emotionally or physically available because of stress from poverty, mental illness, drug addiction, or incarceration (NCH, 2009b).

Trauma, such as physical or sexual abuse, neglect, and domestic violence, is also common among children who are homeless (NCH, 2009b). In fact, Buckner, Bassuk, Weinreb, and Brooks (1999) found that homeless children are three times more likely than poor but housed children to have witnessed violence in their neighborhoods or schools, to have mothers with alcohol or drug problems, or to have mothers who have been arrested. Homeless children compared with poor but housed children are also twice as likely to have been in foster care. Of 777 homeless parents surveyed, 22% said that domestic violence was the primary reason for being homeless (NCH, 2009b).

It comes as no surprise, then, that emotional and psychological development in children who are homeless can be negatively affected. Children who are homeless tend to experience more depression and anxiety than children who are housed (Buckner et al., 1999). Approximately 47% of children who are homeless have been found to have clinically significant internalizing problems, such as depression and anxiety, compared with only 21% of children who are poor but housed (Buckner et al., 1999). Socially, children who are homeless have been found to have less social support and fewer coping behaviors than children who have never been homeless or were previously homeless (Menke, 2000).

Behaviorally, homeless children also tend to exhibit more externalizing problems, such as delinquent and aggressive behavior, than normative samples (Buckner et al., 1999). As early as preschool, children who are homeless have been found to have more behavior problems than children who are not homeless (Koblinsky, Gordon, & Anderson, 2000). Young-blade and Mulvihill (1998) found that the longer preschool children stayed at a homelessness shelter, the more negative their social behavior became. Many of these behavioral problems stem from losses and trauma experienced as a result of homelessness. "The fearful child cannot concentrate in school; will misinterpret comments; and will sometimes regress to immature behavior (a young child may start to bed-wet) or self-destructive coping behavior" (Perry, 2001, p. 36).

Cognitive development in children who are homeless can be affected as well. Flores (2007) found that children who were homeless and attended Head Start programs possessed less conventional knowledge about time than their peers who attended university day care centers. Academic achievement problems have been reported for children who are homeless (Masten et al., 1997; Ziesemer, Marcoux, & Marwell, 1994). Rubin et al. (1996) found that elementary school children who were homeless performed significantly more poorly on academic tests than children who were not homeless. According to the ICP (2007), 75% of homeless children perform below grade level in reading.

These neurological, social, emotional, psychological, behavioral, and cognitive impacts on children who are homeless hinder their developmental growth and place them at risk for ongoing mental health problems. Children who are homeless need mental health interventions to facilitate their developmental growth and resolve mental health problems.

Play Therapy with Children Who Are Homeless

Definitions

Child-centered play therapy (CCPT) is one mental health intervention that has provided positive results for elementary school children who are homeless (Baggerly, 2003, 2004; Baggerly & Borkowski, 2004). CCPT is defined by Landreth (2012) as

> a dynamic interpersonal relationship between a child and a therapist trained in play therapy procedures who provides selected play materials and facilitates the development of a safe relationship for the child to fully express and explore self (feelings, thoughts, experiences, and behaviors) through play, the child's natural medium of communication, for optimal growth and development. (p. 16)

Rationale

The evidence base for the effectiveness of CCPT has been well established by Baggerly, Ray, and Bratton's (2010) description of 12 quantitative treatment control group studies. In addition, a meta-analysis of 93 play therapy and filial therapy studies (Bratton, Ray, Rhine, & Jones, 2005) showed that humanistic, nondirective play therapy had a large treatment effect ($d = 0.92$). In research specific to displaced populations, CCPT has been shown to be effective in reducing symptoms in children who were homeless (Baggerly, 2004; Baggerly & Jenkins, 2009), children exposed to domestic violence (Tyndall-Lind, Landreth, & Giordano, 2001), children who were refugees (Schottelkorb, Doumas, & Garcia, 2012), and children exposed to natural disasters (Shen, 2002).

Self-Reflection

CCPT with a child who is homeless begins with building a safe therapeutic relationship based on the core conditions of unconditional positive regard, empathy, and genuineness (Landreth, 2012; Rogers, 1951). To convey these core conditions effectively to children who are homeless, play therapists must engage in ongoing self-reflection. Concerning unconditional positive regard, the following questions can be illuminating: "Do I deeply believe that every person is worthy of respect, regardless of economic status—even if it is a parent who was evicted in part because of drug abuse? Do I feel guilty over my own economic security when I know that my child client will go hungry tonight in a cold setting?" This type of self-reflection can help therapists determine whether they harbor any disdain or guilt, and can thereby help them avoid a "blame the victim" attitude that diminishes warmth and acceptance of children.

Genuineness, or openness to feelings and attitudes, is enhanced when therapists "listen to self and accept without fear their own complexity of feelings and experiences" (Rogers, 1951, p. 53). When working with children who are homeless, therapists need to monitor their own feelings and experiences related to their racial, cultural, and socioeconomic identity developmental level (Sue & Sue, 2013). Since most play therapists are white and middle-class (Ryan, 2002), it is imperative for such therapists to progress through the white racial identity development stages of resistance, introspection, and integrative awareness (Sue & Sue, 2013). This progression can be accomplished by implementing strategies such as self-exploration, development of friendships with diverse people, and commitment to community change (Sue & Sue, 2013). Genuineness is also strengthened when play therapists reevaluate their foundation for hope: Is it based on financial gain, or on faith and healthy relationships? A therapist whose sense of hope is based on money will inadvertently communicate hopelessness to children who are poor and homeless. Conversely, a therapist whose sense of hope is based on faith and healthy relationships will communicate hopefulness whenever faith and healthy relationships are available, regardless of financial status.

Empathy is conveyed when therapists "sense the feelings and personal meanings which clients experience in each moment and communicate that understanding to clients" (Rogers & Stevens, 1967, p. 54). To develop empathy for children who are homeless, it can be helpful to ponder two questions: "What does it mean to be middle-class?" and "What is it like to live in poverty?" The differences between being middle-class and living in poverty include (1) an intense daily struggle for survival, such as choosing between medicine for a sick family member and a meal for the other family members (NCH, 2009b); and (2) a mistrust of helping professionals who appear judgmental and condescending (Sue & Sue, 2013). Therapists who face the harsh reality of poverty and who accept social responsibility for mitigating its effects on children will begin to understand the struggle of homelessness and empathize with children who are homeless.

Procedures

After a critical self-reflection, we recommend implementing the standard CCPT procedures of (1) allowing the child to lead the play session;

(2) tracking play behavior; (3) reflecting content and feelings; (4) returning responsibility; (5) providing encouragement and building self-esteem; (6) facilitating understanding; and (7) setting therapeutic limits (Landreth, 2012). In work with homeless and displaced children, these procedures are best described in the framework of Maslow's hierarchy of needs: physiological survival; safety; love and belonging; self-esteem; and self-actualization (Daniels, 1992; Maslow, 1968).

The physiological survival need of children who are homeless is met by providing snacks, such as fruit, crackers, and juice, as well as a comfortable place to rest. Such children will arrive at the playroom hungry and physically exhausted, and will not be able to engage in meaningful play until these needs are met. The safety need of children who are homeless is met by creating a safe, private therapeutic setting within the playroom— perhaps the ideal home they are missing (Walsh & Buckley, 1994). Providing play therapy in a quiet setting at the homeless shelter or school adds to children's sense of safety and alleviates transportation concerns. Confidentiality should be explained to children in a concrete manner, such as the following: "This is a confidential or private time for you. If you want to tell others what you did or said, you can, but I will not tell unless you or someone else is being hurt a lot." Personal space and privacy can be emphasized by posting a privacy sign on the door.

A safe therapeutic environment is also created by providing children with carefully selected toys in the following categories: (1) real-life items such as a bendable doll family, a cardboard box top with rooms indicated by strips of tape, a nursing bottle, plastic dishes, a small car, a small plane, and a telephone; (2) aggressive release items, such as handcuffs, a dart gun, a rubber knife, toy soldiers, and an inflatable plastic punching toy; and (3) creative expressive items, such as Play-Doh, a small plain mask, papers, crayons, and blunt scissors (Landreth, 2012). Given the limited budgets of homeless shelters and schools, the least expensive ways to obtain these toys are through garage sales, thrift stores, or dollar stores, or in a play therapy tote bag (available through play therapy toy vendors). However, if funding is available, Landreth's (2012) more extensive list of therapeutic toys is preferable.

Since over 60% of homeless children are African American or Hispanic (NCH, 2009b), ethnically appropriate dolls, artwork, and play food items should be added to the playroom (Glover, 2001). In addition, play therapists are advised to seek understanding of children's cultural backgrounds, beliefs, and values through discussions with parents, reading ethnic literature, and attending ethnic community events. However, play therapists should respect the uniqueness of each child by avoiding stereotypes and overculturalization (i.e., attributing characteristics to ethnicity rather than poverty) (Glover, 2001; Sue & Sue, 2013).

Safety within play sessions is also established when play therapists appropriately and consistently set therapeutic limits to protect people and toys (Landreth, 2012). Therapeutic limit setting through a three-step "A-C-T" process of acknowledging children's feelings or intentions, communicating the limit, and targeting an alternative provides a caring and consistent structure for children to self-regulate their behavior. For example:

> RICHEY: Give me that money. I need it. (*Grabs money from Andy and runs to the other side of the room.*)
>
> ANDY: I'll get you. (*Loads dart gun and aims it at Richey.*)
>
> PLAY THERAPIST: Andy, I know you are mad at Richey for taking your money, but people are not for shooting. You can choose to pretend the Bobo is him and shoot Bobo or tell him you're mad.

The need for love and belonging in children who are homeless is met by consistently implementing Axline's (1969) eight basic principles:

> 1) developing a warm, friendly relationship, 2) accepting children exactly as they are, 3) establishing a feeling of permissiveness, 4) reflecting children's feelings, 5) maintaining a deep respect for children's problem solving ability, 6) allowing the child to lead the session, 7) being patient with the process, and 8) only setting limits as needed. (pp. 73, 74)

Through these principles, play therapists communicate an attitude of love and create an atmosphere of belonging that reaffirm children's inherent value as important persons in society. If children are selected for group play therapy (Sweeney & Homeyer, 1999), they experience a sense of belonging with other children who are homeless, and gain the added therapeutic benefit of universality. These benefits are observed in the following dialogue between 6-year-old Mark and 6-year-old Darron, who both resided at a homeless shelter:

> MARK: I'm going to work so I can have money to pay the rent.
>
> DARRON: Yeah, me too. I don't want to get kicked out of my house.
>
> MARK: I'm going to be a banker to make lots of money for my family.
>
> DARRON: I'm going to be a doctor.
>
> PLAY THERAPIST: You're both excited to make money and keep your family safe.

In this group interaction, the boys validated each other's fear of losing their homes and encouraged each other in finding solutions. The need for self-esteem in children who are homeless is met as play therapists return responsibility to children, encourage them through a difficult process, and give them credit for succeeding on their own (Landreth, 2012). For example, consider the following dialogue between Mark and his play therapist:

MARK: I can't get these [bowling pins] to stand up. (*Grimaces.*)

PLAY THERAPIST: You're frustrated, but you're still trying. [Reflects feeling; encourages.]

MARK: You do it.

PLAY THERAPIST: Mark, I know you're frustrated, but that's something you can keep on trying.

MARK: Well, I got this row up. (*Continues working.*) I got them all up. (*Smiles.*)

PLAY THERAPIST: You're proud you did it on your own!

Through such interactions, children who are homeless learn mastery of situations that seem hopeless and develop the self-esteem they need to overcome future challenges.

Children's highest need, as identified by Maslow, is "a basic human drive toward growth, completeness, and fulfillment" (Corsini & Wedding, 2000, p. 469). The self-actualization of children who are homeless is facilitated through consistent implementation of play therapy procedures such as following children's lead, avoiding judgmental statements, reflecting feelings and content, facilitating decision making, enhancing self-esteem, setting therapeutic limits, and enlarging the meaning of children's play to increase insight (Landreth, 2012). Glimpses of an 8-year-old boy's self-actualization process are seen in the following transcript:

ANDY: I have handcuffs, a cop's badge, a cop's license, and a cop's ID. I have everything I need to be a cop.

PLAY THERAPIST: You have everything you need to be an important person.

ANDY: Now you can't arrest me.

PLAY THERAPIST: You're safe.

ANDY: I'm going to put on my battery charger. Going turbo. Zoom. (*Twirls around and then stands with hands on his hips.*)

PLAY THERAPIST: Now you're powerful!

ANDY: Now that I'm turbo, I may look the same, same clothes, but I'm different. I'm super strong. You can't mess with me. Pow! (*Punches down Bobo doll.*)

PLAY THERAPIST: You're different now. You feel strong and protected.

Through his play, Andy was in the process of changing his self-concept from feeling unimportant and powerless—a common feeling among homeless children—to becoming important and powerful. In the safe, supportive, permissive, and therapeutic environment of play therapy, Andy empowered himself rather than relying on someone else. Ideally, as he incorporated these positive experiences into his self-concept, he would see himself as possessing positive power and a bright future, which would lead him toward self-actualization.

Play Themes and Facilitative Responses

The growth and development of children who are homeless is greatly enhanced as play therapists implement the procedure of enlarging the meaning of children's play. Using toys for their words and play as their language (Landreth, 2012), children symbolically reenact common experiences to resolve conflicts and compensate for unsatisfied needs (Piaget, 1962). To expedite this process, play therapists should enlarge the meaning of children's play by identifying common play themes; linking these themes to children's experiences; and verbally reflecting this understanding of feelings, beliefs, and desires to children. Doing all of this will increase children's awareness and insight. Two unique play themes of children who are homeless appear to be eviction and "I'm rich." However, children who are homeless also display common play themes, such as power and control; aggression; and nurturing (Benedict et al., 1995; Holmberg, Benedict, & Hynan, 1998).

Eviction

Homeless children frequently reenact the experience of being evicted from their homes during their play. Feelings of helplessness, anger, confusion, and loss become evident as children use the toys to relive their eviction. This theme is illustrated in the play of 7-year-old Tyronne, who resided in a homeless shelter and was referred for play therapy by his mother because of his frequent anger outbursts and low self-esteem. During Tyronne's first several sessions, he created disorganized and chaotic battles between toy soldiers and animal families, frequently throwing all the toys together. Therapeutic responses of reflecting his feelings and play content included "The soldiers and animals are so angry that they are fighting," and "They are confused about what to do."

During the 10th session, Tyronne's story became more organized, with the following distinct scene. He carefully set up the furniture and a family of people in the playhouse. He pretended the people were going about the daily routine of cooking, eating, and sleeping, when suddenly the soldiers entered the house, knocked over furniture, and threw the people out of the house. The animals helped the people by checking to see if they were safe and bringing the family back together. Then the animals tried to fight the soldiers to regain the house, but the soldiers prevailed. The play therapist enlarged the meaning of Tyronne's play by recognizing the play theme of eviction, linking it to his experience, and verbalizing reflections such as "The family is scared that the soldiers are kicking them out of the house.

You know what that's like," and "The animals are helping the people, just like you are helped here."

The progression of Tyronne's play themes from disorganized aggression to specific reenactment of eviction reflected identifiable stages of therapeutic progress from general hostility to specific symbolization (Hendricks, 1971; Moustakas, 1955). In his play, Tyronne appeared to be reliving the fear and frustration of his family's eviction, the perceived hostility of the landlord's (soldiers') actions, the nurturance he received from the homeless shelter staff (animals), and the reality of not being able to return home. Providing therapeutic responses along with core conditions helped Tyronne (1) become aware of repressed emotions and beliefs that were clamoring for his attention; (2) reprocess intrusive memories of the traumatic event; (3) gain a sense of mastery and control over his overwhelming experiences; (4) integrate these experiences into his self-structure; and (5) become a more organized whole, thereby moving from maladjusted incongruence to adjusted congruence (Landreth & Sweeney, 1997; Rogers, 1951).

"I'm Rich"

Another common play theme of children who are homeless is called "I'm rich," because children count play money or toss it up in the air and exclaim, "I'm rich!" Children who are homeless appear to be intensely aware of their family's lack of money. For example, one 10-year-old girl stated, "I didn't get to have a birthday party and I only got one present, because we didn't have a house or money." Children who are homeless introject into their self-structure their parents' statements about money, such as "If we just had enough money for rent, we'd be OK," or "If only we won the Lotto, we wouldn't have to worry." In an attempt to gain in fantasy what they do not have in reality, children use the play money to pretend they are rich. Therapeutic responses of enlarging the meaning for the "I'm rich" theme include "You feel happy and powerful with all that money!" and "You really wish you had lots of money so you could have your own home."

Children who are homeless often reveal inaccurate perceptions about money, however. Some children believe that money can only be obtained in unconventional manners. For example, some children toss money up in the air as if it magically falls from the sky, rather than pretending to obtain it through working. Other children pretend to sell drugs to get money so that they can buy sodas and fast food. In addition, some children who are homeless seem to believe that money is more reliable and valuable than relationships. For example, during play, some children may pretend to trick or "kill" a friend to steal the friend's money. Their value of money over relationships may reflect their experience of unreliable parents or other relatives who have left them without basic necessities, and their consequent desperation for survival. Play therapists should communicate this understanding through empathic, nonjudgmental therapeutic responses such as

"You were so hungry you decided to steal the money," or "You know one way to get money fast. Perhaps you've seen that before." Play therapists can also address this complex issue by consulting with parents, teachers, and community leaders about family dynamics, money management, career planning, and social justice.

Power and Control

Children who are homeless have even less power and control over themselves and their circumstances than children who have homes. When children live at homeless shelters, they have little control over when, what, and where they will eat, when they will go to bed, and where they can play. Since a child at a shelter usually resides in one dormitory-type room with the parent(s) and siblings, privacy and space is limited. In addition, prior to becoming homeless, many children have experienced a lack of power and control within communities where drugs, prostitution, and crime are rampant. Consequently, a play theme of power and control is common among children who are homeless. Therapeutic responses of enlarging the meaning help children gain a sense of power and control, as illustrated in the following scenario:

> TRAY: I'm a secret agent for the president.
>
> DAVID: I'm a bodyguard for the princess.
>
> PLAY THERAPIST: You're both someone real important!
>
> TRAY: I'll shoot the bad guys! They can't get me!
>
> DAVID: Me, too. I'll get them first!
>
> PLAY THERAPIST: You're both powerful and in control now!
>
> TRAY: Yeah, we're in charge!

Through such play, children who are homeless assert their sense of innate power and develop their identity as powerful people. Thus, even when their current experience at the shelter limits their power, children will find hope for the future in their strengthened sense of self. Children's empowerment can be facilitated further by encouraging parents and teachers to offer their children as many choices as possible, such as "Do you want to go outside before or after doing your homework?"

Aggression: Abuser/Victim/Protector Roles

Since many children who are homeless have witnessed domestic and community violence (NCH, 2009b), aggression is a common play theme. Children frequently reenact violent scenes by playing the role of the abuser, victim, and/or protector. During this type of play, it is crucial that play therapists maintain a nonanxious presence so as to create a sense of safety for children, as such play can be emotionally overwhelming. As play therapists reflect children's feelings, motives, and physiological responses, such as rapid heart rate and clenched muscles, children begin to associate physiological responses with feelings and to learn to self-regulate. Consider the following scenario:

> MARTY: Don't be messin' with my wife. (*Punches and jumps on top of bop bag.*)
>
> PLAY THERAPIST: You're protecting your wife! You're angry. Your muscles are tight.
>
> MARTY: (*Punches bop bag for several minutes.*) I'm letting you have money to buy a house. But when I see you, you owe me. (*Stands over bop bag and jumps on it.*)
>
> PLAY THERAPIST: You're helping him out, but you're tough and in control.
>
> MARTY: (*Picks up money.*) This money is for my family. You think I'm going to get kicked out of my house? No way! (*Kicks and punches bop bag.*)
>
> PLAY THERAPIST: You're mad! You don't wanna get kicked out of your house. You wanna provide for your family.

Through such therapeutic responses, children will learn to differentiate the feelings of aggression (e.g., anger and rage) from the motives of aggression (e.g., protection and safety). As children become aware of their motives, they can begin to explore alternative, nonviolent strategies for being safe and protected.

Nurturing

Nurturing is another common play theme for children who are homeless. Since basic needs of food and a safe, comfortable bed have not been consistently met for such children, they often symbolically meet this need through play activities such as feeding baby dolls, cooking meals, making beds, and doctoring each other. Consider the following scenario:

> MARY: I'm giving the baby her oatmeal.
>
> PLAY THERAPIST: You're making sure she has enough to eat.
>
> MARY: Here's a blanket, so she won't get cold while she sleeps.
>
> PLAY THERAPIST: You know it's important to keep her warm.
>
> MARY: Time for her checkup from the doctor.
>
> PLAY THERAPIST: You're making sure she's well. You like taking care of the baby.

Through such play, children who are homeless satisfy their own desire for such care; experience the power and pleasure of positive caregiving; and affirm themselves as nurturing persons, thereby integrating nurturing values into their self-structure. Occasionally, however, children will reenact failed nurturance by activities such as pretending to spank a crying baby rather than comforting the baby. When they project feelings of distress and helplessness through this play, therapeutic responses such as "The baby is scared and sad when she doesn't get what she needs" will increase children's awareness of their feelings and affirm that their needs are legitimate. Thus, rather than introjecting the experience of failed nurturance as indication of their lack of worth, they will begin to accept their need for nurturing as an indication of their worth.

Serial Drawings with Children after a Natural Disaster

Serial drawing is a therapeutic approach based on Jungian concepts. It involves having a child produce artwork over time, thereby providing a view of the child's inner world to the therapist (Green, 2007). After a therapeutic relationship and trust are formed between the therapist and child, problems are expressed symbolically in the artwork and healing, and resolution of inner conflicts occurs (Allan, 2004; Green, 2007). The serial drawing technique involves a therapist meeting with a child regularly and asking the child to "draw a picture while we talk." Jung (1931/1969) believed that in times of significant crisis, children can turn inward toward the unconscious for dreams and images that carry within them the potential for healing—otherwise known as the *self-healing archetype*. From Green's (2007) perspective, the play therapist does not analyze the child's images, but rather (1) encourages the child to make the images freely, with little to no direction from the therapist; (2) allows the child to absorb the images fully, so that the images can lead the child wherever he or she may need to go (toward self-healing); and (3) links the meaning of the symbols with the child's outer world at the point the child's ego can accept, and helps the child to build a bridge between "transitional spaces." To reiterate, the serial drawing alone does not heal broken attachment. Rather, the self-healing archetype in children is activated by a curative alliance with a nonjudgmental therapist (Green, 2007). The serial drawing provides for safe expression and exploration of feelings associated with the children's traumatic experiences and dissipated sense of secure attachment.

According to Walsh and Allan (1994), a therapist may employ three different therapeutic styles when utilizing the serial drawing technique with a child: (1) directive (the therapist gives the child specific images to draw related to the trauma); (2) nondirective (the therapist simply says, "Draw whatever you'd like"); and (3) semidirective (the therapist intermittently requests the child to redraw a specific symbol already produced to further explore its inherently healing capacities). In addition to a tolerance for ambiguity, therapists should provide an atmosphere that contains unconditional positive regard, trust, genuineness, warmth, and empathy, all of which may assist children to draw freely in a protected space. To process the serial drawing and amplify its symbols, Allan (2004) suggests that the therapist ask the child one or more of the following questions:

"Does this picture tell a story?"

"I'm wondering if you can tell me what is happening in this scene?"

"If you could give this picture a title, what would it be?"

"If you were inside this picture, what would it feel like?"

"What went on in the story before this scene occurred? What happens next?"

"Could you tell me what you were thinking or feeling as you drew this?"

"What does this [identify a certain object or symbol in the picture] mean to you?"

During the processing (or resolving) of drawings, it is important for a therapist to remember that all verbal and nonverbal communications to the child should reflect support, so the child will come to realize that both good and horrible feelings are acceptable to convey in the therapeutic relationship. Through this acceptance and mutual understanding, feelings of secure attachment slowly begin to emerge as children's feelings, however horrendous, are seen as acceptable; thereby they feel accepted not as *damaged*, but as *whole* psychological individuals.

Case Vignette: Keisha's Serial Drawing

Keisha, a 7-year-old African American female, and her impoverished single mother lived in a dilapidated Section 8 housing unit in a low-lying part of the deep South. As a major hurricane came closer to shore, rising floodwaters seeped into their living room through the home's front door. Riding out the storm overnight, they believed the worst was behind them. Yet the rain and wind continued to pummel the city into the next day. The levees were breached as floodwaters rose to the floor of the attic, completely inundating their house with water and debris. Keisha was to be indefinitely homeless following this massive destruction.

In the days following the storm's passing, Keisha exhibited uncontrollable fits of crying and panic. At night, her mother indicated she would wake up screaming periodically, waking others up at the temporary shelter they were placed in. Keisha was eventually referred to a play therapist for counseling, as she was not coping well with being permanently displaced by the storm. Keisha enjoyed drawing and painting; therefore, the therapist's aim was to sit quietly and allow her to create whatever she wanted.

Keisha moved directly toward the art supplies, which consisted of plain white paper and sharpened colored pencils. These and other art materials, such as paper, glue, and paints, allow children to create free images of what is going on in their lives and express themselves comfortably within the therapeutic dyad. As Keisha drew, the play therapist remained relatively quiet, not wanting to take the focus away from her artistic creation. During play therapy sessions, while a child is drawing, a play therapist does not initiate conversation or take any notes. Instead, the therapist observes the child; the way the child approaches the drawing; the placement of figures; and the types of images, symbols, and themes that emerge in the child's pictures.

In each of the first two sessions, Keisha spent approximately 15–25 minutes drawing a scene. The two scenes looked very similar to each other: The paper was largely covered by dark water, and within the water was a broken vessel with dead fish strewn about. The therapist asked her whether she could describe what it would be like if she was on the boat in the scene. She said, "It would be scary, 'cause it's sunk and everyone's dead." In the third session where the serial drawing technique was utilized, the play therapist asked Keisha whether there was any way the people in the boat could find a life raft or save themselves, and she responded, "Yes, maybe if the sun comes up and saves them." With all of this macabre imagery, the play therapist noticed a bright, shining sun at the top of the scene. Keisha commented how the sun might be a source of healing, and how she missed playing in her backyard in the sunshine with her soccer ball.

After the fifth and sixth play therapy sessions with serial drawing, Keisha began to draw a less macabre scene. She drew and commented that the boat was almost at land, where it would be safe. In children's drawings, the sun can represent a healer, a restorer, or a provider of warmth and understanding for development (Allan, 2004). The ocean or water typifies primordial water, which is the one of the four elements responsible for sustaining life. In a child's drawings, water can represent life and death, or can illustrate the vast, formless unconscious of the child's nascent ego attempting to regenerate.

In one of the last sessions where Keisha used the serial drawing technique, she drew a boat located at the shoreline. Also, people appeared in this scene, all of whom were positioned in the sand with smiley faces. This drawing seemed to reflect Keisha's ongoing sense of coping with her displacement. Her final serial drawing was a bright yellow-and-orange mandala (Figure 17.1). She commented that the sun was happy in this drawing and that she felt happy too. When asked whether she would be OK living in a new home because her old one was no longer there, she responded, "Yes, I'll be OK. We'll find a new home, and it will be OK." Toward the end of the treatment, her affect dysregulation had completely dissipated. She was engaging in regular play with her peers, and the nightmares had stopped.

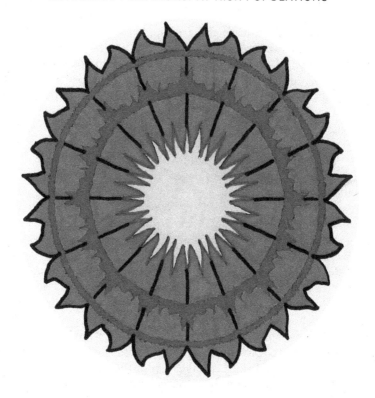

FIGURE 17.1. Sun (a re-creation of Keisha's final drawing).

Conclusion

Play therapy can help children create "home" within their own hearts, thereby giving them the courage to invite others in. Through sensitive and carefully timed interventions within the central arc of a stable, secure relationship with a trained adult, traumatized children begin to abreact the feelings of abandonment and loss that have resulted from homelessness or displacement by a disaster. Through the safe space afforded by a play therapist, many children begin to rediscover a sense of hope and wonder about their world, and begin to develop (or redevelop) healthy, secure attachments with their immediate caregivers and other caring adults surrounding them.

REFERENCES

Allan, J. (2004). *Inscapes of the child's world: Jungian counseling in schools and clinics.* Dallas, TX: Spring.

Axline, V. M. (1969). *Play therapy.* New York: Ballantine Books.

Baggerly, J. N. (2003). Play therapy with homeless children: Perspectives and procedures. *International Journal of Play Therapy, 12*(2), 87–106.

Baggerly, J. N. (2004). The effects of child-centered group play therapy on self-concept, depression, and anxiety of children who are homeless. *International Journal of Play Therapy, 13*(2), 31–51.

Baggerly, J. N., & Borkowski, T. (2004). Applying the ASCA national model to elementary school students who are homeless: A case study. *Professional School Counselor, 8*(2), 116–123.

Baggerly, J. N., & Jenkins, W. (2009). The effectiveness of child-centered play therapy on developmental and diagnostic factors of children who are homeless. *International Journal of Play Therapy, 18*, 45–55.

Baggerly, J. N., Ray, D. C., & Bratton, S. C. (Eds.). (2010). *Child-centered play therapy research: The evidence base for effective practice.* Hoboken, NJ: Wiley.

Becker-Blease, K. A., Turner, H. A., & Finkelhor, D. (2010). Disasters, victimization, and children's mental health. *Child Development, 81*, 1040–1052.

Benedict, H. E., Chavez, D., Holmberg, J., McClain, J., McGee, W., Narcavage, C., . . . Wooley, L. (1995). *Benedict play therapy theme codes.* Unpublished manuscript, Baylor University.

Bratton, S., Ray, D., Rhine, T., & Jones, L. (2005). The efficacy of play therapy with children: A meta-analytic review of the outcome research. *Professional Psychology: Research and Practice, 36*, 376–390.

Buckner, J. C., Bassuk, E. L., Weinreb, L. F., & Brooks, M. G. (1999). Homelessness and its relation to the mental health and behavior of low income school-age children. *Developmental Psychology, 35*, 246–257.

Corsini, R. J., & Wedding, D. (2000). *Current psychotherapies* (6th ed.). Itasca, IL: Peacock.

Daniels, J. (1992). Empowering homeless children through school counseling. *Elementary School Guidance and Counseling, 27*, 104–112.

Flores, R. L. (2007). Effect of poverty on urban preschool children's understanding of conventional time concepts. *Early Child Development and Care, 177*, 121–132.

Glover, G. J. (2001). Cultural considerations in play therapy. In G. L. Landreth (Ed.), *Innovations in play therapy: Issues, process, and special populations* (pp. 31–41). New York: Brunner-Routledge.

Green, E. (2007). The crisis of family separation following traumatic mass destruction: Jungian analytical play therapy in the aftermath of Hurricane Katrina. In N. B. Webb (Ed.), *Play therapy with children in crisis: Individual, group, and family treatment* (3rd ed., pp. 368–388). New York: Guilford Press.

Guha-Sapir, D., Vos, F., Below, R., & Ponserre, S. (2010). *Annual disaster statistical review 2010: The numbers and trends.* Brussels: Centre for Research on the Epidemiology of Disasters. Retrieved from *http://cred.be/sites/default/files/ADSR_2010.pdf*

Hendricks, S. (1971). A descriptive analysis of the process of client-centered play therapy (Doctoral dissertation, North Texas State University, 1971). *Dissertation Abstracts International, 32*, 3689A.

Holmberg, J. R., Benedict, H. E., & Hynan, L. S. (1998). Gender differences in children's play therapy themes: Comparisons of children with a history of attachment disturbance or exposure to violence. *International Journal of Play Therapy, 7*(2), 67–92.

Institute for Children and Poverty (ICP). (2007). *Quickfacts.* Retrieved August 22, 2007, from *www.icpny.org/index.asp?CID_7*

Jung, C. (1969). The stages of life. In H. Read (Ed.) & R. F. C. Hull (Trans.), *The collected work of C. G. Jung, Vol. 8. The structure and dynamics of the psyche* (2nd ed., pp. 387–403). Princeton, NJ: Princeton University Press. (Original work published 1931)

Kagan, R. (2004). *Rebuilding attachments with traumatized children: Healing from losses, violence, abuse, and neglect.* New York: Haworth Press.

Koblinsky, S. A., Gordon, A. L., & Anderson, E. A. (2000). Changes in the social skills and behavior problems of homeless and housed children during the preschool year. *Early Education and Development, 11,* 321–338.

Landreth, G. L. (2012). *Play therapy: The art of the relationship* (3rd ed.). New York: Routledge.

Landreth, G. L., & Sweeney, D. S. (1997). Child-centered play therapy. In K. J. O'Connor & L. M. Braverman (Eds.), *Play therapy: Theory and practice* (pp. 17–45). New York: Wiley.

Maslow, A. H. (1968). *Toward a psychology of being* (2nd ed.). Princeton, NJ: Van Nostrand.

Masten, A. S., Sesma, A., Si-Asar, R., Lawrence, C., Miliotis, D., & Dionne, J. A. (1997). Educational risks for children experiencing homelessness. *Journal of School Psychology, 35,* 27–46.

Menke, E. M. (2000). Comparison of the stressors and coping behaviors of homeless, previously homeless, and never homeless poor children. *Issues in Mental Health Nursing, 21,* 691–710.

Moustakas, C. (1955). Emotional adjustment and the play therapy process. *Journal of Genetic Psychology, 86,* 79–99.

National Coalition for the Homeless (NCH). (2009a). *How many people experience homelessness?* (NCH Fact Sheet No. 2). Retrieved from *www.nationalhomeless.org/publications/facts/How_Many.pdf*

National Coalition for the Homeless (NCH). (2009b). *Why are people homeless?* (NCH Fact Sheet No. 1). Retrieved from *www.nationalhomeless.org/publications/facts/Why.pdf*

Perry, B. (2001). Children and loss. *Academic Search Premier, 110,* 36.

Piaget, J. (1962). *Play, dreams, and imitation in childhood.* New York: Norton.

Rogers, C. (1951). *Client-centered therapy, its current practice, implications, and theory.* Boston: Houghton Mifflin.

Rogers, C., & Stevens, B. (1967). *Person to person: The problem of being human.* Lafayette, CA: Real People Press.

Rosenfeld, L. B., Caye, J. S., Ayalon, O., & Lahad, M. (2005). *When their world falls apart: Helping families and children manage the effects of disasters.* Washington, DC: NASW Press.

Rubin, D. H., Erickson, C. J., Agustin, M. S., Cleary, S. D., Allen, J. K., & Cohen, P. (1996). Cognitive and academic functioning of homeless children compared with housed children. *Pediatrics, 97,* 289–294.

Ryan, S. (2002). *Who are we?: Findings from the Association for Play Therapy membership survey.* Paper presented at the 19th Annual Association for Play Therapy International Conference, St. Louis, MO.

Schottelkorb, A. A., Doumas, D. M., & Garcia, R. (2012). Treatment for childhood refugee trauma: A randomized, controlled trial. *International Journal of Play Therapy, 21*(2), 57–73.

Shen, Y. J. (2002). Short-term group play therapy with Chinese earthquake victims: Effects on anxiety, depression and adjustment. *International Journal of Play Therapy, 11,* 43–64.

Sue, D., & Sue, D. (2013). *Counseling the culturally different. Theory and practice* (6th ed.). New York: Wiley.

Sweeney, D. S., & Homeyer, L. E. (1999). *The handbook of group play therapy: How to do it, how it works, whom it's best for.* San Francisco, CA: Jossey-Bass.

Tyndall-Lind, A., Landreth, G. L., & Giordano, M. A. (2001). Intensive group play therapy with child witnesses of domestic violence. *International Journal of Play Therapy, 10*(1), 53–83.

Walsh, D., & Allan, J. (1994). Jungian art counseling with the suicidal child. *Guidance and Counseling, 10*(1), 3–10.

Walsh, M. E., & Buckley, M. A. (1994). Children's experiences of homelessness: Implications for school counselors. *Elementary School Guidance and Counseling, 29*(1), 4–15.

Youngblade, L. M., & Mulvihill, B. A. (1998). Individual differences in homeless preschoolers' social behavior. *Journal of Applied Developmental Psychology, 19,* 593–614.

Ziesemer, C., Marcoux, L., & Marwell, B. (1994). Homeless children: Are they different from other low-income children? *Social Work, 39,* 658–668.

Index